The Great Brain Robbery
Why Women Have Become Smarter Than Men

Science With an *Attitude*

Dr. Brian Moench

Copyright © 2021 Brian Moench

All rights reserved.

ISBN: 9798578742286

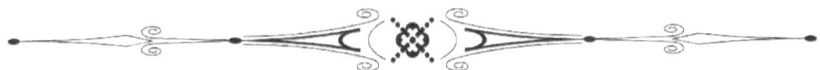

DEDICATION

This book is dedicated to my wife Shauna, who has bravely put up with my attempt to save the world for the last 50, 60, or 200 years, however long we've been married.

ACKNOWLEDGMENTS

This book was made possible only by the dedication of Melodie Charles, who spent far too many hours editing, proof reading, massaging, milking, pureeing, and otherwise reconstructing the material into something with a vague resemblance to a book. And that is not only a testament to her skills, but to how bored she was during the pandemic shutdown.

CONTENTS

Abbreviation,		4
Interesting facts		
Prologue		11
Introduction		21
Chapter One	Women Are Smarter Than Men	29
Chapter Two	How the Brain Works	47
Chapter Three	Why Women Are Smarter Than Men	91
Chapter Four	Environmental Attacks on the Brain	109
Chapter Five	More Environmental Attacks on the Brain	187
Chapter Six	The Great Brain Protectors	257
Chapter Seven	The Alzheimer Paradox-	281
Chapter Eight	Autism: A Male Pandemic	289
Chapter Nine	We Must Put More Women in Charge	305
References		347

ABBREVIATIONS, ACRONYMS, EXPLANATIONS

ADD attention deficit disorder (now classified as a subset of attention deficit   hyperactivity disorder [ADHD])

ADHD attention deficit hyperactivity disorder (now includes attention deficit disorder [ADD] as a subset)

AEC Atomic Energy Commission

AI Artificial Intelligence

ALA alpha-linolenic acid (an omega-3 fatty acid)

ALS amyotrophic lateral sclerosis (Lou Gehrig's Disease)

Alzheimer's Alzheimer's disease

APA American Psychiatric Association

Autism Autism spectrum disorder

BBB blood-brain barrier

BBFL brain's best friend for life

BDNF brain-derived neurotrophic factor

BEIR biologic effects of ionizing radiation

BPA bisphenol A

BPS bisphenol S

C-8 see PFOA

CAT scan computerized tomography scan (this uses X-ray images and computer processing to create cross-sectional images)

CBF cerebral blood flow

CDC Centers for Disease Control and Prevention

CEO Chief Executive Officer

CFO Chief Financial Officer

CPR cardiopulmonary resuscitation

CRA Corn Refiners Association

The Great Brain Robbery – Brian Moench

CSF cerebrospinal fluid

DDT dichlorodiphenyltrichloroethane (an insecticide)

DHA docosahexaenoic acid (an omega-3 fatty acid)

DNA deoxyribonucleic acid (a molecule containing genetic instructions for all organisms and many viruses)

DPT diphtheria, pertussis, and tetanus

DSM Diagnostic and Statistical Manual of Mental Disorders (an authoritative work that defines and classifies mental disorders)

ECT electroshock therapy

EEG electroencephalogram

EMFs electromagnetic fields

EPA eicosapentaenoic acid (an omega-3 fatty acid)

EPA the U.S. Environmental Protection Agency

FCC Federal Communications Commission

FDA Food and Drug Administration

FSA fluorosilicic acid (used in water fluoridation)

FTC Federal Trade Commission

G generation (used with a number to describe the level of wireless technology, mobile internet connection capability)

GABA gamma aminobutyric acid (a naturally occurring amino acid neurotransmitter in the brain)

GBH glyphosate-based herbicide (an herbicide designed to kill weeds; the most famous is Roundup, sold by Bayer

GI gastrointestinal

GMO an organism whose DNA is genetically modified to have a desirable trait

GPS global positioning system

GSH glutathione (a substance produced by the liver)

HBOT hyperbaric oxygen therapy

HFCS high fructose corn syrup

HMO health maintenance organization

HPD hypertensive pregnancy disorders

Hz hertz (a unit of frequency used to measure the number of cycles per second of   currents, waves, and sound)

IARC International Agency for Research on Cancer

Kg kilogram (a unit of weight equal to 1,000 grams)

Km kilometer (a unit of length equal to 1,000 meters)

LC Locus Coeruleus

LNT linear no-threshold

Mcgs micrograms (units of weight equal to one millionth of a gram)

Mgs milligrams (units of weight equal to one thousandth of a gram)

mg/L milligram per liter (unit of concentration by weight of a substance in water, approximately equivalent to unit parts per million)

MHz megahertz (units of frequency equal to one million hertz)

MIT male idiot theory

MIT Massachusetts Institute of Technology

mPFC medial prefrontal cortex

MRI magnetic resonance imaging

NICU newborn intensive care unit

NRC National Research Council

PAHs polycyclic aromatic hydrocarbons

PBDEs polybrominated diphenyl ethers (human-made toxic, persistent compounds used as flame retardants)

PCBs polychlorinated biphenyls (human-made toxic, persistent organic pollutants that had many commercial and industrial uses)

PFC prefrontal cortex (the primary brain site for executive functioning)

PFOA (also C8) perfluorooctanoic acid (a human-made toxic, persistent chemical that is used in products to resist sticking; Teflon is the most famous brand name for such products)

PFOS perfluorooctane sulfonate (a human-made persistent pollutant chemical that is used in products to repel stains; Scotchgard is the most famous brand name for such products)

PGE2 prostaglandin E2

PON2 paraoxonase/arylesterase 2

Pp parts per (denotes small quantities, such as parts per million [ppm], parts per billion [ppb], and parts per trillion [ppt], of substances in the air, water, or soil

PTSD post traumatic stress disorder

REM rapid eye movement

RF reticular formation

RFR radio frequency radiation

ROS reactive oxygen species

RSFC resting-state functional connectivity

SAT a college admissions test that has changed the references in its acronym in response to protests about its not actually measuring what its creators claimed it measured; initially, it was an acronym for the Scholastic Aptitude Test, then it became the Scholastic Assessment Test, then the SAT Reasoning Test, and now there are no words associated with the letters in the acronym SAT

STEM science, technology, engineering, and math

S&P 500 Standard and Poor's 500 Index (tracks and reports risks and returns of the stocks of 500 U.S. companies that have a market capitalization value of more than $10 billion)

TBI traumatic brain injury

tDCS transcranial direct current stimulation (a low-current electrical brain stimulation)

USDA U.S. Department of Agriculture

UPHE Utah Physicians for a Healthy Environment

VOCs volatile organic compounds (these evaporate easily at room temperature; some pollute the environment)

WHO World Health Organization

WMHs white matter hyperintensities

WNV West Nile Virus

Little known, relevant facts

*The abnormal protein clumps associated with Alzheimer's are found in the brains of everyone, even infants.

*Brain cell types are different in males and females. Some cell types are unique to each sex.

*Microscopic particles of both air pollution and plastic contaminate virtually every human being on earth, including all our critical organs, including the brain.

*Women survive traumatic brain injury better than men.

*A person's political orientation, liberal vs. conservative, is reflected in the actual anatomy of their brain. Women have a more liberal brain anatomy.

*The death of brain cells caused by a stroke follows a different mechanism depending on the sex.

The Great Brain Robbery – Brian Moench

*A woman who has a hysterectomy increases her risk of eventually suffering from Alzheimer's.

*From pre-birth to age 6 is the time when brain development is the most critical, where behavioral paths are established, intellectual capability solidifies, and environmental influences, for good or ill, have their greatest impact.

*Having a single woman on a corporate board reduces the risk of bankruptcy by 20%.

*There is virtually no scientific evidence that brain supplements are effective.

*Patients have a better survival rate if their physician is a female.

*IQs in prominent developed countries have recently started to decline.

*95% of baby food in America is contaminated with chemicals and heavy metals known to be neurotoxic.

*10,000 different chemicals have been approved for use in food processing.

*At birth, girls are more developmentally advanced than boys. But as adults, metabolically, women's brains are about three years younger than male brains.

*To create energy, post-menopausal female brain cells will actually start eating parts of nearby neurons; microscopic cannibalism.

*The genetic overlap between zebra fish and humans is 70%. Researchers expect to discover the function of up to 90% of all human genes by studying zebra fish.

*Air pollution is associated with an increased tendency to criminal activity and unethical behavior.

*Different parts of the brain age at different rates.

*The total length of the nerve fiber networks in the brain is approximately 500,000 km, far more than the distance between the earth and the moon.

*In the last decade females have overtaken males in scores on IQ tests in the United States.

*Resting heart rate is the best biologic correlate with anti-social behavior for both genders.

*Women outscored men on 17 of the 19 leadership characteristics.

*Resting pupil size correlates with intelligence, and guess which sex has a larger pupil size.

*Women are better at communicating with dogs (seriously).

*The happiest demographic is single women.

*The cerebral cortex of the female brain has greater complexity and more folds than does the male brain.

*Only about 10% of brain cells are neurons, and there may be as many as 10,000 different subtypes of neurons.

*Most neurotoxins cause greater damage to the brains of boys than girls.

*Radiation wasn't the only neurotoxin widely imposed upon the public by the Manhattan Project.

*The X chromosome has about 900 genes, the Y chromosome fewer than 55.

*Big Tobacco found a way to harm the health of millions of people that don't smoke.

*Exercising your legs is more effective in preserving your brain than "exercising" your brain.

*Religious people suffer more sleep deprivation than atheists and agnostics.

*Rates of Alzheimer's correlate with concentrations of aluminum in drinking water.

*Women have significantly more nightmares than men.

*The four primary cell types of the placenta are different depending on whether the fetus is male or female.

PROLOGUE

I grew up as a free-range kid in a rather weird family, knee deep in contradictions. My mother was a combination of Jim Henson, Leonardo De Vinci, and Teddy Roosevelt. She was an accomplished artist, a school teacher, a producer of children's TV skits and plays, a political activist, and an occasional cook for her eight children, a few of whom she remembered how to spell their name. (I was not one of them—true story)

If we came home from school and something was in the oven, there was a 50% chance it was a papier-mâché Halloween witch's head and not dinner, although dinner and the witch's head would have tasted about the same, thus the need for lots of ketchup at our house. She did know how to make the world's finest gravy, which could make a papier-mâché witch's head taste like entirely adequate stroganoff.

My mother was a towering 4'11" powerhouse of ideas, construction, art projects, and can-do-anything attitude. She always had a creation in progress, like constructing a parade float in our driveway, and a deadline to meet. She could have built the Space Shuttle out of chicken wire, Elmer's glue, flour, newspaper, crepe paper, and paint, and it probably would have worked. As the mother of eight children, she usually had at least two of them hanging on for dear life and/or for something to eat. She breastfed them all on a schedule that she adhered to like clockwork. "What time is it, Mom?" "It's 4:00 p.m., time for Melodie's (my little sister) noon feeding." Because she couldn't see over the steering wheel, she was the most dangerous yet undaunted driver in Salt Lake City, not to mention that in the 1950s, the car she drove was the biggest car in town, a black Packard limousine, with three rows of seats and the maneuverability of a battleship. When I was only a toddler, my mother taught me art, social justice, and a righteous indignation towards people who didn't agree with her, or eventually, me: thus, the need for the battleship.

Prologue

During the 1950s, when most of my friends' mothers were aspiring to be June Cleaver, my mother wrote, produced, choreographed, and made the costumes and scenery for church plays on world peace, the failures of Sigmund Freud, environmental protection, and nuclear war, all in front of some of the most conservative religious gatherings you could find anywhere in the United States. Suffice it to say, many of those audiences left auditoriums with their mouths gaping wide open, as if they had just had experienced electroshock therapy (more about that in a moment).

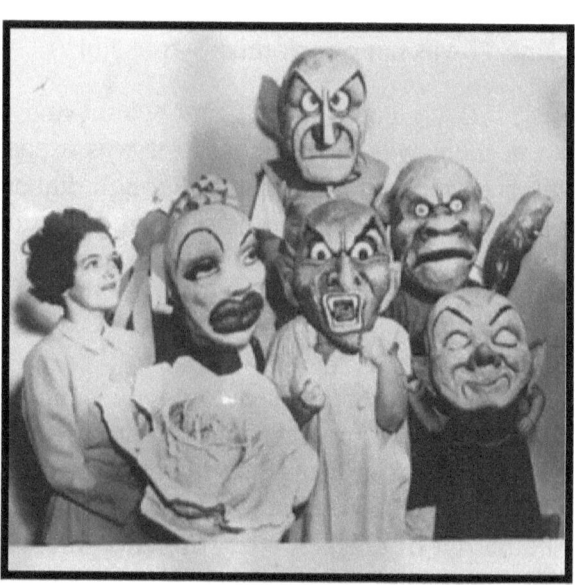

This is my mother with a few of her paper mâché theatrical creations. She is the one on the far left. She donated one of her X chromosomes to me, although I was not allowed to choose which one.

After Richard Nixon was elected President in 1968, my mother became alarmed by what she regarded as the increasingly Machiavellian and corrupt foreign policy of Nixon and Henry Kissinger. There was little of today's platforms for communication; no internet, podcasts, social media, or even cable TV. So when Nixon ran against George McGovern in 1972, she wrote a 20-page essay in long hand explaining the moral and political sins of Nixon's foreign policy and why he should be defeated. She signed it, xeroxed it, and left it on the doorsteps of 100 neighbors, much to my father's dismay. She placed the burden of informing and saving the world on her Tinkerbell sized shoulders. I'll bet my mother was the only person in Utah that subscribed to the New York Times in the 1950s. She was "notorious" long before Ruth Bader Ginsberg was born.

My father was a physician, board certified in internal medicine, but he practiced psychiatry for his career. My mother's plays notwithstanding, he was one of the pioneers of electroshock therapy (ECT) in Utah. He even made his own ECT machine and did the anesthesia and ECT treatment, something that in today's practice requires two physicians. He was affectionately known by colleagues as "the electrician," which was an appropriate moniker for both his profession and his hobbies. He did the electrical wiring of my home. At the insistence of my mother and her sisters, he was reluctantly pressed into service as an obstetrician for a wide swath of a very large extended family that had an aversion to hospitals and were allergic to physicians. He delivered me and some of my seven siblings, several of his grandchildren, nieces, cousins-in-law, cousins out-of-law (of which there were a few), and cousins out of common sense (of which there were many).

He loved poetry, classical music, photography, and beautiful landscapes. According to my older siblings, he was an atheist, but he taught Sunday School in our local Mormon church. He used to quote Cary Grant in the movie, *Arsenic and Old Lace*, saying about the family he grew up in, that mental illness didn't "run" in our family, "it practically galloped." His considerable skills as an amateur plumber, electrician, and auto mechanic were not passed down to me, possibly because of inadequate cognitive skills on my part…actually, definitely because of inadequate cognitive skills on my part. Besides, as a teenager, I was much more interested in girls than I was in anything useful. As a forensic psychiatrist, my father spent his life diagnosing and treating the entire range of human beings—from murderers (as part of court-ordered sanity evaluations) to Mormon missionaries (who should never have left their mothers). In the 1950s, when the doctors at his clinic had medical conferences where they gave presentations to each other about health topics, my father gave them a presentation on nuclear disarmament.

Prologue

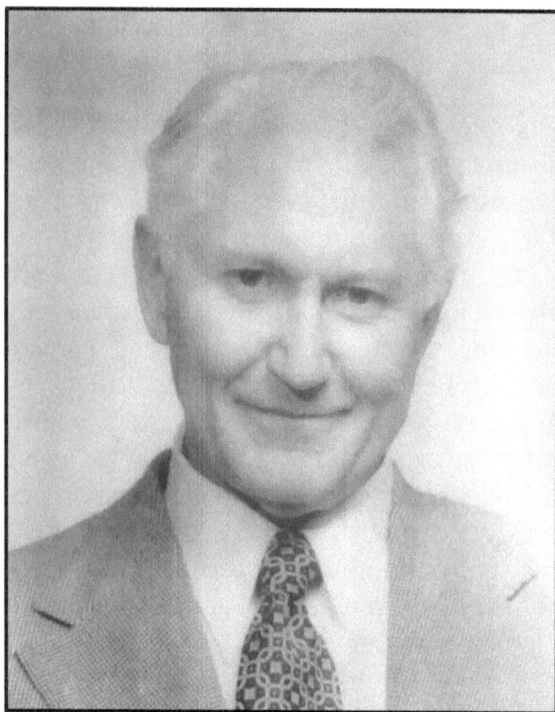

This is my very dignified father, Dr. Louis G. Moench. I inherited one slightly used Y chromosome and none of his dignity. For some reason, he chose not to be photographed wearing one of my mother's masks.

But what seemed at the time to be the strangest thing about our family turned out to be my Dad just paying attention to science better than almost anyone else.

Utah is the closest state downwind of Nevada—at least it was in the 1950s, and I don't think it has moved much since. My father would always check the news for what was happening at the Nevada nuclear testing site. For months at a time, he would prohibit us from drinking milk, formally designated as the holy grail of food in the 1950s by American mothers, including mine. My older siblings said he sometimes called it a "concentrated form of poison." He would have us take iodine in pills or drops. He would sometimes prohibit us from playing outside, especially right after a rain storm. He said there was a dangerous chemical, a name we couldn't pronounce, all over the grass. On those days, he wanted us to wear rubber soled shoes, not leather, because he said the poison would stick to leather. My older siblings said they often overheard my parents talking about bombs, radiation, and prevailing winds. It wasn't until almost 63 years later that I learned Utah had the highest radioactive iodine levels in its milk of any state in the nation, and that the National Cancer Institute had revealed that radiation exposure to America's children like me had been 15-70 times greater than what had been reported to Congress.[1]

I inherited my Y chromosome from my father, obviously. But I inherited my "Why?" chromosome from my mother, as in, "Why did Ronald Reagan nominate that idiot to the Supreme Court?" "Why does the New York Times print this stuff?" "Why does Brian want to stay out until three in the morning with a girl built like Marilyn Monroe?" Obviously, I also inherited an X chromosome from my mother. I used to think the Y chromosome from my father must have gotten me into medical school. After all, he was the scientist, scholar, and jack of all trades. But after researching for this book, I realized it was probably the combination of my mother's X chromosome and my father's interventions to protect me from radiation that left me with enough cognitive potential to get into medical school. My Y chromosome just went along for the ride.

The human brain is our most defining organ. It is by far the most complex and unique biologic entity in the known universe. Throughout the animal kingdom, there are competing versions of every organ system humans have, and many of them are superior to our own. The heart of a shrew can beat 1,500 times per minute. Humans would be dead in five minutes at that rate. A dolphin exchanges 80% of the contents of their lungs with one breath: humans only 17%. A camel has three stomachs with which to store water. The kidneys of a desert rat can concentrate urine 15 times better a human kidney. An ant's neck can withstand the pressure of 5,000 times its own weight without ever going to the gym or taking steroids.

But there is nothing in the animal world that comes close to the superiority of the human brain, especially the female human brain. Given these marvelous thinking machines, it is an incalculable tragedy that we would set in motion anything that

Prologue

would damage or compromise the very thing that sets us apart among everything else in the biological world.

My brain, amazing by animal kingdom standards, pedestrian by human standards, operates on a platform I inherited from my parents—the chromosomes, physical architecture, neurologic pathways, neurotransmitters, the thought processes, and personality eccentricities. But I am also both more and much less than what I inherited from them. Those neurons and chromosomes have been influenced, played with, and in some cases, attacked and tortured by the environment I live in and the toxins I was and am exposed to. In fact, I may be in part the product of whatever environmental toxins my great, great grandfather Louis Frederick Moench's chromosomes were exposed to as a young boy in Neuffen, Germany, in 1850. As a certified male, I was likely impacted more than my five sisters, who never let me forget that they were smarter than I was.

As for medical school, a lot has changed since 1973 when I first entered. In 2017, for the first time, women outnumbered men in the freshman year of American medical schools. I'd say it's long overdue, and this book will explain why.

But too much has also remained the same. Few medical schools teach any formal classes on how environmental degradation, pollution, and the toxic chemicals we are all now exposed to, harm individual and public health. Environmental exposures, both involuntary and voluntary (like smoking and other risky behavior) cause as much as 90% of cancers.[2] How can medical schools not be teaching that? Air pollution is the number one environmental cause of death, causes one in every five deaths worldwide,[3] more than road accidents, violence, fires, and wars combined.[4] Twenty percent of Alzheimer's disease (hereafter Alzheimer's) is caused by air pollution,[5] and about that same percentage of premature births. Common hair products on the market today may contain as many as 5,000 different chemicals, most of which have never been tested on humans for safety. Some have been shown to cause cancer in animals, and others are endocrine disruptors,[6] mimicking potent endogenous hormones like estrogen, and capable of acting as carcinogens and reproductive toxins. The average person now excretes at least 2,282 exogenous chemicals in their urine,[7] and many of them have a wide range of hazardous effects. One study found 287 chemicals in the umbilical cord blood of newborns; 158 within that batch are known to be toxic to the brain.[8]

In 2020, I was asked to give the first ever lecture to students at the University of Utah Medical School on the consequences of our ubiquitous exposure to environmental neurotoxins. That was a small step in the right direction. Hopefully this book is a second step in the right direction.

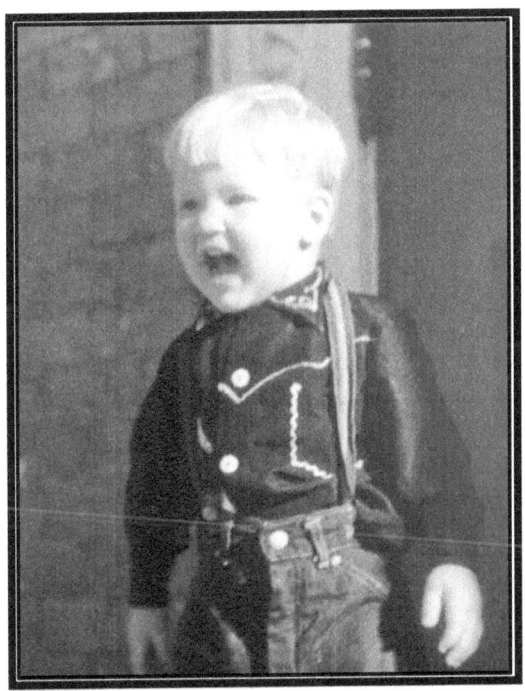

This is a picture of me in 1953 at age three, lecturing the other toddlers in the neighborhood about global warming.

Prologue

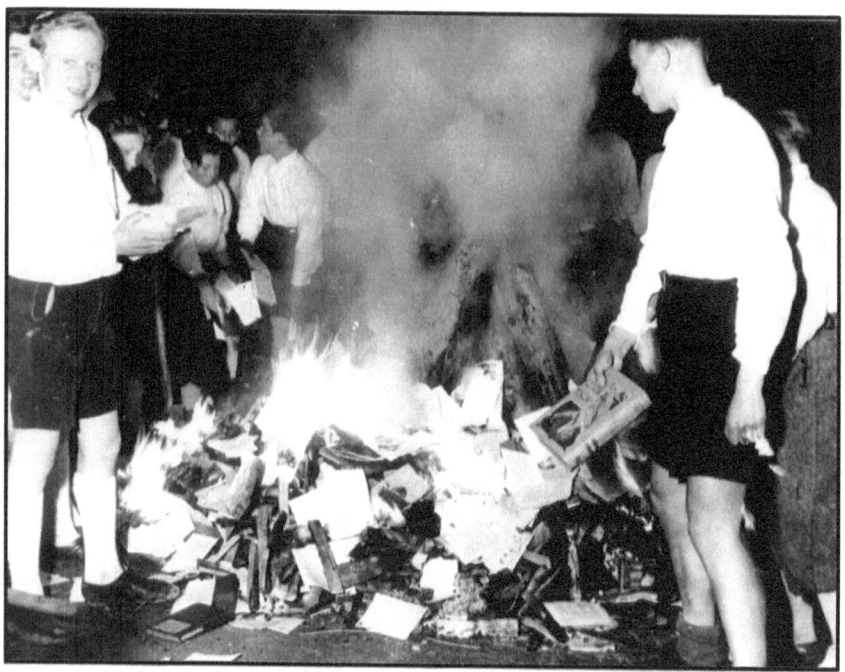

The Great Brain Robbery has been the number one book at MAGA book burnings, three years in a row.

INTRODUCTION

Congratulations! By purchasing, stealing, borrowing, plagiarizing, or burning this book, you have just demonstrated that you are a proud owner of the most complex of biological entities in the known universe—a human brain. But before you start celebrating your exalted status, you might pause for an obvious caveat. While the U.S. Declaration of Independence says, "all men are created equal," it does not say that all brains are created equal. And we know that to be true because as everyone knows, Boston Celtics fans are smarter than Los Angeles Lakers fans, because when it comes to NBA championships, they're are not interested in quantity, they're only going for quality. People who read the *Atlantic* think they are smarter than people who read *People* magazine, and people who grew up reading *Mad Magazine* have been clinically proven to be the most stable of geniuses.

At the risk of being accused of being politically incorrect and a traitor to my own gender, we now have solid evidence that women are smarter than men. For those of you who question the premise of this book, I'll give you three lines of scientific evidence. First, there was never a popular TV show called *Jane Ass*. Second, an extremely scientific study was just published yesterday in the *Journal of Irreproducible Mind-Numbing Trivia* proving one out of every three men is just as stupid as the other two. And third, you have never heard a woman declare, "Hold my beer and watch this." It is well known that Donald Trump said those exact words when he famously descended that escalator in 2015 and announced that he was going to insult half the country and run for president. Actually, Donald reportedly doesn't drink, so it was probably, "Spray my hair, and watch this!"

Now, are all men morons, idiots and goofballs? No. I'm proud to be counted in the same gender as this man.

Introduction

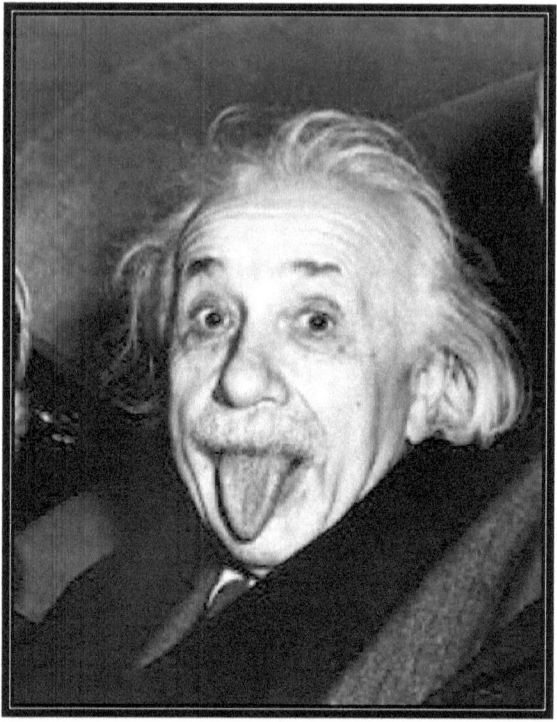

Are all women geniuses? Of course not. After all, some of them decided to marry men.

In February 2008, David Monk, a 46-year-old British man, assisted by two friends and a considerable quantity of alcohol, decided that the perfect way to end a day of skiing in the Italian Alps was to go sledding.[1] They soon realized that their manly adventure would require an important accessory that none of them were in possession of—a sled. In a stroke of communal genius, they secured the services of a foam pad that was installed to stop skiers at the bottom of the slope from crashing to their deaths, concluding that, under the circumstances, it would make the perfect sled. They then climbed to the top of the hill and launched themselves downward, quickly achieving the speed necessary to elicit the intended amount of thrill seeking, interrupted eventually by a crash into the same metal poles that had been laid bare by stealing the foam pad/sled. David died, leaving a presumably heart-broken wife and two fatherless children. Another one of the sledders was hospitalized with severe head injuries. In mourning his death, his friends described David as a "brilliant guy."

His "brilliance" notwithstanding, David was awarded, posthumously, a Darwin Award, which is given to "those who improve our gene pool by removing themselves from it in the most spectacular way possible."

The *British Medical Journal* is one of the oldest, stodgiest (that is a word—I looked it up), most prestigious medical journals in the world. When it arrives in the mail, a handlebar mustache and a monocle are attached because otherwise you're not allowed to read it. In the 2014 Christmas edition was an article with an audio version about testing the "male idiot theory" (MIT). Most people think that MIT is the acronym for the highly prestigious Massachusetts Institute of Technology. Now that you know there are two MITs, you can rightly brag at a dinner party that you also are also a graduate of MIT, with no one the wiser.

The official name of this MIT study is, "The Darwin Awards: sex differences in idiotic behavior."[2] Now, you may think that the term "idiot" doesn't need further definition, but that just means you're one of the idiots. Which puts you in good company, or least my company, because I didn't know either until I read the study. According to people with intelligent-sounding British accents involved in the study, idiots are specifically people who take senseless risks, not taking into account what the consequences would be, for rewards that are almost nonexistent. In other words, Americans.

Winners of the Darwin Award "must die in such an idiotic manner that 'their action ensures the long-term survival of the species, by selectively allowing one less idiot to survive.'"[2] So no common morons unable to chew gum and simultaneously ambulate need apply. For example, don't think that you will achieve a Darwin Award if you just shoot yourself in the head while demonstrating that your gun is unloaded. That is too common —you've got to be more creatively stupid than that. But, if a person shoots himself in the head to prove that the gun IS loaded, that is a much specialer (also a word—I got away with it in a Scrabble game once)

Introduction

achievement in idiocy and might at least earn you a nomination for the award. If your stupidity is legendary but not successful in precipitating your demise, you also don't qualify. For example, take the man who lost control of a belt sander while using it as a masturbation device and ripped off his testicle. Determined to get full use of his work tools he then repaired the injury with a staple gun, saving his other testicle (true story). He is now the new Surgeon General of Padusky Falls, Idaho (full disclosure, this book was not written under oath).

The official criteria for achieving the Darwin Award are:

1. The candidate must be eliminated from the gene pool.

2. The candidate must show an astounding misapplication of common sense.

3. The event must be verified.

4. The candidate must be capable of sound judgment.

5. The candidate must be the cause of his or her own demise.

The Darwin Awards are open to all ethnicities, cultures, and socioeconomic groups. According to the paper, 88% of Darwin Award winners were men. It should also be noted that about 3% of the nominees were couples, most of whom were "adventurous couples in compromising positions." The English translation of that is, these idiot men pressured their female counterparts into attempting procreation while risking their lives. For example, one couple parked their car in the right lane of the largest freeway in Brazil, in a dense fog, and began "the deed," soon to be run over by a large truck. So, I'd say that "couples" winners of the Darwin Award are really just male winners with an additional victim of their male stupidity.

Limitations of the study acknowledged by the authors include a likelihood that women nominate men more often, and men's deeds are more likely to be reported and witnessed, i.e., women are less likely to do the, "Hold my beer and watch this," thing. Alcohol seems to be an important element in award-winning events, much like a performance-enhancing substance in Olympic athletes, and men are likely to drink more. Males are much more likely to be admitted to an emergency room with virtually every kind of accidental injury—no surprise there. Men seem to be more willing to enlist the help of gadgets and machinery in carrying out absurd life-threatening adventures. It also could be, however unlikely, that the Darwin Awards Committee has a gender bias.

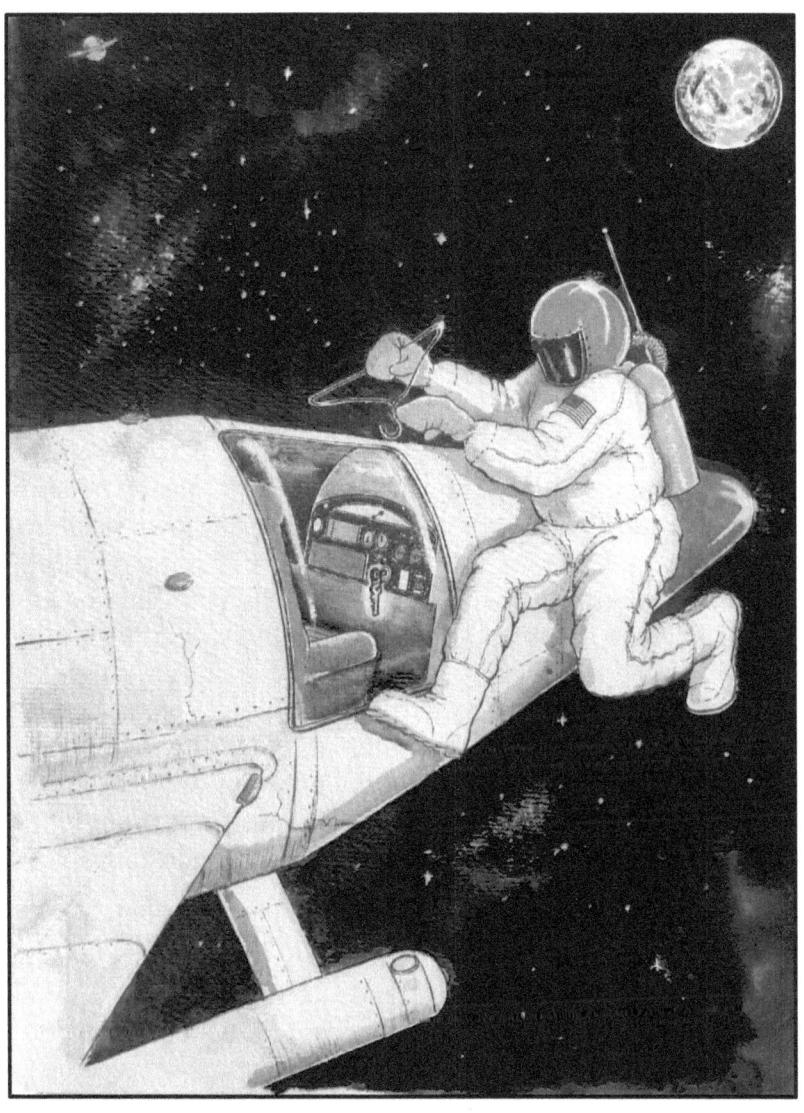

2004 Darwin Award Winner, Rocket Scientist Category

Introduction

Perhaps my entire gender should receive a group Darwin Award. A survey taken in late March 2020, during the initial stages of the COVID pandemic, showed that elderly men (the group that can't figure out how to unmute themselves for a zoom call) were the least concerned about catching the disease, less concerned than women their own age, and even less than younger people of either sex. This was despite the fact that elderly men are far and away the group at greatest risk for a serious or fatal outcome.[128]

But there is more scientific evidence of the superiority of women's thought processes than the tragic ending of the life of David Monk, other Darwin Award winners, and elderly men. Knowing this is true and having the supporting evidence are critical if you want to alienate yourself from friends at a cocktail party, are looking for a way to get thrown out of your next family reunion, or want to orchestrate some make-up sex after starting a fight with your spouse.

Contrary to what you've been told, perception is not everything. Men perceive themselves as smarter than women, and women are far more likely to underestimate their own intelligence than men,[4] despite notable progress in the last 70 years, among both sexes, in perceiving women as equally intelligent. But women are still less likely to speak up in business meetings, and they are more reluctant to engage in negotiations for raises, or career advancements. Women are less likely to be chosen as leaders in business, in politics, and in academia. Even when women achieve the rank of Chief Executive Officer (CEO) they are more likely to be ultimately forced out. One such ex-CEO, Carly Fiorina, says, "When a man is in a job, he is presumed to be competent; a woman isn't given that presumption."[5]

The fact that women are less likely to be chosen means, of course, that men are more likely. Evidence suggests that the primary reason men are overly represented when leaders are picked is that men are much more likely to be overconfident, convinced of their own abilities beyond what any objective criteria would warrant.[6] This perception of gender intellectual differences may seem insignificant at the individual level, but in the aggregate, it plays a significant role in the direction of careers chosen by women compared with men.

Researchers asked nearly 1,200 people to read a job posting and then refer two people they knew for the job. Half of those subjects were led to believe the fictitious job required high-level intellectual ability. The other half were told the job would require instead, a worker who was motivated and would bring "consistent effort." There was no difference in how often men and women were recommended for the motivation and effort job, but women were recommended 38% less often than men for the job that required high intellect.[7] This type of gender-perception bias is found in children as young as 5 years old.

The most interesting finding in the study was that women were just as likely as men to recommend men for the fictitious intellectual job. Because companies heavily value suggestions by current or former employees, they are already dealing with a pool of candidates heavily tilted in favor of men.[8] Business research shows that when a group of employees successfully performs a group task, and it's not clear that individual members deserve disproportionate credit, both men and women are likely to assume it was a man who played the decisive role.[9]

Men are the embodiment of the Dunning-Kruger Effect.[10] If you're not familiar with the term, that refers to people manifesting a cognitive dissonance that they are more intelligent and capable than they actually are. To put it bluntly, it is the overestimation of one's ability because one is not smart enough to know one's limitations. To put it more bluntly, it is stupid people who are too stupid to know how stupid they are. A more common term for this is "husband." The effect is named after the researchers that observed and first wrote about the phenomenon, David Dunning and Justin Kruger. Other researchers refer to it as the *male hubris, female humility* effect. But perhaps their research just rediscovered what Charles Darwin wrote in his book, *The Descent of Man*, "Ignorance more frequently begets confidence than does knowledge."

Introduction

The New York Times interviewed a sixth-grade math teacher, Melissa Kondrick, in Pleasanton, California, who made this observation: "We will have boys shouting out the answer, and if they're wrong, they don't care. If a girl gets it wrong, they will not answer another question. You'll see them shut down."[11] This observation makes it a little easier to understand the white supremacy group choosing the oddly juvenile name, "Proud Boys." Harvard University Press published a book in 1982, *In a Different Voice*, by psychologist, Carol Gilligan that was widely hailed as a "feminist classic," and by the publisher as starting "a revolution, making women's voices heard, in their own right and with their own integrity, for virtually the first time in social scientific theorizing about women. Its impact was immediate and continues to this day, in the academic world and beyond." Gilligan wrote about her experience that male students are much more willing to interrupt class discussions with questions and comments than female students. Because of the inhibition that girls felt in a classroom with boys, some have advocated for same gender classrooms.

Speaking of males not caring enough if they're wrong, in October 2020, a group of researchers from MIT (the college) announced that they had designed a nuclear fusion reactor that is "very likely to work." Since when is "very likely" a high enough standard for a nuclear reactor? I'm pretty sure "very likely to work" were the exact words used by the guys that built both the Hindenburg and the Titanic. Dunning Kruger guys and nuclear fusion should never be allowed to play together.

But Darwin didn't title his book *The Descent of Men and Women*. Perhaps he foreshadowed the research of Dunning and Ehrlinger that showed women performed as well as men on a science quiz but underestimated their own performance. This is likely to unnecessarily discourage women from pursuing scientific careers, and it also contributes to women being selected less often for jobs and careers where intelligence is a necessary qualification.

As to why women are smarter than men, in this case, Bill Clinton's political strategist James Carville was wrong. It's not "the economy, stupid;" it's "the environment, stupid," and it's "biology, stupid," although neither of these has yet to emerge as a winning presidential campaign motto. Follow me now, as I descend into a rabbit hole of science, political incorrectness, fascinating information, and an important take-home message. And I deny under oath that my wife twisted my arm to make me write this book.

Beyond having internet access, which makes me an expert in whatever issue I'm angry about at the moment, I do have some qualifications to write about the human brain, having observed a few in action and even more during inaction. In the course of my career as an anesthesiologist, I successfully put to sleep about 40,000 of them. But my goal with this book is to keep your brain awake, alarmed, a bit entertained, and angry about what has happened to you.

The conclusions in this book are drawn from researchers that study and work with gender on animals and humans from a traditional perspective, i.e., that there are two genders, male and female, people with XY chromosomes and people with XX chromosomes. For completeness' sake, I should mention that a small number of males have 47 chromosomes, such as an XYY genotype, referred to as Jacob's syndrome, and others who are XXY, known as Klinefelter's syndrome. Jacob's syndrome patients often don't get diagnosed as such because, although they commonly have some specific physical characteristics, like larger head size, scoliosis, and widely spaced eyes, those physical characteristics usually do not fall outside the normal range. Klinefelter males have small testes with a reduced production of testosterone. Triple X syndrome affects about one in 1,000 females, and they, too, may go unrecognized because physical characteristics are not very distinctive. All three of these disorders are often associated with neurological developmental delays, impaired brain function, and higher rates of autism. When a female has one of two X chromosomes missing or partially missing, it is referred to as Turner's syndrome, and there are usually distinct physical characteristics like short stature and webbed necks. Their intelligence is usually normal but can be impaired.

Introduction

The research I have cited, and therefore the theme of this book, makes no attempt to address the neurologic, intellectual, or behavioral status of individuals with these chromosomal abnormalities. I acknowledge that there is a movement to de-emphasize biologic sex in favor of "gender," which is more of a description of cultural, sociologic, or behavioral differentiations. I am aware that some people believe gender is more of a spectrum, or that it can be fluid, ambiguous, "transgender," or that individuals can be dimorphic, i.e., experience a dissociation between physical sexual identity and mental gender identity. My book does not attempt to address the brain function of this subset of the population and my references to "men and women" or "male and female" implies only their biological, i.e., chromosomal sex. Research conclusions or assumptions regarding individuals with a gender identity different from their biologic sex, gender dysphoria, or transgenderism, is beyond the scope of this book.

This book in no way is intended to be disguised as a political book, and politics is not part of my agenda in writing it, other than hoping that it may lead to better public policy which requires entering the political area. Nonetheless, the current political atmosphere in the United States is a jarring manifestation of poor judgement and lack of critical thinking on a mass scale. I will be picking on Donald Trump occasionally in the following chapters because no other person in my lifetime or in American history has been so influential in ushering trickle-down stupidity into the public arena, injecting it into the everyday lives of Americans, and weaving it into government policy. And he may be the most conspicuous and easily understood example of the theme of this book.

> I know I should say that writing this book was a labor of love. It was indeed labor, but instead of love it was more like child birth, extremely painful, traumatic, and included at least one person naked, screaming, sweating profusely and hating life.

Chapter One

WOMEN ARE SMARTER THAN MEN

"Half this game is ninety percent mental.

—Danny Ozark, manager of the Philadelphia Phillies

"When it comes to ruining a painting, he's an artist."

—Movie mogul Samuel Goldwyn on an abstract artist

"Chemistry is a class you take in high school or college, where you figure out two plus two is 10 or something."

—Dennis Rodman explaining team chemistry

Although he died in 2008, George Carlin was gracious enough to leave behind a review of this yet-to-be written book in a single sentence. "It's all bullshit and it's bad for you." I thank Carlin for that excellent review, and he's absolutely right. And if he had been allowed a follow-up sentence, he would have explained a bit more. "And it's really bad for men." If you'd like to know more about why that is the case, read on.

Harvard University is the mythical paragon of American intelligence, of academia, scientific research, truth, enlightenment, self-righteousness, suffocating condescension and malignant self-absorption (Ted Cruz went there). It was deliciously ironic, then, that Lawrence Summers resigned as Harvard's president in 2005 after publicly suggesting in a controversial speech that an innate gender disadvantage could explain why women lag behind the success of men in scientific careers. Some have come to Summers' defense saying that his comments have been misconstrued and that he was addressing the number of women in scientific careers more than declaring women innately handicapped in scientific aptitude compared to men. But it was certainly a political mistake, if not a factual one. A president of Harvard University, of all people, should know that female students earn higher grades than males in all age groups, in elementary and high school, and at the university undergraduate level—6.3% better grades. This disparity was found in even the traditionally male-dominated subjects—science, technology, engineering, and math (STEM), although in those courses the difference was less.[1]

Using almost every measure of academic success, girls are outperforming boys in almost every country. Studying over 1 million students in 30 different countries, Daniel and Susan Voyer, at the University of New Brunswick in Canada, found that from 1914 through 2011, girls achieved better grades than boys in all subjects at all levels. However, girls' advantages in math and science did not emerge until middle school or junior high, and their advantage across the board followed a curve, peaking in middle school, then decreasing in high school and college.[2]

The authors postulated that the reason for girls' performing better in school might be that parents assume that boys are better in math and science, and so the girls might have been more encouraged by their parents. They also theorized that girls simply work harder, study more, and make more of an effort to understand the material as opposed to boys, who focus on performance, test results, and final grades.

In STEM subjects, boys and girls were equally represented in the top 10% of their classes, but girls were overly represented in the top 10% in non-STEM. Explanations for this included the theory that boys' averages were the end result of both more gifted students and more intellectually handicapped students. But researchers did not find that to be true.

In a major national standardized test measuring engineering and technology skills, girls outperform boys, and their advantage has increased over the past five years.[3] Girls widely outperform boys in reading tests and achievement. A Stanford study examining 260 million state tests from grades 3 through 8, from 10,000 U.S. school districts, found that girls performed a half a grade better in reading by the fourth grade, and a full year better by the eighth grade.[4] Across all cultures and in all developed countries, women buy more books and read more, especially fiction. Undoubtedly, this contributes to their better performance in school.[5]

One narrow area where boys seem to have a slight advantage over girls is the math Scholastic Aptitude Test (SAT), a test that has claimed to measure less what is actually taught in school than complex problem solving. Girls do better with numerical skills and problem solving that involves set procedures. Girls' math accomplishments happen in the backdrop of their having a less positive attitude towards math and less confidence in their math abilities,[6] and boys being more likely to join math clubs and enter math competitions.[7]

Digging deeper into math tests, the Stanford study also found that the one geographic area where boys did better than girls in math, was in rich, white, suburban school districts. This suggests that the difference is attributable to social expectations or how they are treated in school rather than a reflection of innate gender differences. In economically poor districts, girls outperform boys in math. This observation will be relevant as we discuss, in subsequent chapters, the likely causes of the gender discrepancies.

In the 21st century, girls are more likely to attend college and to graduate from college.[8] Women now earn more bachelor's, master's, and doctoral degrees than men.[9] Females have an advantage in the ability to plan for the future.[10] They are superior in their ability to sustain focus and performance during longer tests, regardless of the subject.[11]

IQ tests were first introduced to American society and education about 100 years ago. At that time, women scored about five points lower than men. Between then and now, IQ test results in modern societies have steadily risen for both sexes (until just recently) but they had been rising faster in girls than in boys. By 2012, that rise among females finally reached the point where they had overtaken males by a slim margin.[12]

Several recent studies have found that poverty is associated with loss of IQ. That is not the same as low intelligence curtailing a person's career potential. It means that being or becoming poor actually impairs a person's cognitive abilities. Alice Walton, an economist, believes that the research suggests that poverty can lower a person's IQ by an astonishing 13 points.[13] She gives this example: poor individuals facing a difficult financial problem experience "a cognitive strain that's equivalent to a 13-point deficit in IQ or a full night's sleep lost."[13] In the aftermath of the pandemic-caused economic collapse, widespread financial stress is undoubtedly taking a massive toll on the cognitive ability of millions of Americans.

For a multitude of reasons, women struggle financially more than men do. So as women test better, achieve more academically, perform intellectually better than men on average across a total population, this is occurring with essentially with one frontal lobe tied behind their back because of economic handicaps.

In a study of 100 men and women given memory tasks to perform at 2 minutes, 15 minutes, and 24 hours later, women performed better.[14] In just about every way possible to test memory, females have a broad advantage in episodic and verbal memory. Females access their memory faster than men and are able to attach a date for an event more accurately.[15] They demonstrate superior autobiographical memory, random word recall, story recall, auditory memory, object location memory, and facial recognition memory, especially for female faces.[16] Females have an advantage over males in encoding memory of their own life events, whether their characterization of those events are positive, negative, or neutral.[17] Their memory advantage is independent of overall intelligence. Females are even able to attribute detail to imagined future events.

Perceptions of women's intelligence and capabilities have significantly evolved just recently. A 2018 analysis of gender stereotypes in the U.S. since the Second World War found 86% of adults consider men and women equally competent, 9% considered women more competent, and only 5% felt men were.[18] These perceptions transcended differences in sex, race, ethnicity, college education, marital status, and employment status. Further, the lead author of the study said, "communal stereotypes have changed, but increasingly towards portraying women as more compassionate, affectionate, and sensitive than men." However, "Men are still viewed as more ambitious, aggressive, and decisive than women, and that agency stereotype has not substantially changed since the 1940s."[19]

This assessment was prominently manifested during other surveys of behavior during the COVID pandemic in 2020. Women were twice as likely to wear masks in public than men, according to a study conducted by the Centers for Disease Control (CDC).[20] Bank robbers' willingness to wear masks make them more socially responsible than the average man. Men were more likely to consider wearing a mask as a "sign of weakness" and were less likely to believe they could be endangered by the virus. This is despite the fact that men have twice the mortality risk from COVID as women, according to several studies in different countries.[21]

Men were also less likely to observe COVID hand washing advisories. Recalling the criteria for being considered for the Darwin Award—the candidate must show an astounding misapplication of common sense, must be otherwise capable of sound judgement, and must be the cause of their own demise— we might consider giving American men a class action Darwin Award for risking their lives by not wearing a mask. According to most pundits, the more rational approach to pandemic public policy and behavior was a major reason for a shift of women voters from the Republican Party to the Democrats in 2020.

While this irrational and aggressively anti-social behavior is more common in men, it is not exclusively so. By February 2021, the COVID-19 pandemic had killed at least 510,000 Americans and has surpassed the number of U.S. soldiers killed in WWI, WWII, and the Vietnam War combined. President Trump recovered from his COVID infection and resumed holding large political rallies with thousands of people packed closely together, and few of them wearing masks. These were aptly named "super spreader events" because they are exactly the kind of behavior that the CDC and virtually all other medical experts warned the entire country against as a necessary means of controlling the pandemic. The pandemic spiked again, particularly in the same battleground states where

Donald Trump had held these rallies. Ignoring for the moment the mindset of the former President, the attendees of both sexes should all be given Darwin Awards for risking their own lives (and ours) to satisfy whatever psychological need they had for attending.

No one would be surprised to know that men commit more crime than women by far. As of 2017, 93.3% of inmates in federal prison were men.[22] The presumed causes would simply be the Y chromosome, testosterone, and social factors, but there is very little research to offer a more scientific explanation. One study found a correlation with a lower resting heart rate measured at age 11 and a crime history as young adults.[23] The lower the heart rate, the more likely a person is to have a criminal history, in both sexes, in all races, and irrespective of social adversity factors. At age 11, girls have a higher resting heart rate. Other studies have found that heart rate is the best biologic correlate with anti-social behavior for both genders.[24] No one seems to know why heart rate inversely correlates with antisocial behavior, even controlling for other factors, but girls do have higher heart rates.

Numerous studies have found that delinquency and criminal behavior is associated with significantly lower intelligence. Criminal activity in adolescence and adulthood is inversely correlated with intelligence studies in childhood, as early as age three. This was especially true of verbal intelligence, an area where girls have a strong advantage over boys. In Chapter 4, I'll offer another contributing explanation.

When confronted with stress, such as a job interview, women are better able to stay calm under pressure and adapt to highly emotionally charged situations. For the same reason, women make better police officers than men. Peru and Russia are two countries that have begun a process of switching over to female police forces because they are better at remaining calm when facing a potential volatile circumstance.

In an era where police brutality is a major national issue, having more female police officers and fewer male officers should loom large in the debate. Research has shown that female officers can handle violent suspects as well as males, but only 11% have ever fired their weapon while on duty, compared to 30% of male officers,[34] despite the fact they are generally at a physical disadvantage. Female officers are much less likely to use force in the course of their duties and are more likely to display empathy to de-escalate potentially violent encounters. They are less likely to injure suspects. When female officers paired with male partners took the lead, force was less likely to be used than it was when the male officer was in charge. Male officers are far more likely to be the subject of citizen complaints, and they cost their cities far more in payouts over lawsuits.[25]

The domestic stereotype of women's performing better than men when pressured to multitask, i.e., orchestrate child care, fix meals, run a household, etc., has not been confirmed by recent research. However, other research does suggest that prior to menopause, when estrogen is still abundant in women, they are indeed able to perform two tasks at once that use the same area of the brain, while men and post-menopausal women are less able.[26]

Women have superior leadership skills. The Harvard Business Review says, "Women scored at a statistically significant higher level than men on the vast majority of leadership competencies we measured.... In fact, they were thought to be more effective in 84% of the competencies that we most frequently measure."[27] Women outscored men on 17 of the 19 leadership qualities that differentiate excellent leaders from average or poor ones. The only two categories where men scored slightly higher than women were "technical or professional expertise" and "develops strategic perspective." Nonetheless, only 4.9% of Fortune 500 Chief Executive Officers (CEOs) and 2% of the Standard and Poor's (S&P) 500 CEOs are women, and that number is actually declining.[27] You might say that the stupidity of men is confirmed by the fact that they don't put more women in charge (see Chapter 9).

Traditionally, the vast majority of artists and inventors have been men. But studies have also found the artistic works of men are judged as being more creative than similar works by women.[28] There is marked disparity in how much the artistic works of men sell for compared to similar works of women. Other studies found that even among children, there was a wider variance in creativity in boys than among girls. Boys did more out-of-the-box thinking in finishing artwork, but girls excelled in "adaptive creativity," i.e., ingenuity within expected parameters.

An exhaustive study from multiple academic centers of 250,000 songs produced and released over 45 years concluded that in the area of music, women are more creative than men, i.e., "created more novel songs—works that are more musically fresh and unusual—than male artists."[29] The researchers believed the difference to be cultural influences rather than raw ability. They observed, "For the same levels of performance, women tend to receive more negative evaluations than men, and they have to outperform men to receive comparable evaluations. To overcome this 'double standard,' female minorities work harder." They also believed that their research indicated that female artists benefited more from an increased willingness to collaborate with others. But females consistently didn't have as much confidence in their work as men.

If more women were truck drivers, our roads would be much safer. Men currently hold most driving jobs and are much more likely to drive dangerously. A study from the UK found that for 5 of the 6 studied types of vehicles, men posed a much higher risk to others than women. For passenger cars, the risk of a male driver was twice that of a female driver per kilometer (km) driven. For male truck drivers, the accident risk was four times higher, and for motorcycles, men had nearly a 12 times higher risk.[30]

There must be a tail pipe embedded somewhere on the Y chromosome, because whenever a male gets behind the wheel of something, they immediately get "reckless brain syndrome." Men are 3.4 times more likely than women to get a ticket for reckless driving and 3.1 times more likely to get arrested for drunk driving.[31] Among teenagers, boys have twice the rate of death in an auto accident as girls do.

Car insurers have long charged women lower premiums than men, providing clear evidence that men are higher-risk drivers and are responsible for the majority of traffic accidents worldwide, although more drivers are men than women. Generally, the ability and the interest in self-preservation has to be considered a top priority of beings with higher intelligence, and women are simply better at it than men.

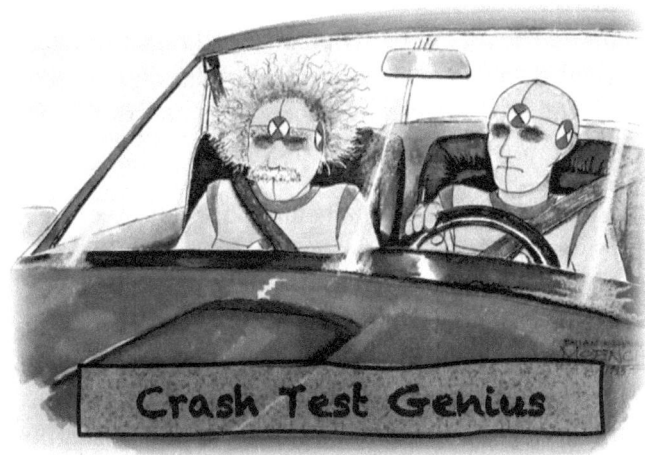

In matters of finance, women save more money and are better investors. A study by Fidelity spanning a decade, and another three-year study by Openfolio found that female investors outperformed their male counterparts,[32] and their portfolios were lower risk.

Women are better at computer coding. Researchers compared acceptance rates of contributions from men versus women in an open-source software community and found that women's contributions were accepted more often than men's if the gender of the contributor was not known.[33] If the gender was known, then men had a higher acceptance rate. Another study found that girls created much more sophisticated coding systems when designing 3D games than boys did.

Women have more refined senses than men. Females can see more colors and are better at discriminating among colors. Women think of colors as azure, periwinkle, lavender, aqua, moss, mauve, chartreuse, and eggshell. Men think of colors as red, white, and blue, or in some cases just red and not red. That is one reason why women have as many clothes and shoes as they do, and men simply can't understand why.

If you have ever heard "the eyes are the window to the soul," replace that with "the eyes are the window to the brain." The key physical feature of the eye is, of course, the iris. The color of the iris is likely related to numerous genes rather than just one, and those genes also play other roles. The same melanin that makes skin dark is related embryologically to the melanin that makes an iris dark, i.e., brown. Melanin also acts as an insulator for neurons. The more melanin insulating a nerve, the more efficiently and faster the nerve can transmit electrical signals.[34] There is some research to suggest that the same genes that are involved in developing the frontal lobes are also involved in establishing the color of the iris.

As a side note, having blue eyes is an evolutionary physical trait that probably emerged as a genetic mutation, possibly from a single individual somewhere around 29,000 years ago.[35] The genetic mutation prevented the activation of melanin in the iris, introducing for the first-time, blue-eyed homo sapiens. Lack of melanin also made their skin lighter. Blue eyes reflect more light; brown eyes absorb more light. Blue eyes can change after birth and throughout childhood, even changing to brown. A baby with brown eyes, however, will keep that color throughout life.

Some neurologic traits are firmly correlated with eye color. Women with blue eyes complain less of post-operative pain,[36] but both men and women with blue eyes are more susceptible to alcoholism.[37] Blue eyes are also associated with diseases and disorders like type I diabetes and hearing loss. Numerous studies have found certain personality traits are much more common among blue-eyed individuals, such as introversion and inhibited behavior, wariness of new experiences, and being more risk averse. And my wife just informed me that Hitler had blue eyes, so forget everything I just wrote that invoked scientific data, and we'll just go with her anecdote.

The eye can also be the window to one's overall state of health, in that it is the only part of the body that allows direct vision of the body's blood vessels and nerves (albeit with specialized equipment). At the center of the iris is, of course, the pupil. The size of the pupil is related to more than an automatic response to the amount of light needed to optimize vision. Activation of the sympathetic nervous system, the "fight or flight" response, dilates the pupils in response to the endogenous release of epinephrine. Anything that causes excitement will cause your pupils to dilate. A dilated pupil has been considered alluring and a mark of beauty for centuries. Women of Renaissance Italy and Victorian England used to put the extract of berries from a poisonous plant, belladonna, in their eyes to dilate their pupils for cosmetic effect. In fact, the name Belladonna means "beautiful woman." It could have been a big price to pay, in that prolonged use could also cause blindness. It is suggested that belladonna poison is what Shakespeare had in mind when he had Juliet drink something that made her appear dead in Shakespeare's *Romeo and Juliet*. [38]

The size of the pupil is also related to mentation. Pupil size precisely tracks changes in memory load, dilating as a response to memory banking, and in turn, constricting with the recall of each memory item. Numerous studies have shown that resting pupil size correlates with intelligence.[39] The larger the pupil, the greater the cognitive ability, specifically "fluid intelligence" more than working memory. If you have to ask what is "fluid intelligence," that is an indication that you don't have much of it. Don't feel bad; just like you, I thought it meant drinking "smart" water, or smart drinking of water, or perhaps just another word for coffee.

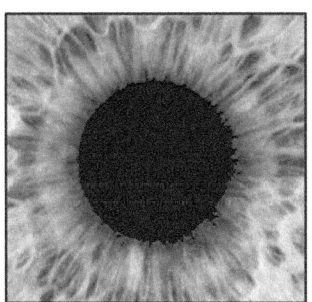 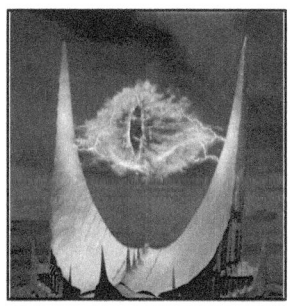

My wife's pupil is on the left, mine is on the right.
Notice how hers is slightly larger than mine.

According to the psychologist that coined the term, Raymond Cattell, fluid intelligence is "the ability to perceive relationships independent of previous specific practice or instruction concerning those relationships." In layman's terms that is simply reasoning and problem solving.

The author of one of the first studies to find this association believes it is due to greater nerve signaling with the neurotransmitter norepinephrine, which in turn, increases functional connectivity throughout the brain. A healthy eye with a normal-sized pupil is referred to as "emmetropic." You know what this is all leading up to. Women with emmetropic eyes have larger pupils than men with emmetropic eyes, yet another indicator that they are more intelligent. [56]

The difference between the brains of males and females is also manifested in differences in the patterns of eye movement when they perform visual scanning. As a person reads a book or gazes at a picture, the eyes are involved in tiny movements called saccades, punctuated by pauses called fixations. This eye movement exposes characteristics about the brain that are subconsciously dictating this pattern. One researcher described it this way: "Who a person is relates to how they move their eyes."[40] The ability to focus on what's important is revealed in eye movements. People who are more curious, enjoy learning, and pursue new experiences move their eyes much more, the amplitude of their saccades is greater, and they score higher on intelligence tests.

One study provides an example. Researchers analyzed the eye movements of subjects in passive viewing of pictures. Females engaged in more exploratory gaze, had higher saccade amplitudes, and conducted lengthier scan paths. They also spent less time in "fixation," prompting the researchers to speculate that was the result of their inspecting pictures more quickly. In fact, researchers blinded to the sex of the subject could accurately predict the sex 70% of the time based only on the revealing eye movement patterns.[41] When viewing human faces, women explore the image more thoroughly and are better than men at facial recognition,[42] partially due to different eye movements. They pay more attention to the eyes, while men pay more attention to a face's nose.[43]

Compared to men, women have nearly 50% more neurons in their olfactory bulb, the brain's smell center, which not only gives them a more acute sense of smell, it enhances their ability to differentiate, identify, and remember scents and odors.[44] This explains the classic meme of women's being bothered by someone else's smelly socks, a problem my wife wouldn't know anything about had she not read about it in *Reader's Digest*. Given the close relationship between the senses of smell and taste, it is not surprising that women have more refined palates, a superior ability to recognize different tastes.[45] This is at least partly attributable to more taste buds in their tongues. This is likely at least one reason why men support the fast-food industry more than women, and their food choices, by any measure, are usually less healthy and more meat oriented.[46] Suffice it to say, it is not women who are keeping Taco Bell and Arby's in business.

Women generally have better hearing than men. Specifically, they are better able to hear sounds at higher frequencies, above 2,000 hertz (Hz), although men may be better at locating the sources of sounds. Men are more likely to hear using just one side of their brain, whereas women are more likely to use both hemispheres.[47] Men are more than five times more likely to lose their hearing compared with women. Some of that difference may relate to sociological factors like occupations and lifestyle choices (like listening to loud music) well known to damage hearing, but that does not account for all of that disparity. Women also have better tactile acuity, i.e., sense of touch. For example, women can detect differences in the textures of a fabric better than men, but it is probably due to a higher concentration of nerve endings in their smaller hands rather than originating from differential brain anatomy. The one sense where men seem to have an advantage is in some aspects of sight, specifically detail and rapid movement.

In the happiness game, on average, women throughout the world are at a disadvantage. They have lower incomes, are still less educated, are more likely to be divorced, and are, as a group, less healthy. Women have an increased risk of being diagnosed with clinical depression. Nonetheless, surveys suggest that despite these disadvantages, women on average report as much or more life satisfaction than men.[48] Other researchers think that a more comprehensive analysis suggests that women have more negative feelings about day-to-day activities, and that the level of happiness they report may not represent how they actually feel.[49] How many times a person laughs during the day may be a better indicator. That's why I'm trying to punctuate this otherwise rather depressing book with scientifically proven humor and surgically precise sarcasm.

Numerous other studies have shown that the happiest adults are unmarried, childless women. In rather sharp contrast, married men are happier than single men. Attitudes toward marriage vary significantly between women and men. Only 37% of men believe they can have a fulfilling life without marriage, but 59% of women do.[50] So it seems that women are essential to everyone's happiness, and men, not so much.

The "women are smarter" premise and the "single women are happier" premise also fit, at least loosely, with evidence that smarter people of both sexes are happier when not being around other people. Recent research has found that people who have more social interactions with close friends are happier; no surprise there. But there was one major exception. When very smart people spend time with others, it actually reduces their level of happiness.[51] It's lonely at the top of the intellectual heap, so I've been told. If nobody likes you and you don't like anyone else, you can rationalize it by claiming that's because you're just too smart for everyone. Good luck with that argument at your next family reunion, job interview, or online dating pitch.

The movies and TV are also proof of female superiority. Who were the stars of *Alien, Mulan, Thelma and Louise, Frozen, Wonder Woman, Rosemary's Baby, and Barbie*? Certainly not men. And they didn't even need Meryl Streep to play any of the leads. Who were the intelligent ones of the hit series (and almost a documentary), *The Flintstones*? Wilma and Betty, not Fred or Barney.

Finally, if you still don't find it convincing that women are functioning with superior brains, then consider this. Women speak fluent canine better than men, i.e., women are better at interpreting dogs' attempts to communicate through barking and growling (from a real study).[52] So when a man says to a dog, "Who's a good boy?" he's really just asking about himself. When a woman says it, she's actually talking to the dog.

THE FARCE IS WITH THEM: THE DEATH OF CRITICAL THINKING

Having made an airtight case that women are mentally superior to men, I will now poke a small hole in that balloon with this caveat. In the run-up to the 2020 election, millions of Americans took a leap back into the Dark Ages with the wholesale abandonment of rationality, embracing a medieval universe of hideous conspiracy theories known as QAnon. The various theories swirled around a leading narrative that prominent Democrats, deep state elites, and Hollywood celebrities are running a sex-trafficking ring for Satan-worshipping pedophiles financed by Jewish kingpins (a revival of the 2016 "Pizzagate"). Some versions went even further—the perpetrators were murdering the children to drink their youthful blood and engage in cannibalism. Similar anti-Semitic conspiracy theories have infected European society on and off for centuries. They erupted during Nazi rule of Germany in the 1930s and were used to "justify" the Holocaust.

The frosting on this degenerate, malevolent cake is that Donald Trump is supposed to be miraculously and heroically working behind the scenes to bring all this evil to an end in a blaze of glory. Much like the Second Coming of Jesus Christ, Donald Trump was going to sweep up all these evildoers in the "Storm," a violent whirlwind of righteous retribution (note that he used that specific word as his campaign slogan), ending with the criminal elites being ceremoniously paraded off to jail, or much worse, killed in mass executions. Many Trump supporters that invaded the Capitol on Jan. 6, 2021 viewed what they were doing as ushering in that "Storm," and some had the apparent intent of executing Nancy Pelosi, Vice President Mike Pence, and other political enemies or weak-kneed supporters of Trump.

Speaking of knees, from the same political contingency so overcome with patriotism that they couldn't tolerate black athletes kneeling during the national anthem, came the thousands who "proved" their patriotism by waving and making love to the American flag while attempting to overthrow the American government, assassinate its leaders, and bring an end to the principles and institutions that define our government. This mindset is hardly born of critical thinking.

The current public maestro of QAnon and host of what I expect will be a new PBS special, *Quack History Month*, is new House member from Georgia (and a real Georgia peach), Marjorie Taylor Greene. Her latest conspiracy jewels included claims that school mass murders, like the one at Parkland, Florida, where 16 students and a teacher were slaughtered, didn't happen and were false flag operations intended gin up public support for gun control. She claims that the apocalyptic wildfires in California were caused by a Jewish cabal that included the solar company Solaren, and the Rothschilds banking family. They accomplished their massive arsonist feat by using space lasers.[53] She has called for the public execution of some of her Democratic colleagues,[54] the assassination of Barack Obama, and a "bullet to the head" of Nancy Pelosi. After widespread calls for her expulsion from Congress, she says she received confirmation of continued endorsement by our former President, and that in a single day, Jan. 29, 2021, she took in $1.6 million dollars in campaign contributions from 60,000 supporters who apparently like her malicious insanity.

Like many other conspiracy theories, this absurdity started on testosterone-fueled platforms such as 4chan and 8chan and by noted conspiracy puppeteers such as Alex Jones. But it mutated and spread rapidly, not so much by testosterone, but primarily by women, especially mothers, on mainstream social media (Facebook and Instagram), where women wade deeply in the flooded streams of anti-vaxxer and anti-lockdown paranoia. It has been whitewashed with a soft veneer of maternal protectionism. At QAnon rallies, most of the crowds are females, and most of them mothers; many bring their children to the rallies. Many of the signs read some version of "Save the Children." And who doesn't want to save the children?

I'd love to "save the children" from this breathtaking stupidity. Annie Kelly, a researcher on anti-feminist and far-right digital culture, wrote in the New York Times, "Conspiracy theories are no less dangerous [even] when they claim to be driven by maternal love."[55]

I do not intend for this commentary to drift into an issue of pandemic-provoked rupturing of normal psychology and sociology guard rails and the ascendency of political cultism. That will undoubtedly be the theme of numerous other books. What I wish to remain focused on exclusively is the complete and utter lack of critical thinking required to embrace such dangerous nonsense. For presumably rational adults to immerse themselves in the assumption that, without a shred of evidence, vast numbers of other people (some identified, most not) are engaged in such hideous evil and duplicity, is a skin-crawling affront to anyone capable of rational thought and a gesture of inhumane contempt for the people they accuse. But to take violent action toward and even plan the murder of those same people as they did on Jan. 6, 2021, obviously risking their own lives and wellbeing in the process, is abject abandonment of rationality for emotionally driven gullibility.

Even the very conservative American Enterprise Institute is alarmed[56] at the number of Republican women that have swallowed QAnon conspiracies "crook, slime, and stinker." Over one-third of them believe that QAnon conspiracies are accurate. On conspiracy theories only, I'll give these women an "F" compared to men; I will give men an "F+." With both of them, "The Farce is with Them."

Women Are Smarter Than Men

The book was thought up right here in America. Sale is permitted only after a five day wading period. The book was first written in 2021and upgreated in 2024 using artyfishal intellijunts and otto correct. If you sea any airs, oar nodis any missed steaks in the book, you can contact our kustumer cervix department, and talk two a friendly purse sun with a 4un aksent hoo can help yoo get a gnu book write uway.

Chapter Two

HOW THE BRAIN WORKS

> "Things are more like they are now, than they have ever been."
>
> —Attributed to both President Dwight Eisenhower and President Gerald Ford

> "Wherever I have gone in this country, I have found Americans."
>
> —Alf Landon, who ran against President Franklin Delano Roosevelt

> "We're ordering a lot of supplies. We're ordering a lot of, uh, elements that frankly we wouldn't be ordering unless it was something like this. But we're ordering a lot of different elements of medical."
>
> —President Donald Trump on why he didn't order medical supplies for the pandemic sooner

Let's face it, in an organ beauty contest, the human brain is probably going to place dead last, behind even the pancreas. The runaway winner would be the heart, but only because few people have seen an actual heart—not so pretty in real life. People put the heart on bumper stickers, letters, emojis, greeting cards—everything. We have a quasi holiday devoted to hearts, Valentines 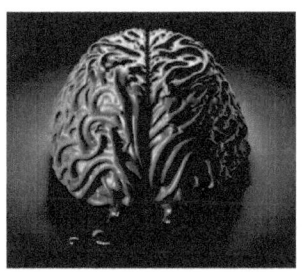 Day. And of course, boxes of chocolates come in the fake shape of a heart. But nobody sends chocolates in the shape of the real love organ, the brain because it looks like a haystack of worms.

How the Brain Works

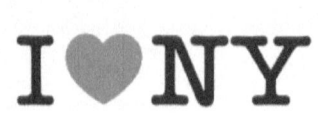

If you are fond of New York, you buy something with this on it.

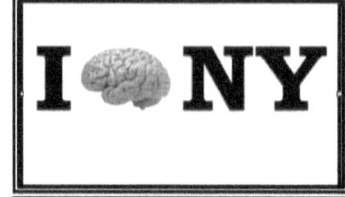

But you can't even find something like this.

We have given the heart credit it doesn't deserve, allowing it to usurp what is clearly the brain's territory, and that is to think, feel, and emote. No one falls in love because of their heart, which has nothing to do with it. We have allowed centuries of brain discrimination simply because the brain is ugly. We should all be ashamed. It's time we gave the brain its due.

The heart performs the rather mundane task of beating about 3 billion times during an average lifetime. Granted, a heartbeat is what keeps you alive, but your brain is the only reason why that even matters. The brain performs thousands, if not millions of mundane tasks. But in addition to the mundane, it allows a human the ability to do such diverse things as carve the *statue of David* out of a single block of marble, make the necessary calculations to travel the solar system and the universe, and create destructive devices so unimaginably horrific that they could end most life on earth. As marvelous as our brains are, as Robynne Boyd wrote in the *Scientific American*,[1] our brains remain a mystery even unto themselves.

There is a popular myth, even more popular than Bigfoot, that humans only use 10% of our brains' intellectual capacity. Over the course of 24 hours, imaging technology has demonstrated that virtually the entirety of our brains is in use, even during sleep and general anesthesia. Researchers have found that the only thing that can completely shut down the brain is watching The Real Housewives of New Jersey.

For people fortunate enough to have one, an adult human brain weighs about 3 pounds, unquestionably the most important 3 pounds, even in men. Within those three pounds is everything that constitutes your claim as a member of the human species. As important as opposable thumbs are, opposable cerebral hemispheres are even more important to being one of our species. In order for you to understand later chapters, this chapter is intended to make you an armchair neuroscientist. Once you finish the chapter, you have my permission to open up your own practice. Given that we live in an era when science, training, expertise, evidence, and common sense are no longer valued or even accepted, you should do a booming business.

As I wrote this, there were people in my home state of Utah trying to break into hospitals to secretly videotape what they assumed to be empty intensive care rooms. These COVID sleuths were determined to shine the light of truth to the world, because, as everyone knows, people who are critically ill and needing life support drive themselves to the hospital given that ambulances haven't been invented yet. Therefore, the COVID-19 pandemic is a hoax. Those people would be good candidates to be your first patients.

Your brain is an energy hog; it is the most metabolically demanding organ in the body. That seems odd given that your heart must beat constantly, around once or more per second for your entire life. If you look at a beating heart on the operating table, you can see how much work is being done by that amazing organ. But the brain still requires more energy.

About 20-25% of your total body's energy consumption is spent operating your brain. Per pound, at rest, your brain consumes about ten times more calories than your largest muscles. Reading this book just increased that energy consumption, which will help you lose weight, an entire nanogram at least. If you are someone that calculates calories burned compared to calories consumed in an effort to stay in good physical shape, you might consider spending an hour solving differential equations...while running on a treadmill. Intense focus on a rigorous mental task, like taking the SAT, does increase the metabolic rate of the brain, but not by much.

But there is something of a biological disconnect between the energy demands of the brain and the energy stores available to it. To meet those energy demands, the brain is primarily dependent on cerebral blood flow (CBF), which is why CBF is in a constant state of flux, directed toward the most active parts of the brain. Any problems achieving adequate chronic blood flow are closely related to age-related cognitive decline, and acute blood flow interruptions, lasting only a few minutes, are the direct cause of strokes.

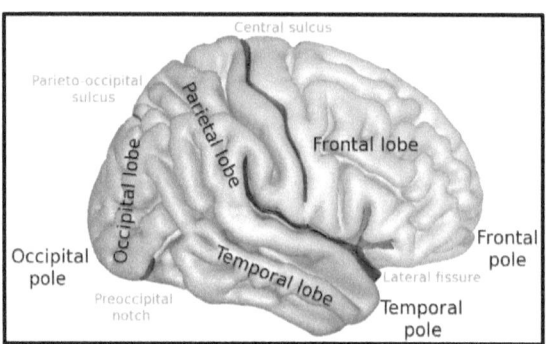

Primary lobes of the brain looking at the outside of the hemispheres.

GROSS (or in politically correct vernacular, "aesthetically challenged") ANATOMY

Starting from the bottom, because that is the chronological sequence of development, there are three embryonic divisions of the brain. The hindbrain consists of the spinal cord, brain stem, and cerebellum. The medulla oblongata in the hindbrain is what keeps you alive in the short term via control of your heart rate and blood pressure, and keeping your lungs expanding and contracting—all automatic functions. This part of your brain keeps life's essential activities going without your having to spend time, energy, or conscious commitment to the occasionally useful endeavor of not dying. The term, "lizard brain," is often used derisively (and that is an insult to lizards), but it originated in reference to the oldest part of the brain, i.e., the brain stem, because of its primary role in managing primitive survival instincts like flight or fight.

It's actually to the credit of God or your evolutionary ancestors that you don't have to consciously think about breathing and telling your heart to beat, because you'd have a really hard time accomplishing the really important things in life, things like tweeting conspiracy theories to people you don't know. The medulla oblongata also contributes to keeping you alive long term by engineering your swallowing reflex without your having to even think about it. For example, that critical, unconscious reflex is what allows you to down a food item that clearly violates the Geneva Convention, i.e., a corn dog, just for a few votes in the Iowa caucuses. Every once in a while, you should send some flowers and a thank you card to your under-appreciated medulla oblongata.

Let's say you're in bed having a wonderful dream that you have just been granted a big promotion. That dream happens, thanks in large part, to the pons part of your hindbrain. Then, your alarm goes off, and the auditory cortex within your temporal lobe kicks in. The neurons in your Locus Coeruleus (LC; more about that later) have been quiet during rapid eye movement (REM) sleep, but now they light up like a microwave with a fork in it (so I've heard). You check your pulse to see if you are, in fact, alive. If you are, you know you have to go to work. If not, you can sleep in a lot longer.

Another part of your brain, the cerebellum, allows you enough physical movement and balance to get out of bed, avoid tripping on your treadmill, and not fall on your face. The cerebellum takes orders from the boss (the cerebrum) and figures out how to implement those orders. The cerebellum makes calculations about which muscles need to be triggered in order to achieve any certain movement, whether it's fine-muscle movement or the large-muscle demands of rising out of bed and making it to the bathroom before realizing too late that, thanks to the COVID pandemic, you're out of toilet paper. The cerebellum is also involved in marshaling the memory involved in achieving a learned or a habitual movement. The ability to walk depends on information stored in the cerebellum.

Actually, the cerebellum, called the little brain, has been historically underrated and underappreciated, kind of like New Zealand. Conventional wisdom was that the cerebellum was primarily just involved in movement. New research, however, has found a much bigger part in overall brain function. It plays a diverse role in processing information from our five senses as well as pain, movements, thought, and emotion.² It is probably integral to higher functions like language, tool use, and construction. Evidence of its importance is that the cerebellum is home to 80% of the brain's neurons, despite being only the size of a tennis ball, about 10% of the total brain mass. For its size, it has even more folds than the rest of the brain, creating 80% as much surface area as the cerebral cortex. This anatomic trait suggests that the cerebellum, long thought to primarily control muscle movement, has played an even more significant role in the evolution of our uniquely human brain functions, like our highest cognitive capability and complex behavior.²

Once you're out of bed, you might call on the services of your midbrain, the uppermost part of the brain stem, to brush your teeth, basically without thinking about it. While your midbrain may be front and center at this point, by now most of the neurons in your entire brain are already up and running. Next up are your occipital lobes at the back of your cerebral hemispheres, where sight is processed as you look in the mirror for evidence of what the hell happened to you last night. As your wife asks you to pick up your underwear, put your dirty socks in the hamper, and let the dog out, your auditory cortex notices that the children are fighting and late for school, and your phone starts ringing with telemarketer calls—then your natural secretary kicks in, the Reticular Formation (RF). The RF screens out less important incoming information so that your brain is not overloaded with good news. In the year 2024, Americans' RFs were clearly working overtime, doing an excellent job of not overloading them with good news.

As you consider shaving, showering, and developing your strategy for the day's activities, you begin to activate your forebrain, consisting primarily of your cerebrum, which includes all the wrinkly stuff that makes your brain look like a huge, bloated walnut. Also like a walnut, your cerebrum is split into two halves or hemispheres, with a deep canyon between them. The "walnuttier" you are, the better. The two hemispheres communicate with each other with a massive bridge, the corpus callosum, lying at the bottom of the canyon.

The hemispheres specialize in different characteristics. The left hemisphere is the seat of your ability to communicate or your failure to communicate. "Honey, when's our anniversary?" "Yesterday." This is a sign that things aren't going well in your left hemisphere and are about to not go well for you whatever hemisphere you live in, left, right, north, or south.

The right hemisphere is where your ability to engage in logic and abstract reasoning and understand math and science originates. If you believe in God and believe that God made humans, you have to reconcile that, for no good reason He (She?) arranged all the nerves carrying signals from the body to the brain to cross over to the opposite side. The end result is that the right side of the brain controls the left side of the body and vice versa. The purpose of that was to add another two years to the residency of neurosurgeons.

Each cerebral hemisphere can be divided into regions or lobes. The occipital lobes in the back of the brain control sight, and their links to other memory parts of the brain allow to you to remember what you looked like while you were on top of the world at age 12, just before acne.

Moving toward the front of the brain, the temporal lobes are next to the occipital lobes. The temporal lobes process your hearing, such that when your wife says the toaster is on fire, you conclude you can continue texting. By integrating your memory bank with the current sensations of touch, taste, and sight, you conclude that the toaster is indeed on fire and that she can handle it as does everything else. The warm and fuzzy nostalgia over what music you were listening to when you attempted a first kiss with your teenage heartthrob also comes from your temporal lobes. If you remember that as a traumatic experience from which you never quite recovered, that is all thanks to the part of your temporal lobes called the hippocampus, a really happening place in the brain.

The hippocampus is part of the limbic system, a cortical region regulating learning, memory encoding, memory consolidation, emotion, and spatial awareness and spatial navigation (not a reference to Star Trek). It plays a large role in goal-oriented behavior and the flexible use of information to achieve that goal.[3]

From animal studies, we learn that damage to the hippocampus leads to hyperactive behavior and a loss of the ability to learn inhibition from previous experience. Anonymous (alas, probably not Einstein) could have been referring to a damaged hippocampus when he/she famously said the definition of insanity is doing the same thing over and over again and expecting a different result.

"Amygdala" sounds like the name of the red-headed girl in my second-grade class that had the best pigtails and could beat up every boy in the class, by which I mean me. But it is the real name of the part of the brain she would have activated to beat up every boy in the class. Your amygdala is the next-door neighbor of your hippocampus. It's shaped like an almond and about the same size, and it is responsible for emotions and behavioral responses to emotions—things that don't involve a lot of thought, like motivation, aggression, fear, and voting. Thinking you can outrun a charging grizzly bear would be a good example of using your amygdala, while not using your cerebral cortex.

A good example of the role of the amygdala and other key parts of the brain comes from a character-building event of my youth, and will be referred to henceforth as "The Great Escape." As a 20-year-old Mormon missionary in 1970, I was driving a car full of other missionaries returning to Boston from New Brunswick, Canada. It's a 13-hour drive, and much of it is on a very lonely road through hundreds of miles of forest. The landscape was flat, the scenery repetitive, and despite forest as far as the eye could see, it took on an unrelenting bleakness. And did I mention it was mind…numbingly…boring? It almost felt like we were on another planet all by ourselves. We didn't see evidence of other human life forms, i.e., potential converts, for hours on end. And we were tired. You can sense I'm trying to justify some upcoming bad behavior.

We were caravanning with another car filled with equally bored missionaries. As representatives of God with numb minds are wont to do, we decided to break up the monotony by trying to get ourselves killed. The other car was being driven by a missionary who was essentially a reformed car thief who had extensive experience in "fast and furious" type driving to avoid being captured by the police. Given these circumstances, you can easily see why we concluded God would be supportive if we turned the long trip into a daredevil race between the two cars of Mormon "elders" (an anachronistic and inaccurate title for 19 to 21-year-old missionaries) dressed like the Blues Brothers minus the sunglasses.

At first, the race went rather well for me, as I put the pedal to the metal, quickly hit 110 mph, and took the lead, much to the satisfaction of everyone in our car and no doubt to God, given that the missionaries in our car were obviously more righteous. The two racing cars full of missionaries then jockeyed for position on the road, and I assumed I had gotten the upper hand. A few minutes later, however, the other car being driven by Elder Ex-Car-Thief came zooming by, leaving a cloud of dust, passing us by using the unpaved left shoulder of the road, going 115 mph. At that point, however, my amygdala kicked into high gear with a well-earned fear of "meeting our Maker," and I decided I didn't want the ten missionaries involved to end up as permanent residents of the Boston cemetery. But other important parts of my brain kicked in shortly after. Stay tuned, the story continues later.

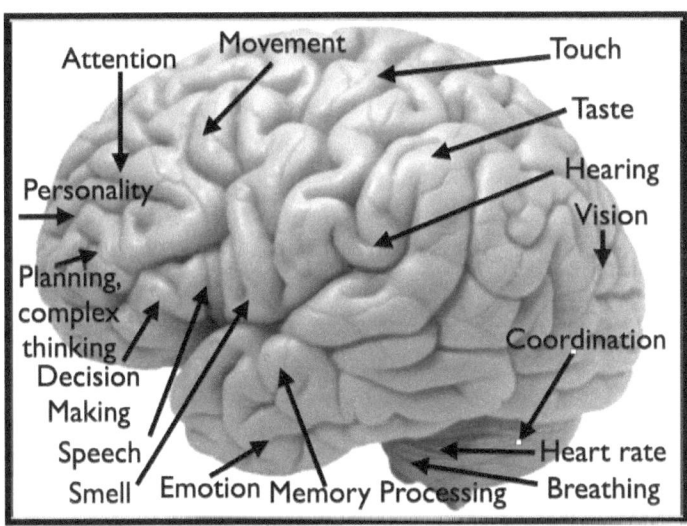

Functions of the brain by region

Several studies have shown that there are some subtle differences in brain anatomy depending on a person's political views. Young adults who identify themselves as strong conservatives have a larger right amygdala. Liberals have increased gray matter in the anterior cingulate cortex. Psychological tests find that conservatives demonstrate stronger physical and emotional reactions to threat (think grizzly bears, the police, and grizzly bears dressed like the police), conflict, and system justification, i.e., support for the existing social order. In contrast, liberals are less dogmatic, more open to nuance, novelty, and uncertainty. Thus, the brain regions activated by risk and conflict correspond to structural differences between liberals and conservatives.[4] This raises again the issue of whether the anatomy is a cause or the effect of the political orientation, and many researchers believe it's both.

Some of the anatomic differences between men and women are the same as those between liberals and conservatives, so it may not be much of a surprise that over the last several election cycles, women have been aligning themselves more with Democrats than Republicans (with the notable exception of the QAnon contingency as previously mentioned).

Moving forward, your parietal lobes have a lot on their plate, some of which is a matter of the food on your dinner plate. They provide you with information on taste, temperature, and touch as well as reading and mathematics. For example, your parietal lobes are the ones that allow you to read the menu and salivate while you order an extra-deluxe, quadruple bacon cheeseburger with fries, while doing the math on how much the ambulance ride to the hospital will cost that follows the heart attack from the extra-deluxe, quadruple bacon cheeseburger. My mother must have had huge parietal lobes, just because of the one thing she made really well—gravy. Her gravy was worth a ride to the hospital.

At the front of the brain are the frontal lobes, named by someone with very little imagination. In some people, the main function of the frontal lobes is to prevent the hollow sound of a ripe melon when someone taps on your forehead. In other people, the frontal lobes are the seat of executive functioning, which is rational thinking, creativity, planning, and integration of strategy, voluntary movement, and short-term memory. Tom Brady's analyzing a cover

2 defense and calling an audible at the line of scrimmage, Jeff Bezos's developing a business strategy to eliminate all other businesses on the planet, or an emergency room nurse's triaging a COVID patient with multiple failed organ systems, are all examples of executive functioning.

Within the frontal lobes are key regions such as Broca's area, named after 19th century French neurosurgeon Paul Broca, who discovered its function. This small area lights up just before words are spoken. By connecting with the temporal cortex, the center of sensory information processing, and the motor cortex, which controls the mouth, lips and tongue, Broca's area allows thoughts to be transformed into language and expression. The classic stroke outcome of a person losing the ability to translate their thoughts into decipherable speech is known as Broca's aphasia.

Carl Wernicke was a 19th century German neurologist who put his name in the books by establishing the association between diseases and certain areas of the brain. Wernicke's area, located behind Broca's area in the posterior part of the temporal lobe, is where we process written and spoken language. Damage here leaves a patient with receptive or Wernicke's aphasia. The patient can still speak but doesn't make sense and can't comprehend the speech of others.

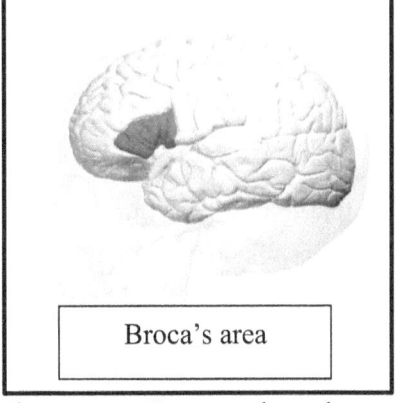

Broca's area

Wernicke's area

The fusiform gyrus is the specialized part of the brain that allows to you read this book, with its wealth of information. The humor in the book is processed in the inferior frontal cortex, in fact, the extremely inferior part of the frontal cortex.

On the surface of the cerebrum and cerebellum is a thin outer layer, about 1/4 of an inch thick, called the cortex. Whoever came up with that name was using their cerebral cortex, because that's the Latin word for "bark." The various regions of the cortex (bark) of the cerebrum are arranged in an orderly fashion corresponding to the location of body parts. Within those anatomic areas neurons that perform similar functions tend to be grouped together. For example, neurons that control frequently performed, related movements are positioned close together like the lips and the tongue. In contrast, the positioning of various parts of the body in the cortex of the cerebellum is much more random, like a jigsaw puzzle that falls out of a box. A piece of the shoulder may be next to the foot. An eyebrow may be represented next to your elbow, your lip may be next to your toes, something most of us can only achieve when we put our foot in our mouth metaphorically.

The brain's bark is also known appropriately as gray matter. This area appears grossly as "gray" because nerves in the cortex do not have the insulation (called myelin) that makes most other parts of the brain appear white. If you have ever described someone's nerves as "raw," that is exactly what's going on in your brain's bark. The highest level of thought processing happens in the cortex. The bark of the brain is where Einstein, Marie Curie, and Newel Taylor (who helped saved my grade in calculus...thank you, Newel) had neurons that the rest of us can only fantasize about.

Buried inside the forebrain are highly specialized areas—the thalamus, hypothalamus, pituitary gland, and olfactory bulb. The thalamus relays sensory input from multiple body parts to the cerebral cortex. A typical sensory impulse travels from the body surface toward the thalamus, which receives it as a sensation. This sensation is then passed onto the cerebral cortex for interpretation as touch, pain, or temperature.

The hypothalamus is about the size of a marble and is responsible for the sweaty palms you get when the boss asks you to step in her office, when you asked someone out of your league to the homecoming dance, or when I faced the next stage of The Great Escape. While going 110 mph, my cerebellum allowed me the fine motor skills to avoid careening off a cliff, and my occipital lobes allowed me to spot a small speck in my rear-view mirror getting larger and larger. My hippocampus then offered this penetrating insight: if the object in the mirror was getting larger, then it was getting closer and closer to me. My frontal lobes then weighed in with this lightning bolt—if I was going 110, then whoever now had their flashing lights on behind me was going even faster. My frontal lobes then handed the ball back to my hypothalamus, which said to my frontal lobes, "Be afraid, be very afraid." Lateraling the ball back to my frontal lobes for some outstanding executive functioning that comes with being 20 years old, I decided I'd better slow down, having concluded that my life might very well be over shortly. To be continued.

The hypothalamus is also the origin of basic physiologic sensations like hunger, thirst, and with the help of your amygdala, driving with your middle finger out the window at other drivers. In women, the hypothalamus controls the menstrual cycle and reproductive impulses.

Next door to the hypothalamus is the thalamus, the gatekeeper of information exchanged between the cortex and the spinal cord. Sensory impulses from throughout the body are sent from the spinal cord to the thalamus, which relays it to the cerebral cortex for interpretation.

The next phase of The Great Escape was a sigh of relief when I saw a car being driven by a member of the Royal Canadian Mounted Police speed past me, chasing the other missionary car that was now ahead of mine and still going about 110 mph. I smiled and smugly assumed the other missionaries were in big trouble and that God was running interference for me because of my obvious righteousness. The joy I felt came from the activation of my entire limbic system, which included multiple brain regions —the hypothalamus, hippocampus, amygdala, limbic cortex, and the precuneus --- all communicating with each other. Happy people seem to have a larger than average right precuneus, which serves to integrate the emotional and cognitive contributors to happiness.[78] My right precuneus must have been bursting with joy and rapture. But The Great Escape didn't end there.

MICROSCOPIC ANATOMY

Precuneus is the dark (red) shaded area.

The brain starts to develop at the embryonic stage about 3 weeks after conception. Primitive neural cells begin to divide at about 6 weeks' gestation, differentiating into the two most common types of brain cells, neurons and glia.[5] By the ninth week after conception, the brain is identifiable as a tiny, round structure. As soon as they are produced, neurons travel to various parts of the brain, where they begin to establish connections with other neurons as part of basic neural networks, the brain's interstate highway system. By this time the fetal brain is starting to develop the neurotransmitters that allow neurons to communicate with each other.

People often use the term, "neuron," when they are referring to brain cells. But that ignores the many other types of cells that populate the brain's infrastructure. There are different types of neurons and multiple types of support cells. In fact, researchers have found 17 different types of brain cells. An entire baseball team of different brain cells exists inside your skull, including plenty of substitutes and relief pitchers. Only about 10% of those brain cells are neurons.[1] As for neurons, there may be as many as 10,000 different subtypes of neurons. As with other cells, each type of brain cell has the same set of genes (like the players on the team all wearing the same uniform), but different cell types are formed because they activate different genes. And again, just as different players on the team excel at different skills—pitcher, catcher, groin scratcher—different skills are activated by the genes in the various types of brain cells.

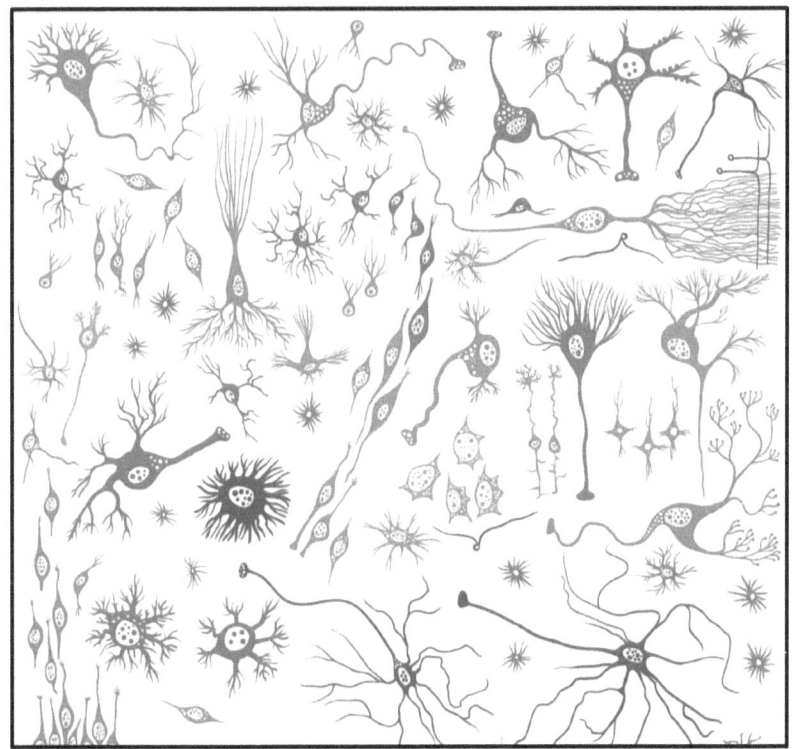
Just a few of the many different types of neurons and other brain cells

Neurons may be the all-stars on the team, but like other all-stars, they are rather needy and are surrounded by an entourage. Nearly as important are glial cells that provide neuron support. Astrocytes, microglia, and oligodendrocytes are just some of the other cell types whose main function is to support neurons. Microglia act as the local garbage collector, vigilante, and mortician by scavenging dead or dying cells or even actively engaging in phagocytosis, which is a medical dictionary word for killing live cells. It turns out, population control is critical for a brain to remain healthy, as is neutralizing the toxic contents of dead cells.

Connections occur between neurons via their branches, called axons, and dendrites. Dendrites look like short tree branches, and axons look like long telephone wires. Axon-to-axon and axon-to-dendrite connections are called synapses. Incoming signals are received by the dendrites; outgoing signals are sent via axons. A fatty substance called myelin is wrapped around axons, much like the insulation for an electrical wire, making the propagation of the electrical impulse more efficient.

As with other organs, the energy needed for the brain to operate is provided by oxygen and glucose delivered by blood vessels. When neurons are active, local microscopic blood vessels called capillaries dilate to deliver more oxygen and glucose to meet the demand, in much the same way that doing curls in the gym increases blood flow to the biceps. This phenomenon is the key to brain imaging studies.

At the center of the brain is a network of cavities filled with cerebral spinal fluid (CSF) called ventricles. The fluid is produced and recycled several times each day. The ventricles cushion the brain from trauma and movement, remove metabolic waste products, and deliver needed hormones. During brain formation, the ventricular wall is where new neurons are born.

Hydrocephalus is a well-known disorder characterized by excessive CSF production, forcing an increase in the size of the ventricles, which can damage brain tissue and harm brain function and growth. It is most common in infants and in adults over 60 years old.

Abnormally large ventricles, "ventriculomegaly," without hydrocephalus, occurs in other brain disorders. For example, 80% of schizophrenic patients demonstrate ventriculomegaly as an indication not of excessive CSF production but of failure of neuronal growth or loss of neuronal mass. Some environmental exposures can cause ventriculomegaly of this type. Increased prenatal ventricular volume may be an early anatomical feature indicating impaired development of the cerebral cortex and can be a marker of increased risk for psychiatric disorders, attention deficit hyperactivity disorder (ADHD), autism spectrum disorder (hereafter "autism"), and intellectual impairment. (See chapters 4,5, and 8 for environmental causes).

While cell proliferation, also known as neurogenesis, is obviously important to normal brain development, surprisingly, cell death and "pruning" is important as well. Many cells only serve a transient function. The brain develops thanks to external environmental influences and exposures to internal and physical stimuli, which combine to determine which connections should be pruned and which should be kept. If a neuron fires and establishes a useful connection, it will likely survive. If a neuron's connections seldom see any action, it is likely to regress and be pruned. Once formed, up to 50% of neurons, with their axons and dendrites, may ultimately be eliminated in some areas of the brain beginning around age 2. Much of the synaptic pruning occurs between childhood and adolescence.[6] You can think of this as brain cells engaged in a suicide mission for the benefit of the troops; taking a hit for the team. After birth, production of neurons slows dramatically and continues only to a very limited extent.

Most human brain growth occurs in childhood. The brain reaches about 90% of its adult volume by the age of 6,[7] and that corresponds to about 90% of its overall, permanent organizational and architectural structure. After birth, the primary growth occurs in the connections made between neurons (referred to as the "synaptic big bang") rather than in a continued increase in the number of neurons. This stage of brain development is also referred to as "the connectome."

From intrauterine life to the age of five or six is the time when brains are made or broken, where behavioral paths are established, where intellectual capability solidifies, and where environmental influences, for good or ill, have their greatest impact. Exposures to environmental neurotoxins interfere with the young brain's ability to differentiate between important neural connections and less important or useless connections, disrupting the connectome.

The multi-folding, or wrinkles of the mature human brain, is assumed to be an evolutionary adaptation to accommodate dramatic growth in the size of the brain while having to fit into a cranial vault small enough to fit through the birth canal. If you think you should have had a bigger head, blame the size of the pelvis of Mitochondrial Eve, the mother of all homo sapiens, who lived about 200,000 years ago. The hundred-dollar word for folding is "gyrification." That gyrification is worth far more than a hundred dollars, because it allows the cerebral cortex a surface area three times as large as the interior surface of the skull.[8]

The formation of ridges (gyri) and valleys (sulci) in the brain surface allows for compact wiring that promotes and enhances efficient neural processing. The increased surface area allowed via gyrification implies a larger amount of cortical gray matter, which presumably yields a greater potential for neuronal connections and complex brain function.[9] Thanks to gyrification, the surface area of the human brain is approximately ten times greater than that of the brain of a macaque monkey. That gyrification is undoubtedly an incomparable, intellectual asset, and increases with maturation from childhood to early adulthood.

In a study of identical (monozygotic) and fraternal (dizygotic) twins,[10] researchers determined that, while genetics are important in the pattern of gyrification, especially in early development, environmental factors contribute significantly to the eventual surface morphology of the brain.

The brain ages much like the rest of the body. In infancy, the brain is relatively smooth, but from then until early adulthood, those folds deepen. When we reach our 30s and 40s, brain volume starts to decrease. That decline accelerates around age 60. Certain parts of the brain take the largest hit in brain contraction. The prefrontal cortex, cerebellum, and hippocampus are the "biggest losers," to use TV vernacular. Thinning of the cortex follows a similar pattern corresponding to age, with the frontal and temporal lobes being the biggest losers in those sweepstakes. It is thought that the last parts of the brain to develop are the first parts to deteriorate.[5]

Speaking of losers, back to The Great Escape. I lost my joy and rapture after only a few seconds. When I rounded the next bend, I saw the other car of missionaries pulled over to the side of the road, and the Mountie was standing in the middle of the road motioning me to stop and pull over. He had nabbed both cars, and my precuneus must have gone totally dark. The Mountie ordered me out of the car and was so angry he was having a hard time making his Broca's area work; he was almost speechless. Finally, his speech neurons rose to the occasion and he preceded to berate me for racing and "unbelievably reckless" driving. The neurons in my amygdala went into overdrive and sent signals through their synapses to my cerebral cortex to create visions of me dying naked and starving in a Canadian jail. When the Mountie asked who we were and what we were doing in Canada I told him we were missionaries, i.e., God's emissaries. He exploded with, "What do you think the Big Guy Above would think about your driving?" I resisted the temptation to say, "He would have thought we were pretty good for amatuers."

I don't know that researchers have established the "repentance lobe" of the brain, but mine must have lit up like the proverbial Christmas tree. But then the Mountie used his prefrontal cortex and decided throwing American missionaries in jail might trigger a nuclear war, so like Tom Brady looking over the defense, he decided to play it safe. Apparently, Mounties can collect money for fines on the spot. So instead of jail, he issued me a ticket and fined me $60 (the equivalent of about $440 in 2024 money). I mustered a little frontal lobe action myself and pled the case that we were poor missionaries and didn't have that kind of money (which was true). He said in that case, he would follow us to the next gas station where we would have to charge $60 on our church's credit card and give him the cash.

Now I'm sure all Mounties are honest, but that didn't feel right to me. And it really didn't feel right, given that just like Paul's epiphany on the road to Damascus, I had my own epiphany on the road to Boston, that when the church financial clerk discovered the $60 charge, it would no doubt lead to a month of group flagellation or worse—prayer. Nonetheless, there were few things I could leverage to strengthen my position, so I did as I was told. Thirty minutes later I had $60 in my hand ready to hand over to the Mountie, but then my prefrontal cortex said, "Wait!" To be continued.

With the change in anatomy with aging, the brain's function also deteriorates. Declarative memory (recalling names, numbers, and facts), and working memory (utilization of new information) start to decline in our 30s. Procedural memories (movement skills like riding a bike, swinging a golf club, or leaving your blinker on while you're driving) tend to be retained well into older adulthood. It's not all bad news, however. A few brain functions can actually improve in early to middle-age adulthood. Verbal abilities, math, and abstract reasoning can all improve in early middle age.

The macro loss of brain volume corresponds to changes at the microscopic level. Like paint aging with long-term exposure to the elements, individual neurons shrink, their dendritic branches retract and lose complexity, and the insulating myelin sheaths start to deteriorate. The number of synapses drops, which impairs many aspects of brain function. Neurogenesis also declines with age, as does the production of chemical transmitters like dopamine and the receptors to which those chemicals become attached. Just like your skin starts to sag with age, your brain sags, too, literally, in that the tension on the cerebral cortex decreases.[11] This is particularly true in patients with Alzheimer's. Unfortunately, unlike plastic surgery for sagging skin, plastic surgery for a sagging brain hasn't worked out well, although no doubt someone in Hollywood will try it.

HUMAN BRAIN VS. A COMPUTER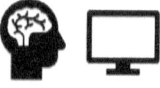

Many people have compared the human brain to a computer. Stephen Hawking reportedly said, "The development of full AI [artificial intelligence] could spell the end of the human race." Elon Musk thinks AI is a greater threat to humans than nuclear war.[12] I think Elon Musk is a bigger threat than nuclear war. And he is missing the obvious—AI could start a nuclear war. As of 2017, however, human brains still have a competitive advantage over computers for multiple reasons.

The human brain can do a billion-billion calculations per second on just 20 watts of power, one third of what a 60-watt lightbulb uses.[13] For a super computer to do that would require a million times that energy. Some estimates are that by the year 2040, computers will exceed the thought process capability of humans. I wouldn't bet the farm on it.

Neurons can fire about 200 times per second. Computer processors, on the other hand, are capable of operating at billions of times per second. Information on fiber-optic cables travels about one million times faster than on neurons. The gray matter of brains contains a density of 10^9 synapses per microliter, similar to the .3 x 10^9 transistors per microliter in a computer. Where a modern microprocessor chip has 10^9 transistors, the human brain contains about 10^{14} synapses in the neocortex (and a brain uses about as much power as a microprocessor).[14]

A state of-the-art microprocessor would have approximately 30 km of total wire connecting its transistors. In comparison, the total length of the nerve fiber network in the human brain, primarily in the form of axons, is approximately 500,000 km, far more than the distance between the earth and the moon.[15]

Computers are governed by an internal clock that synchronizes their calculations. The internal clock speed of a computer is usually measured in megahertz (MHz), i.e., a million ticks per second. Clock speed is a rough estimate of the speed of a computer. Given that the neocortex contains about 10^{10} neurons, each of which fires nerve impulses at about 10 Hz, that would provide capability for 10^{11} instructions per second, which is about 100 times more than the one million instructions per second (MIPS) of a modern microprocessor (assuming multiple computing units).[16] Accounting for all this infrastructure, on a task like facial recognition, the human brain is about 100 times faster than a computer. In an effort to mimic this digitally, in 2013 scientists needed more than 82,000 processors running on one of the world's fastest supercomputers to mimic just 1 second of a normal human's brain activity.[17]

However, computer capability is expanding rapidly. The European Union's Human Brain Project is an effort to construct a virtual human brain and has probably come the closest to reach that goal of any serious endeavor so far. After working on it for ten years, in 2018, the project members assembled a super computer with one million processing cores and 1,200 circuit boards, located at the University of Manchester in the United Kingdom.[18] The researchers claim that this virtual brain can per perform 200 quadrillion actions simultaneously. Steve Furber, a professor of computer engineering at the University of Manchester, said this achievement, as record breaking as it is, only rises to the level of duplicating the capability of a mouse brain. Even computers like this are far from being able to think on their own. He said, "Even with a million processors, we can only approach 1 percent of the scale of the human brain, and that's with a lot of simplifying assumptions."[18]

Recently, a study found that the human brain can hold 10 times as much information as previously thought. Scientists now believe that the capacity of the human brain is about a "petabyte."[19] If you are counting bytes, that is 1,000 terabytes, which as of 2016, was nearly equal to all the information stored on the internet. It has been predicted that a computer will reach the processing capacity of a human brain within the next few decades, but experts doubt that computers will ever equal the complexity of the brain, if for no other reason than that the human brain has so far proven incapable of figuring out how the human brain works.

Back to The Great Escape. The Mountie had his human brain on quite a roll, like he was performing Hamlet on Broadway with his full-throated soliloquy on my driving criminality. I deserved it. With the $60 still in my hand, I adopted a full head-down position, literally and figuratively, shut my brain's Broca's area off, and just let the auditory cortex of my temporal lobe listen to his monologue without protest. The longer this went on, the more the Mountie became enamored with his own performance. But he got so carried away that he forgot to ask for the money. (His hippocampus got overwhelmed by the amygdala in his limbic system.) Finally satisfied that he had reached the climax and had thoroughly eviscerated me with his tongue acting as the whip under the direction of his posterior middle temporal gyrus, Broca's, and Wernicke's areas, he decided to exit stage right. He ceremoniously climbed into his car. It was worthy of a standing ovation, but we were already standing, so when he turned his back, I stuck the $60 back in my pocket so I could applaud. To be continued.

MALE VS. FEMALE BATTLE UNDER THE MICROSCOPE

In keeping with the style of current communication, and to make this book youth friendly, I thought I'd try crafting this next section in 140 characters, glyphs, emojis, acronyms, and hashtags. But after a few sentences I gave up when I found out emojis haven't been invented yet for "prostaglandin," "ventriculomegaly," or for:

CV$%67∫y−2dy=∫7x3dx−y−1=74x4+Cy=−174x4+JW@31

<++ proto bych rád vyjádřil svůj dík —>&8#,

which is either the password to my flip phone or Finland's nuclear launch codes. The brain's approximately 100 billion neurons are linked with each other by synapses. Synapses are less than a thousandth of a millimeter across and act like microscopic bridges transporting electrical impulses from one neuron to another by releasing chemicals into the tiny gap between neurons, which propagates the impulse. A single neuron may make tens of thousands of connections with other neurons. Taken together, there are more than 125 trillion synapses in the cerebral cortex alone, approximately equal to the number of stars in 1,500 Milky Way galaxies. "A single human brain has more switches than all the computers and routers and Internet connections on Earth," according to researchers at Stanford University.[20]

The population of synapses is not static. Periods of rapid growth during fetal development, infancy, and adolescence transitions to equally massive bursts of "pruning," during which underused and/or redundant synapses are eliminated, and then ultimately, with advanced age, to a steady, persistent decline. This is a great example of the mantra, "use it or lose it."

Of course, some of us achieve better performance from greater complexity within that marvelous organ than others do. The anatomic differences in the brains of men and women help explain some of that disparity. That is not to say that there is a typical male brain or a typical female brain. What that statement means is that certain anatomic characteristics are more often found in one sex or the other, such that examining a brain's architecture allows one to predict to which sex that brain will belong with an accuracy rate of about 80%.[21]

On average, men have about 10% larger brains, even when discounting their larger overall physical size. But despite men's believing that size matters, size alone often doesn't matter, and doesn't bestow upon males a particular advantage.

Examination of fossil skulls indicate that Neanderthals had larger brains than homo sapiens.[22] In case you're a fan of the hair style the "man bun," Neanderthals had an "occipital bun." The occiput is the back of the brain, and it processes vision. Together with larger eyes, the occipital bun allowed visual acuity to become a premium asset for Neanderthals. They would have been great at hitting a 100-mph fastball or returning a 157-mph first serve from tennis giant John Isner. But great vision may have come at a price. The Neanderthal brain minus the occiput was about 15% smaller than the brain of homo sapiens, including a smaller cerebellum. A Neanderthal might have been able to return Isner's serve but probably couldn't have kept score. He might have hit the 100-mph fastball but may not have been able to figure out how to run the bases.

The cerebellum may be the key to the superiority and survivability advantage of homo sapiens compared to Neanderthals. With less space committed to the occiput, homo sapiens were able to evolve larger cerebellums, and we are just learning about what an advantage that is. We learned from modern humans that "cognitive flexibility, attention, language processing, episodic and working memory capacity were positively correlated with size-adjusted cerebellar volume."[23] In fact, an inferior and smaller cerebellum may have been responsible for Neanderthal extinction.

Studies attempting to correlate intelligence with overall brain size show a very weak association, if any. Nonetheless, intelligence per unit of overall brain volume is actually slightly higher in females, suggesting they use available energy more efficiently, and that the female brain is more densely packed with neurons. Furthermore, the larger male brain requires more energy input, which is a disadvantage. Normal aging and shrinking of brain volume are accompanied by a decrease in brain metabolism and energy requirements.

There is strong evidence that men and women have different biochemical and anatomic pathways for performing the same brain functions—utilizing memory, recognizing faces, generating emotions, problem solving, and decision making.[24]

I have no doubt that female Mormon missionaries would have handled the next stage of The Great Escape differently from how I did, given that the purpose of our missions was to convert and baptize people. We waved to the Mountie, thanked him for his earth-shaking call to repentance, and as soon as he drove out of sight, all ten of us used our left frontal lobes (where logic and analytics supposedly percolate), jumped back in the cars, and barreled down the highway at 90 mph to get to the U.S./Canadian border as fast as we could. We made it through customs three hours later, it turns out just before the Mountie clocked in for the night, realized he was $60 short, and put out an all-points bulletin out for our arrest at the border. The other car of missionaries made it through customs but was eventually detained by Maine police. But some sweet talking by our Elder Ex-Car-Thief got them off the hook.

No one in our car was capable of sweet talking so much as a bunny rabbit, so I used the right side of my frontal lobe, the site where creativity mythically blooms, and I saw visions of a carload of missionaries having to shoot our way back to Boston à la Bonnie and Clyde. Then my analytics lobe took over again, and I realized that we had no guns, that our only semblance of bullet-proof vests consisted of paperback copies of the Book of Mormon, and that it would be a bit more difficult to convert people if we were also shooting at them. So, we took all the back roads from Maine to Boston to avoid the Maine Highway Patrol. In the end, we escaped responsibility for our behavior, just as Jesus would have wanted.

The coup de grâce was that a month later, back at mission headquarters, we received a notice in the mail thanking us for paying our fine. Long after I returned home from my two-year mission, I learned that anyone driving those two cars risked being arrested.

Fifty years later, I'm still "WANTED" in Canada. The Great Escape will no doubt be made into a feature-length movie, starring Timothy Chalamet as me.

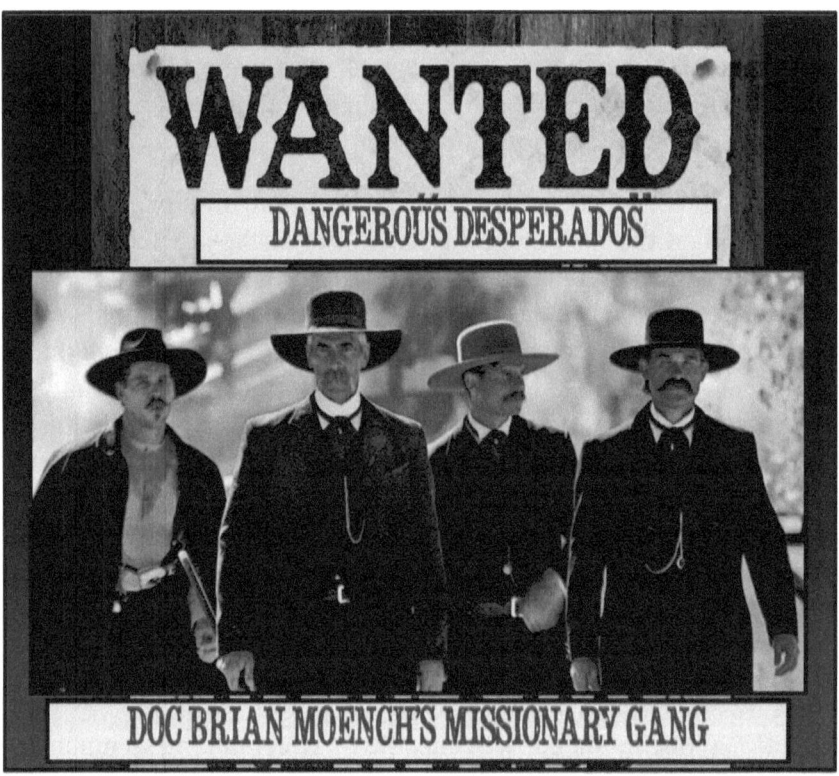

The cerebral cortex consists of six layers of different types of brain cells. The mean cortical thickness found in both hemispheres is significantly larger in females compared with males. This is most likely the result of increased density in the number of neurons. Females also have greater cortical complexity and more gyrification, which increases cortical surface area.[25]

And, of course, that yields some of the world's worst pick-up lines, such as; "Do you have a Band-Aid? I just scraped my knee falling for the youthful superiority of your anterior cingulate neuronal density." "Do you know CPR? Because being an old guy, your gyrification is taking my breath away! Seriously some one call an ambulance." "I was wondering if you had an extra heart because I'm going to need a transplant now that all six layers of your cortical complexity just stole mine." This also lends itself to more sophisticated and politically correct insults, such as instead of calling someone a moron, you say, "Hey, person with whom I disagree, you should consider the possibility that your frontal lobe synaptic transmission is devoid of sufficiency!" and then see how the moron responds.

In the area of language processing, near the Sylvian fissure (named after Franciscus Sylvius [1614-1672], German/Dutch physician and anatomist), females have an average of 11% greater neuronal density.[26] That's undoubtedly one of the reasons why women don't say things like, "Hey, person with whom I disagree, you should consider the possibility that your frontal lobe synaptic transmission is devoid of sufficiency!"

In 2001, Harvard researchers found that the frontal lobes, where problem solving and decision making are thought to take place, are larger in women, as are the limbic cortex where emotions are generated. They also found that men had larger parietal cortexes and amygdalae, which, as we mentioned, are involved in spatial perception, aggressive survival instincts, and emotional, sexual, and social behavior.[27]

Have you ever wondered why women can remember and despise every one of their male partner's ex-girlfriends going back to kindergarten? Well, keep wondering; scientists haven't figured that one out. For many years it was thought that, compared to men, women have larger hippocampuses, an explanation for why women had stronger emotions about memories. Newer studies have thrown that into doubt.[28]

Controlling for age, the largest brain magnetic resonance imaging (MRI) study done to date found that women had thicker cerebral cortices, which are thought to be associated with greater overall cognitive skills and intelligence.[29] Men, however, had larger volumes of some subcortical brain structures, "including the hippocampus (plays broad roles in memory and spatial awareness), the amygdala [see previous description], striatum (learning, inhibition, and reward-processing), and thalamus (processing and relaying sensory information to other parts of the brain)."[30] Adjusting the data for men's overall larger brain volumes, the difference in size in subcortical structures was reduced such that men retained a size advantage in 14 areas and women in 10.[31] An argument can certainly be made that those ten areas where women have a size advantage are the most crucial parts of the brain for higher intelligence. There was also greater variability among men in cortical thickness and brain volume.[31]

Women have a higher ratio of gray matter to white matter, but men have 6.5 times as much gray matter in certain intelligence areas, and women have nearly ten times as much white matter in those same areas. Those differences were largest in the frontal lobes.

The corpus callosum, the white matter bridge between both hemispheres that allows them to communicate with each other, is thicker in women.[32] Anatomically, women's hemispheres are more symmetrical than men's, and that not only affects how a brain looks (who doesn't want a "good looking" brain?), it also affects how a brain functions.

There is more interhemisphere activity in female brains, and more intrahemisphere activity in male brains. Recent research on neural connections shows that the sexes have different patterns of connectivity between neurons. Females have increased connectivity between neurons in the cortices of the right and left hemispheres, and in contrast, males have increased connectivity within hemispheres, from the front of hemispheres to the back, including the cerebellum.[33] Researchers believe this corresponds to clinical differences that women are better at intuitive and logical thinking, at emotional processing, and at reading others' intentions in social interactions. The male pattern of connectivity would offer an advantage in coordinating perception with action and developing physical skills,[34] especially those that involve visual acuity, recognizing small details from a distance, and rapid movement. This might provide a "hunter/gatherer" evolutionary explanation for why men are willing to watch NASCAR; otherwise, it remains one of the great scientific mysteries.

In one of the largest functional brain imaging studies ever done, measuring blood flow to 128 different brain regions in nearly

27,000 patients, researchers found distinct differences in the brains of women compared with men.[35] They found that female brains were more active in the pre-frontal cortex, the site of our ability to concentrate and maintain impulse control, as well as the limbic system beneath the temporal lobe, which controls mood and deals with anxiety. The visual and physical coordination centers of men received more blood flow.

This physical finding of blood flow patterns corresponds to clinical findings that women demonstrate more empathy, intuition, collaboration, and self-control (See Chapter 9). The blood-flow pattern in the limbic system is also consistent with the clinical manifestation of women's being more susceptible to anxiety, depression, insomnia, and eating disorders. Societal influences, no doubt, also play a role in these common mood and behavioral disorders, given the misogynistic pressures on women who are routinely valued more for their physical appearance than their mental attributes, which often includes denial of career opportunities. The study does not answer the obvious chicken and egg question raised, however. Does the blood-flow pattern create the difference in functionality, or is it merely a reflection of that difference?

That women are more empathetic than men is demonstrated by a substantial body of research.[36] Women are better at "feeling your pain," and men are better at inflicting it. Some of that may be sociologic influences, but it is likely biological as well. That difference is found early in childhood and increases with age up to adolescence.[37] Women react more emotionally than men do when they perceive pain in someone else.[38] Researchers concluded this from using a functional MRI scan to measure the blood flow to the sensory areas of the brain associated with pain, while the subject watched someone else get stuck by a needle. The area that mimics the pain in someone else showed a larger response in females. Studies have found that females felt empathy when someone else suffered pain, even when the same person had behaved unfairly toward them in the past. While this undoubtedly is an admirable and useful character trait for life in general, I can attest, from personal experience, that it translates poorly into playing the game of football (a game that, nonetheless, shouldn't be played by anyone other than females, see Chapter 6). In the regions of the brain that control empathy, women have a greater volume of gray matter.

There may also be differences in the brains of males and females at the microscopic level. In mice, researchers have found brain cell types that are solely found in males and others that are solely found in females.[39] Like the arms of a starfish, the previously mentioned neuronal dendrites and long extensions called axons connect with other neurons through synapses. The configuration of dendrites and the number of synapses are different in males compared to females. Astrocytes, one of several types of glial cells, are bushier in parts of the male brain, with longer extensions and more numerous processes than those in the same regions of the female brain.[40]

Microglia cells are the ground troops of the brain's immune system and constitute 10-15% of all the cells in the brain. They not only rush to protect the brain from attack by multiple insults, they also act like members of the old forest service perched in watch towers looking for plumes of smoke. Microglia surveil the brain, ready to put out fires anywhere they sense a threat. The density of microglia varies in different parts of the brain and differs according to gender.

Early in the embryonic stage, male and female microglia actually start to behave differently. What goes on with the brain's microglia is a microcosm of how the brains of males and females differ at the macro level. Female microglia behave as if they are miniature mothers, driven by stereotypical maternal instinct. They are more likely to activate genes engaged in nurturing and the repair of neuronal damage. Male brains have more microglia, and their microglia have higher voltage levels in their membranes, which means they're at a higher state of alert, even when they're in a relaxed state.

You could have guessed this, but male microglia wear themselves out more quickly. They act more like cowboys, more likely to charge into an area of concern and just "start shooting," because their genes are more prone to initiate programmed cell death (apoptosis) rather than repair. As one researcher described: "It almost seems as if the male cells are more willing to take risks than the female ones. They almost always react faster, but as a result, they sometimes seem to put themselves in danger."[41] They even look different. Male microglia look more bloated, with larger cell bodies.

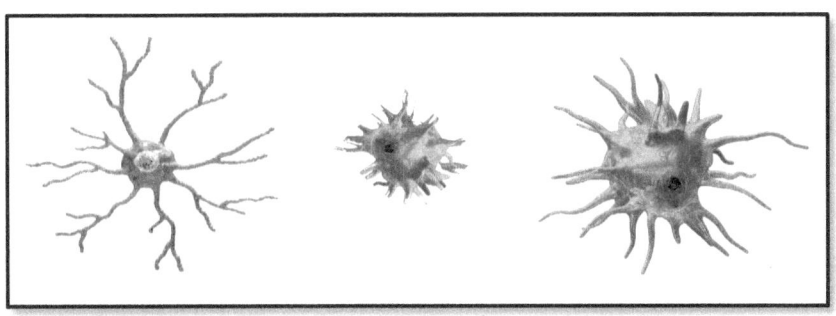

Female microglia   Male microglia   Activated microglia

Male microglia are more immature (in every sense of the word) compared to their female counterparts and are more active in the male brain, producing higher concentrations of an inflammatory mediator, PGE2 (prostaglandin E2) in certain areas of the brain. Enhanced microglia activity suggests male brains have more clean-up work to do. Put another way, men have dirtier minds than women, which would surprise no one in the metaphorical sense, but perhaps surprising as a description of their microbiologic state of mind. This probably plays a role in increasing vulnerability to developmental disorders such as autism.[42] So if you're a woman, and you need a powerful comeback in any argument with a man, try this: "Dude, my microglia can phagocytize circles around your prostaglandins." Boom, mic drop!

In fact, boys have a higher percentage of all non-neuron brain cells, suggesting male neurons are more fragile, needier, and have higher baseline levels of inflammation, a likely contributor to neuropsychiatric disorders.[43]

The term blood-brain barrier (BBB) refers to a specialized group of cells that line the inside of the network of microscopic blood vessels that permeate the brain. The BBB incorporates unique physical, transport, and metabolic properties in the accomplishment of a very important task. These specialized cells tightly control the movement of ions, foreign molecules, and cells between the blood and the brain tissue to a greater degree than any other blood-vessel network in the body. Think of the brain as a castle and the BBB as a huge wall and a moat filled with alligators, protecting the brain from invasion by toxins and pathologic organisms that may exist in the circulatory system.[44] Unfortunately, the BBB doesn't protect the brain from being attacked by pathologic conspiracy theories, Facebook, or The Bachelor on TV.

The BBB does not fully form until about 6 months after birth, so almost from conception until then, the development of the brain is particularly at risk from chemical exposure. There are two characteristics that are associated with a deterioration of the protective function of the BBB, and by now I'll bet you can guess what those are—age and the male sex.[45] This micro anatomic distinction between the sexes plays a large role in the vulnerability of the male brain to disease and many environmental toxins.

Now for a little twist. In laboratory animals, when put under stress before being given a task, males perform comparatively better than females. Furthermore, there is an anatomic correlate; the dendrites of the neurons in males increased proportionally to their improved performance, and in females, the opposite occurred. However, the females' deteriorating performance under stress only occurred during certain times of their hormonal cycle. If the ovaries were removed, the sex differences disappeared.[46]

In contrast, in studies where animals are placed in a situation of enrichment, like Madison Ave penthouses, gold toilets, credit cards with no limits…no, actually cages filled with toys and other animals for socialization (the opposite of stress) the experience increased the branches of dendrites, i.e., the opportunity for greater neuron interaction. In males, however, the same experience had no effect on dendrites; in fact, the enriched situation may have actually caused the branches to shrivel up.

Male and female lab animals think differently from each other. For example, if you put male rats in a water maze (and who doesn't after a few beers?), they will default to using the geometric configuration of their environment to navigate the maze. Female rats will simply ask directions. You knew that was coming. Actually, no. Females navigate the same maze using a different method—landmark clues.[47] Studies of humans show the same type of gender differences in tests of navigation, giving license to the standard clichés. Navigational learning was more impaired in male rats than females when noise was added as a distraction.[48]

YOU REAP HOW YOU SLEEP

"I bought one of those new 'memory foam' mattresses, but it didn't improve my memory at all. Then I couldn't remember where to send it back." That is the inscription over the Tomb of the Unknown Comedian, who, admittedly, deserved to die over that one. Actually, he should have given it more time, because if it had improved his sleep, it likely would have also improved his memory.

Physical health, mental health, and cognitive potential are all closely tied to adequate and healthy sleep patterns. Virtually all animals sleep, and all animals need sleep. Sharks may not go completely unconscious, but they do have rest periods, often in groups. Total, prolonged sleep deprivation can be lethal. Workers involved in healthcare and other emergency situations and night-shift workers of many other occupations know the physical and mental taxation that sleep deprivation exacts on humans.

A sleep study in fruit flies (stop laughing; fruit flies work hard and deserve a good night's rest, too), found that the toxic metabolites of oxidative stress, reactive oxygen species (ROS), accumulated in the gastrointestinal (GI) tract of the sleep-deprived fruit flies before they died. But when the fruit flies were given anti-oxidant molecules to neutralize the ROS, they enjoyed a normal lifespan (not quite sure how a fruit fly manifests "enjoyment").[49] This fruit fly research is actually serious science, strengthening the connection between the brain and the GI tract, which is very relevant to what is discussed in Chapter 8.

The average person experiences between 3 and 6 sleep cycles per night, each one averaging roughly 90 minutes. The American Academy of Sleep Medicine recognizes four stages within those cycles. REM sleep is what most people have heard of. But there are also three stages of non-REM sleep that precede REM sleep in the cycle. The slow wave, or deep, delta sleep stage of non-REM sleep is thought to represent the deepest sleep, during which insight and creativity are nurtured. REM sleep, featuring eyes moving quickly from side to side behind closed eyelids, is a lighter sleep and is characterized by more brain activity. This is when the most vivid dreaming occurs. Newborns spend about half of their sleep time in REM sleep.

During REM sleep, the axons of neurons form new synapses, important to interneuronal communication, consolidating memory, and learning. It is during sleep that brain repairs are made and toxic byproducts are cleared. Every night while you're asleep, your brain's disaster clean-up crew arrives, with microscopic plumbers, carpenters, and electricians, to scrub up, unclog, rebuild, and reconnect the mess you made of it during the day.

For the first two to three years of life, sleep plays a role in assisting the growth and development of the brain, including the pruning of neurons and connections. At somewhere around 30 months of age, sleep changes its role from building and cutting connections during REM sleep to neuron repair during REM and non-REM sleep. REM sleep declines with age in both sexes, leaving less capacity for repairs.

Adequate sleep helps teenagers beyond just staying awake in class. It also helps them cope with social challenges, disappointments, and discrimination, including racial bias.[50] Poor sleep patterns and sleep deprivation are associated with impaired cognition among middle-aged adults.[51] Slow-wave sleep is especially important for clearing beta-amyloid proteins. In all age groups, slow-wave sleep activity is greater in women than in men,[52] but as with REM sleep, there is a decline in slow-wave sleep with age, especially for women after menopause.

Whether you are in an anger management program, or your behavior is sending others into an anger management program, you should pay attention to your sleep patterns. College students report experiencing more anger following nights of reduced sleep. Other sleep studies have found the same thing—decreased adaptation to frustrating or irritating circumstances among people who are relatively sleep deprived.[53]

If you are a religious person, specifically a Catholic or a Baptist, compared to an atheist or an agnostic, you are more likely to suffer sleep deprivation. Seventy-three percent of these non-religious people report getting seven or more hours of sleep. Only 63% of Catholics, and 55% of Baptists report getting that much sleep. Irreligious people also have less difficulty falling asleep.[54] I'm going to interpret that study as proof that worrying about heaven and hell just makes us arrive at either place sooner.

Adequate sleep also yields a more optimistic mental attitude, which for Catholics and Baptists, must translate into greater confidence about getting into heaven.[54] I will refrain from further prejudicing your reaction to this, but if you conclude this means religion is bad for sleep and therefore bad for your brain, makes you less intelligent, bad for your health, and good sleep increases your chance of getting into heaven, I will only suggest that "results may vary."

Inadequate brain rest through sleep has multiple other health consequences beyond the harm it can do to your brain. It increases the risk of obesity[55] and cardiovascular disease,[56] and may increase your risk of cancer.

Sleep is crucial to learning and forming long-term memories. The brain is actually very busy during sleep, specifically repeating what we might have learned or experienced during the day. Episodic memory accumulating during the awake state initially gets stored in the hippocampus. During sleep, the information gets transferred to the cerebral cortex for long-term storage.[57]

"Memories are dynamic, not static. In other words, memories, even old memories, are not final. Sleep constantly updates them. We predict that during the sleep cycle, both old and new memories are spontaneously replayed, which prevents forgetting and increases recall performance," said Maksim Bazhenov, PhD, lead author of a recent sleep study and professor of medicine at University of California, San Diego.[58]

Memory replay during sleep allows neurons to store multiple potentially interfering memories, which helps protect against memory loss, making it possible for different memories to coexist.[59] That allows a person to remember movements developed for one skill, like playing the guitar, and, a separate skill, like singing at the same time. Or putting your makeup on and driving through the garage door at the same time (no further comment on that on). Adequate sleep helps to consolidate and protect newly encoded memories.

Researchers from the University of California at Berkeley suggest that it is possible to estimate when a person is likely to get Alzheimer's based on sleep patterns. Examining the sleep experience and habits of 32 older, healthy adults, they showed that those who started out experiencing more fragmented sleep and less non-REM, slow-wave sleep had the greatest increase in beta-amyloid, the abnormal protein that is a hallmark of Alzheimer's, during the length of the study. Sleep is known to help "deep cleaning" of the brain of beta-amyloid deposits.[60]

The best studies of gender and sleep suggest that among people with or without sleep complaints or physical illnesses, women sleep better than men.[61] Other research suggests that women need more sleep, probably around 20-30 minutes more sleep per night, and in fact, they sleep slightly longer than men.[62] Researchers explain the difference, believing that women simply use their brain more, and their brains are more complex,[63] which increases their need for sleep and recovery time. Women more often have to be multi-taskers, typically having to rear and care for children in addition to working. Women typically have to do more unpaid work and get less high-quality leisure time compared to men. Consequently, women often have a harder time shutting their brain down to transition to sleep.

Hormones play a role for women in their need for more sleep. Women experience significant fluctuations of those hormones during their monthly menstrual cycle. The surge in progesterone, typically in the last two weeks of the cycle, creates a demand for more energy. Adrenal function is stressed, and the production of the neurotransmitter serotonin falls. Lack of sleep often aggravates PMS symptoms. The prefrontal cortex (PFC) is particularly vulnerable to sleep deprivation. [64]

The PFC is important in directing complex cognition, pro-social behavior, and temporizing risk taking. Data gathered from 11 medical institutions from 11,395 physicians found that even modest sleep deprivation was associated with a 53% increase in self-reported, clinically significant medical errors. High levels of sleep deprivation nearly doubled that association.[65] This data is hardly surprising to anyone in the medical professions. People who have slept less than 7 hours in the previous 24 hours have a higher rate of both causing and being involved in auto accidents. There is even greater risk for those who have slept much less.[66] Drivers who reported less than 4 hours of sleep in the previous 24-hour cycle were responsible for accidents at an astounding 15.1 times higher rate than drivers that slept between seven and nine hours.

Even one single night of sleep deprivation affects men and women differently. In men, it increases their impulsivity and risk taking. In women, it decreases their risk taking but increases their selfishness in economic tasks.[67] Neuroimaging studies have found that the brain mechanisms and areas of activity used by men and women to solve the same problems are different, so it is easier to understand how brain performance after sleep deprivation might not only be different in the two genders but might be modified in opposite ways.

Sleep deprivation is almost guaranteed collateral damage of raising babies and young children, which can play a major role in postpartum depression for women. Our first child was more colicky than the classic colicky baby. She cried almost nonstop for the first 24 hours after we brought her home. My wife and I nicknamed her Rosemary's Baby, because we wondered how we had brought this misery upon ourselves. She didn't sleep through the night for the first nine years of her life. Years and three more children later (what were we thinking?), I often would wake up in the morning and find all four children in bed with us. But during all those years, it was my wife that suffered the most sleep deprivation, even though I spent every fourth night on emergency call at the hospital. In fact, sometimes I looked forward to being on call because it was often a more restful night than being at home. In both sexes, the more a person uses their brain, the more sleep they need.

Women have more vivid and emotionally charged dreams than men, in large part secondary to hormonal fluctuations during their menstrual cycle. REM sleep, the fourth and final stage of the normal sleep cycle, is when the most dramatic dreams normally occur. Women spend more time in REM sleep compared to men, and this seems to be particularly true during pregnancy.

Women report significantly more nightmares than men (probably because they're often married to men). More dramatic dreams also lead to more prolonged recall of dreams. According to dream experts, the most common dreams that women have involve having their teeth fall out, being chased, flying, falling, and the classic being naked in public.

Dreams are thought to be a reflection of what our brains do during the day. Men dream of sex twice as often as women. When they're conscious, they also think about sex twice as often as women. The number of women surprised about that could fit dancing on the head of a pin.

I'm sure you remember this question on Jeopardy. "How often men think about sex." And the answer is, "What is every seven seconds?" (You may have missed that episode). But the popular meme that men think about sex every seven seconds is wildly exaggerated, the quintessential "old wives tale," intended to smear the character of men among old wives. Let's clear up this misconception right now once and for all. The actual research shows that men think of sex only 19 times a day.[78]

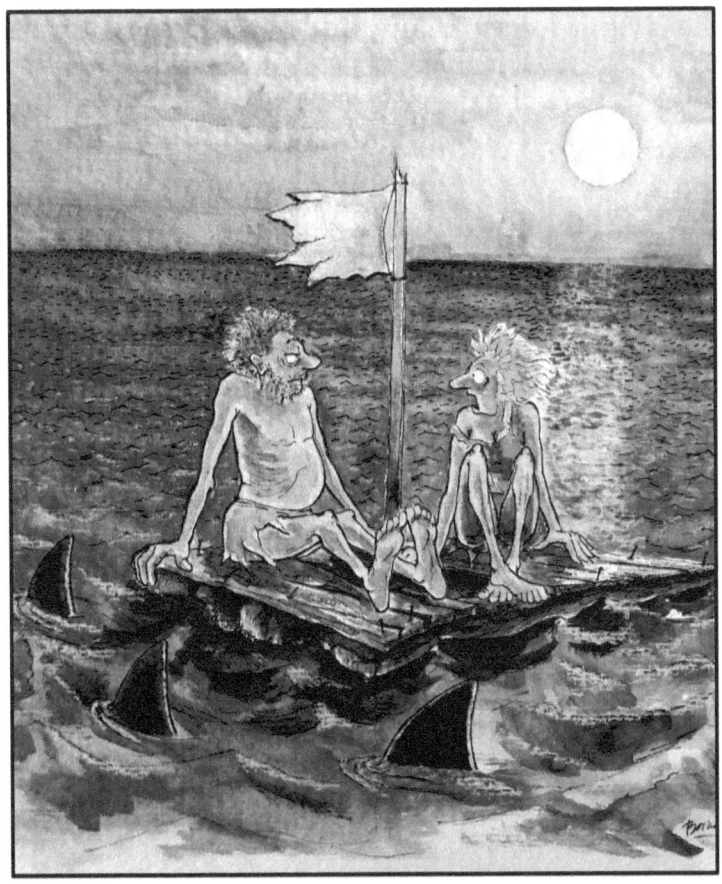

"What!!!? Are you serious? I can't believe you'd even ask!!!"

When it comes to falling in love, those statistics are flip flopped, with women dreaming about falling in love twice as often as men.[68] That may be one of the most overt pieces of evidence that, for both men and women, sex and love are not the same thing. They may not even reside in the same universe.

Dreams are a means of processing, integrating, and addressing our everyday lives, priorities, and anxieties. Twice as many women as men consciously try to find relevance to their daytime lives in the recall of their dreams. REM cycle dreams have been shown to be associated with a dramatically enhanced capacity to correctly engage in problem solving,[69] which translates into women's having that advantage over men. Sleep is very beneficial to solidifying pre-sleep learning.⁷⁰ Other studies have found that women appear to be more resistant to sleep disruption than men[61] and to the damage of inflammatory chemicals like cortisol, that are released with sleep deprivation.[71]

Excessive sleep also is associated with cognitive decline. Middle-aged or elderly people of both sexes who report sleeping more than ten hours per day show more cognitive decline than those sleep an average of seven hours.[72]

Oxytocin (not to be confused with Oxycontin, which opened the floodgates for the country's narcotic epidemic), is both a neurotransmitter and a hormone, best known for being activated during childbirth (sometimes needed as an intravenous medication during obstetrical procedures), and breast feeding. It is produced in the hypothalamus, then transported to and released by the pituitary gland. Both sexes produce it, and in both, it helps foster the nurturing instinct of parents toward their children, even those nicknamed Rosemary's Baby. Women produce more oxytocin than men.

When it is released into the bloodstream, oxytocin increases uterine contractions and progression of the birthing process. But when it is released into the brain, it further promotes a wide range of emotionally laden thoughts and behavior—typically prosocial behavior, acceptance of others, empathy, relaxation, trust, relationship building, and psychological stability. It also reduces anxiety and the stress response. The hormone is much more thoroughly researched in females, but new research in males suggests it affects their behavior in a similar, positive way.

Oxytocin is released in the first several months of a romantic relationship, and during male erection, sexual activity, and orgasm. It is triggered in a female by nipple stimulation. It has, therefore, been given even as many nicknames as the male penis—the love bucket, the cuddle monster, the teddy bear, baby magic, Love Potion No. 9, the cruise ship lollipop...feel free to make up your own.

Intranasal oxytocin enhances positive self-perception, and in social situations increases openness, trust, and feelings of altruism.[73] It also enhances the interpretation of emotions behind the facial expressions of others, even to the point of making people overly sensitive to the emotions they inaccurately perceive in others, like feeling way too much of your pain.[74]

It has long been known that pregnancy hormones enhance maternal instincts and interest in childcare behavior. Recently it has been found that fatherhood also produces hormone changes that help fathers behave in much the same way. These hormone changes include decreases in testosterone and increases in oxytocin. Research shows that when given oxytocin, fathers of one- to two-year-old children showed evidence of increased empathy and attention toward their children, detected by brain scans.[75] Oxytocin even helps men behave "more responsibly to their partner." For example, researchers took a group of men in monogamous heterosexual relationships and gave them a dose of oxytocin, then showed them photos of their female spouse/partner or of randomly selected women. MRI scans of their brains showed higher activity when showed pictures of their partners when given oxytocin.[76]

In another study, men given either a placebo or oxytocin were then placed in a room with an attractive female researcher. Test subjects who were in a monogamous relationship and given oxytocin were more comfortable when the female researcher kept a greater distance from them.[77] From the research, it seems that women should be pouring a little chaser of oxytocin in their husband's coffee in the morning. More oxytocin in women is likely why women have a greater capacity to handle many types of stress better than men, including making better police officers (see Chapter 1)

Because of differences in gross anatomy, micro anatomy, physiology, chemistry, and hormonal production and transport generally, the brains of men function quite differently from the brains of women. In many respects, this gives females an advantage in intellect, emotional stability, and socialization.

How the Brain Works

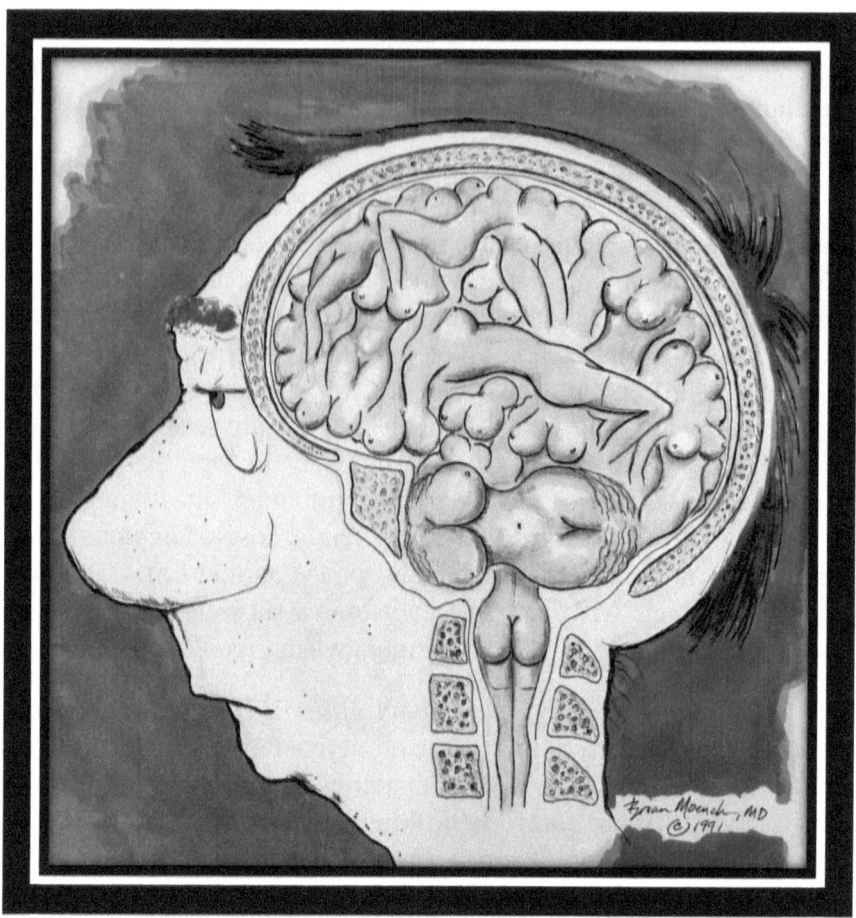

MRI scan of the male brain

The Great Brain Robbery – Brian Moench

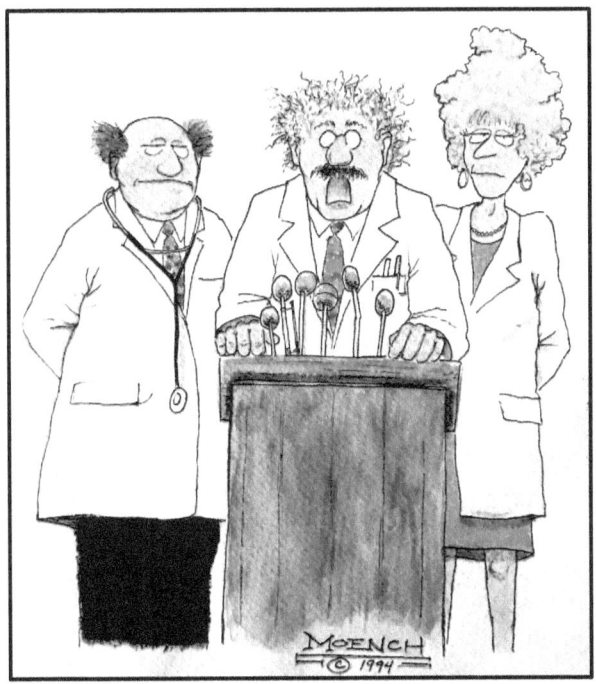

Government scientists have just completed the most comprehensive study of sexual activity ever done in this country. Here's what they found about the differences between men and women.

1. Men finished the survey first and then fell asleep.
2. Indeed, some women can have multiple organisms.
3. A variety of positions are important to men, like shortstop, quarterback, tight end.
4. Most Americans still practice monotony.
5. 99% of women are glad they're not Melania.
6. 20% of men are important.
7. Most women thought sperm banks charged a substantial penalty for early withdrawal.
8. Half the country suffers from ED; electoral dysfunction.
9. 84% of men don't know how to put on a condominium.
10. 25% of women had no idea Jesus was part of the "second coming."

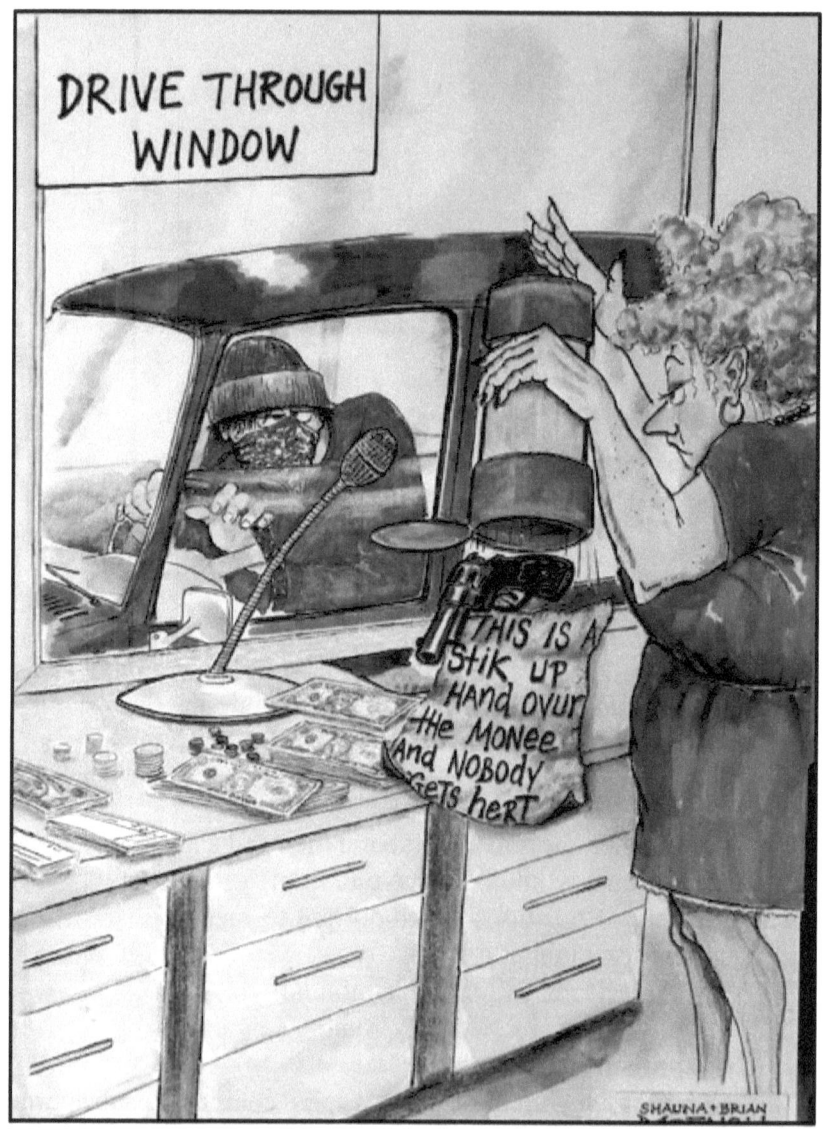

During the pandemic, Florida Man robs a bank responsibly.

Chapter 3

WHY WOMEN ARE SMARTER THAN MEN

"He's even using children. It reminds me of Saddam Hussein when he used kids."

—Texas Representative Steve Stockman on President Obama's push for gun control after the massacre at Newtown

"I actually don't like thinking. I think people think I like to think a lot. And I don't. I do not like to think at all."

—Kanye West

"No, I think gay marriage is something that should be between a man and a woman."

—Former California Governor Arnold Schwarzenegger

One of the most popular memes on the internet is *Florida Man*, referring to any number of breathtakingly stupid things done by some man somewhere in Florida. They include such gems as: "Florida Man Steals $300 Worth of Sex Toys While Dressed as Ninja." "Florida Man Tries to Pick Up Prostitute While Driving Special Needs School Bus." "Florida Man Arrested for Calling 911 After His Cat Was Denied Entry into Strip Club." "Florida Man Removes Facial Tattoos with Welding Grinder." "Florida Man posts his *Wanted* photo on Facebook, never suspecting it would lead to his arrest."

The memes have spawned a comic book, a documentary, a docuseries, podcasts, and band names, among countless other awards. The @_FloridaMan Twitter account has 400,000 followers, which I'm told is a lot. There is a Florida Man Music Festival and *Florida Man*, a one-man play. In Tampa, a tour guide leads Florida Man walking and drinking tours, (more like stumbling and falling tours). *The Onion* has a similar running spoof, *Area Man*, just to make sure Florida doesn't have all the fun. *South Park* has an action figure called *Alabama Man* to spoof macho toys. One chilling thought is that outcomes of our national elections often hinge on the disposition, or in many cases the machinations of the "swing state" of Florida, and Florida is filled with Florida Men.

I am deliberately choosing to ignore some political incorrectness here. Some might accuse me of piling on what is cheap entertainment at the expense of others, some of whom are no doubt victims of painful sociologic back stories beyond their control, like poor education, mental illness, or possibly drug abuse. But I use these examples merely to highlight other arenas in which the judgement and thought processes of men prominently lag behind women.

To that point, a meme of *Florida Woman* exists but with far less material to draw from. In fact, many of the examples seem to be women resorting to extraordinary and creative ways to retaliate against men. In addition to many other contributors to these failures of judgement, all of which are beyond the scope of this book, there is substantial evidence that environmental toxins play a role in a ubiquitous compromise of the intellectual abilities of all of us. Darwin Award winners and Florida Men everywhere are only the most entertaining examples of the cognitive shortcomings of 21st Century human beings, and males more than females. A brief lesson on genetics and molecular biology will help you understand how we got here.

Everyone gets roughly 40 trillion cells[1] to work with to put together their bodies—their bones, muscles, skin, all types of tissues, and all their critical organs, including the brain. Think of them as 40 trillion miniature *Legos*. About a trillion of those cells reside in your brain, about 100 billion of which are neurons.[2] Every neuron has at least ten, maybe up to 50 other cells providing support, resources, structure, and protection for those precious neurons. How all those human bodies and human brains end up obviously varies greatly, but most people start out with about the same number of building blocks.

The Great Brain Robbery – Brian Moench

There are hundreds of different types of cells throughout the body, each type with their own function within the organism. Inside the nucleus of a cell (the command post), are 23 pairs of chromosomes. The chromosomes are comprised of deoxyribonucleic acid (DNA).

DNA is part of my DNA. Yes, you read that right. In junior high, I retired from a short career in juvenile delinquency and launched my career in science. However, the only science award I ever won was in the seventh grade at Evergreen Junior High School, for a Styrofoam model I built of the DNA double helix. Full disclosure: my father told me everything to do and how to make the model. But I did choose what color to spray paint the Styrofoam. I took the coveted third-place award out of four science projects. I embellished that achievement slightly when I told my grandchildren I won the Nobel Prize.

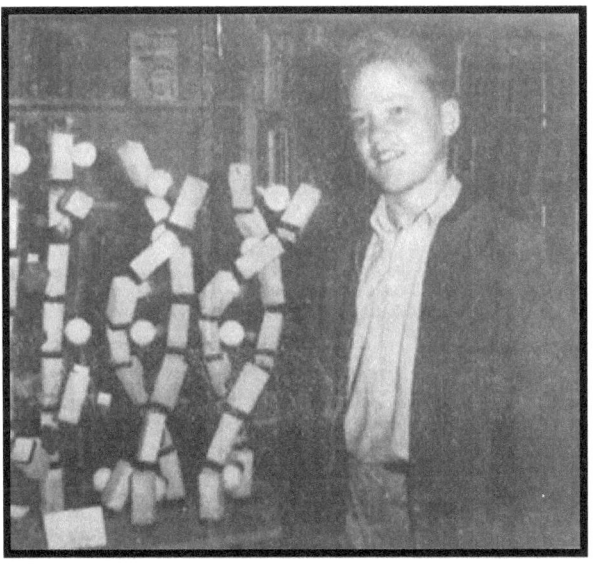

Winner of the 1963 Nobel Prize for Spray Painted Styrofoam
Brian Moench, age 13

DNA is composed of millions of small chemicals called bases, and like baseball, there are four bases—adenine, thymine, cytosine, and guanine. Those bases form millions of tiny bridges between two spiral staircases made of phosphate, and those paired staircases are your chromosomes. Sections of chromosomes are called genes, and humans have about 21,000 genes (about the same number as a mouse, so humans aren't that special), and 3 billion bases per chromosome. Genes are the biologic messengers passed from parent to offspring. Just as your brain is an energy hog, your brain is also a gene hog, in that about half of your total genes are committed to neurological development.

The same DNA sequencing is found in every cell, whether it is a bone cell or a neuron (except mature red blood cells, which don't have any, and the sperm and egg, which have only half). That's somewhat intuitive when you consider that we all start life as a single cell. The reason a bone cell looks different and performs a different function from a neuron is a difference in which of those genes are activated or inactivated. Turning genes on or off can be influenced by the epigenetics (chemical bath) that surround those genes. Think of genes as a collection of instruments sitting idle in front of sheet music. Epigenetics are the musicians that come to play the instruments, and genetic expression, or the phenotype, is the symphony produced by their interaction. If anything adverse happens to any of the components, Beethoven's Fifth won't sound right. And by the way, a fifth of Beethoven won't drink right either.

The expression of a gene has one result: the production of a protein molecule—a note in the symphony. While genes contain the blueprint and tools for appropriate, healthy organ function, genes are basically inert molecules. By themselves, they do not participate directly in biological processes. They do not create blond or black hair, health or disease, intelligence or Darwin Award behavior. There is certainly a relationship between the information in a gene and how that organism looks, feels, thinks, and behaves, but it is only the beginning of the process. The blueprint in the gene sequences must be extracted, recoded, and translated into proteins that drive cell action. It is the proteins, the notes in the symphony, that create the depth, complexity, and harmony of the music. Humans are only as good as the proteins that their genes produce.

Mutations or exposure to toxins, analogous to someone stealing the sheet music or busting up the instruments, can rearrange those bases, that is, break up the covalent bonds (a bond created when two atoms share a pair of electrons) that connect them to each other, causing genetic damage. Those musical instruments (genes in this analogy) can be repaired, but there's no guarantee that will happen. The damage can be passed on to subsequent generations, affecting their health. Less potent but more common toxins can trigger epigenetic changes that also impair genetic function, as if the musicians break a string or their fingers. But these can also be passed on to four or even five generations.

A more academic description of epigenetics would be heritable changes in gene expression occurring without changes in DNA sequence. The most well studied example of these toxins causing chemical harm is their adding of simple molecules called methyl groups, (one carbon atom connected to three hydrogen atoms—CH_3) to the chemical bath that surrounds chromosomes. Those methyl groups can attach themselves to genes like a blood-sucking mosquito that never lets go, changing or impairing their function for life.[3]

Like drunken musicians, epigenetics can make the most exhilarating genetic sheet music and the finest instruments turn Mozart's music into hillbilly country western. The role of most environmental toxins is that of epigenetic spoilers of what would otherwise have been a brain that functions as a fine work of art.

"Fetal programming of disease" is a term coined to describe the effect environmental influences have on the epigenetics of an individual at the most fragile stage of life— in a mother's womb. Much of your risk for a wide variety of chronic adult diseases is tied to events that occurred while you were in the womb, courtesy of fetal programming and epigenetic damage that occurred before you were born. Just like genetics, the epigenetic footprint you carry may have been passed down from your great grandparents or even further back. Researchers studied nematode worms (observing worms can be extremely exciting and is not recommended if you have a pacemaker), and found that environmental influences caused epigenetic changes that were passed on through 14 subsequent generations.[4] If that epigenetic persistence reflects what is possible in humans, that means your health is being affected, for good or ill, by what your ancestors were doing in pre-Revolutionary War America.

All embryos start out as female. Dwayne "the Rock" Johnson? Yup, started out as a female. Lebron James—female. Hitler—female. Likewise, no matter what the underlying chromosome profile is, the brain will act as a female brain until or unless it is exposed to testicular steroids. During critical developmental windows of intrauterine life, permanent anatomical and physiologic changes take place directed by the presence or absence of the male hormone, androgen.

Non-neuronal cells and chemical inflammatory mediators are increased in parts of the androgen-driven male brain compared to that of the female. Overall, during development, the male brain is comparatively under some degree of siege from higher levels of excitation and inflammation.[5] The development of the fetal male brain occurs almost as if it were on fire.

Greater inflammation has distinct disadvantages in brain development, laying the foundation for increased risk of neuropsychiatric disorders and impaired function. This inflammation is the likely common denominator behind the sex differentiation found in early onset brain disorders, males having a significantly higher frequency and/or greater severity in disorders like autism and ADHD. Mental disorders that are thought to originate during fetal development but are not manifest until adolescence or early adulthood, like schizophrenia, occur much more commonly in boys. Boys have a higher risk of the full range of speech disorders, including disorders of the motor component of speech, i.e., inarticulation, apraxia, stuttering, and neurologic disorders like dyslexia and Tourette's syndrome.

However, by middle age and older, schizophrenia is more often diagnosed in women. Other disorders that typically emerge later in life, such as depression, are twice as common in females, perhaps due in part, to males' having more than a 50% greater production of serotonin, the neurotransmitter once thought to be in short supply in depression.

Genes normally involved in male brain development are overly expressed in patients with autism. But these are many of the same genes activated in the production of neuroinflammation.[6] Males also are at a disadvantage because of their sex chromosomes. Nearly all of your 40 trillion cells have a set of your sex chromosomes. The Y chromosome of all male homo sapiens comes from a single male ancestor who lived 100,000-300,000 years ago.[7] If you're looking for a person to scapegoat for how you turned out, you're not likely to find that person at your next family reunion.

The X chromosome is a large chromosome with far more genetic information than its Y counterpart. Geneticists have lost all respect for the Y chromosome. Aretha Franklin's song "R-E-S-P-E-C-T" was not written by geneticists about the Y chromosome. If your chromosomes went to junior high, the Y chromosome would be the skinny, nerdy kid with glasses that gets harassed in the halls and is given a wedgie in the locker room by bullies, in this case, ironically, by the X chromosomes.

Geneticists believe that the X and Y chromosomes started out with about the same number of genes—about 1,000. But evolutionary history has not been kind to the Y chromosome. Over hundreds of thousands of years of evolution, the Y chromosome has lost most of its genetic material. Today, the Y chromosome has fewer than 55 genes, the X chromosome 800-900. Some geneticists think the Y chromosome is now little more than a shriveled up, genetic wasteland.

Try this for a take-down of any man who needs some humble pie fed to his male privilege. The Y chromosome is the only chromosome that is not necessary for human life. The *Dumb and Dumber* movies are proof of that. Actually, most movies produced by Hollywood are proof of that. In fact, some scientists even predict that at the rate the Y chromosome is shrinking, it may ultimately disappear within as little as 100,000 years (true, not a joke). We're all going to die from the climate crisis long before that. Other researchers believe that the human Y chromosome has more like 5 million years left,[8] as has been the case in other species. But even that is a mere blip in an evolutionary time frame, given that life on Earth started about 3.5 billion years ago.

Even newer research suggests that the loss of genes from the Y chromosomes has stopped, and perhaps only one gene has been lost on the Y chromosome in the last 25 million years.[9] For now, one of those remaining genes carries the master switch gene, *SRY*, which directs the male testes and the secretion of testosterone, turning the embryo into a male.

About 20% of men can lose Y chromosomes from their cells as they age. This is the most commonly acquired genetic mutation during human life. By the age of 70, more than 40% of men lose Y chromosomes from some of their white blood cells, referred to as "mosaic aneuploidy," i.e., some, but not all cells have the wrong number of chromosomes. This degenerative variant is linked to increased mortality risk, including from cancer.[10] Smoking, air pollution, and likely other environmental exposures can exacerbate and accelerate loss of the Y chromosome.[11] Genetic decay of the Y chromosome occurs because, in contrast to the two X chromosomes in a female, there is very little exchange of genes between the X and Y chromosome during reproduction. Genes on the Y chromosome are unable to participate in genetic recombination—the exchange of genes that occurs in each generation, which helps to eliminate degenerative gene mutations. Without that benefit, Y chromosomal genes deteriorate over time and are eventually lost from the genome.

Men that father a child after age 40 are significantly more likely to produce a girl, meaning they preferentially are delivering an X chromosome for conception as they age.[12] No one knows exactly why that is, but given the vulnerability of the Y chromosome and its ultimate disappearance in cells of many elderly males, it seems likely that that vulnerability must play a role.

The Y is the only "Lone Ranger" chromosome in the human genome, meaning the only one for which there are not two copies. That means mutations and deletions in the Y chromosome more easily persist and continue being passed on from one male to the next through multiple generations. However, some genes that are displaced from the Y chromosome may not be destined for homelessness or a genetic black hole; they may be able to join other chromosomes. Some geneticists also point to an ability of genes on the Y chromosome to engage in "gene amplification," the acquisition of multiple copies of genes that promote healthy sperm function and mitigate gene loss. Mammals and a few non-mammalian species also have Y chromosomes, and these protective defense mechanisms are found in those species.

The Y chromosome has also developed another defense mechanism, palindromes, DNA sequences that read the same forward as backward—like the words, "did," "level," and "rotator," which can protect them from further degradation. But the loss of the Y chromosome is a risk factor for early death of men from all causes as well as for Alzheimer's, schizophrenia, diabetes, cancer, heart disease, and an impaired immune system.[13]

If A=B, and B=C, then A=C. If air pollution causes of loss the Y chromosome, and loss of the Y chromosome contributes to Alzheimer's, therefore, air pollution may make men more vulnerable to Alzheimer's than women. But that is only a small part of the evidence. More about that in Chapter 5.

With his single X chromosome, the male lacks a healthy copy of the X genes to fall back on. If there is anything amiss on the X chromosome of the male then, with no back-up, that male will show some aberration when he ages and matures. For example, more men are color blind than women, a trait thought to be tied to a defect in the X chromosome. With two X chromosomes, a woman has a "back up" chromosome that can compensate for a defective one.

There may be some inherent loss of key proteins for brain development or repair mechanisms in boys. The X chromosome is loaded with genes involved in brain development and cognition, although one of the female's X chromosomes is normally largely inactivated in the areas of brain development.[14] The X chromosome also has more functioning immunity genes than the Y chromosome, which makes a baby girl more resistant to life-threatening infections.[15]

When the first blast of testosterone from the Y chromosome comes along at about the eighth week after conception, what starts out as a female brain now morphs into a male brain. While at this stage of development, the fetus is adding about 250,000 brain cells per minute, the male fetus is actually killing off some cells in the communication centers and growing more cells in the sex and aggression centers.[16] In other words, at 8 weeks after conception, the male is already preparing to drink beer, watch football, and leave the toilet seat up.

A female fetus will also be exposed to testosterone about the same time, albeit at much lower doses. If the male testosterone surge doesn't happen, the female brain continues to grow unperturbed. Differences between male and female newborns and infants and what they do with their brains appears very early. Among one-day-old newborns, girls prefer to watch a human face, and boys prefer to watch objects like a mobile.[17] That should tell you everything you want to know about the two sexes. In one-year-old infants, girls spend more time looking at their mothers than boys do. As early as one year old, girls prefer chick flicks. Given a choice of what kind of film to watch, baby girls more often choose to watch a film with a face, and boys more often choose to watch a film with cars.[17] And that is why women should rule the world. More on that later.

Girls have a well-documented advantage in acquiring verbal skills, including a superior ability to learn new languages. By the age of 16 months, girls have the use of an average of 95 words, but boys only average about 25 words.[18] Girls are able to construct word combinations on average about 3 months earlier than boys.[19] About 70% of late talkers are boys, and only about 30% of early talkers are boys.[20] Girls speak in complex sentences earlier than boys.

As a new parent, I was introduced to the prodigious vocabulary, not to mention chutzpah of little girls. One day I found our two-year-old daughter standing up on the back of a toilet, with the medicine cabinet open, helping herself to the medicine bottles. Horrified at the prospect of her snacking on a lethal handful of Tylenol gummies, I said, "What are doing up there?" She replied as you might expect a two-year-old defense attorney to do. "Daddy, don't you trust me?" I said, "It's not that I don't trust you, but you can't be up there." She replied, "You just go away, Daddy, and I'll trust myself." I knew then that the picnic part of parenting had come to a screeching halt, and that she would end up either in law school, robbing banks, or, God forbid, a member of Congress.

The advantage that girls have over boys in developing communication and language skills has been confirmed over several decades of studies in countries throughout the world. Girls' brains have comparatively more volume in the areas involving language, the temporal and parietal regions. Boys have more volume in the parietal cortices where visual-spatial functioning originates.

Numerous studies have looked at sex hormone levels, either in amniotic fluid or soon after birth, and how they correlate with anatomical development of known language areas of the brain. Estrogen has been found to be consistently, positively associated with the growth of language areas in the brain, and communication skills and testosterone levels have shown to have an inverse correlation. Indeed, fetal testosterone levels are inversely correlated with language development and the manifestation of empathy,[21] and are directly correlated with autistic traits.[22]

Testosterone levels are inversely correlated with babbling at 5 months of age.[23] A higher testosterone concentration in intrauterine development is correlated with a smaller vocabulary assessed at age 2.[24] Higher estrogen levels measured at 5 months corresponded to superior language skills in both boys and girls at ages 4 and 5.[25]

Research from several years ago found that as adults, the average woman uses a total of about 20,000 words per day, the average male 7,000. The surprise there is that there are 7,000 ways to say, "Sup, Bro?" Newer research has challenged that historic assumption, finding that both sexes use about the same number of words.[26] By age 20, the average person has a vocabulary of about 42,000 words (not counting the words, "Ok, boomer"), increasing to 48,000 by the age of 60.[27]

A certain gene called *FOXP2* plays a large role in language development. In a small sample size of 4-year-old children, the amount of the protein that gene produces was significantly lower in boys than girls.[28] Studies of children 8 to 11 years old found a direct correlation between the levels of testosterone in the amniotic fluid during the pregnancy and diminished gray matter in specific language areas of the brain.

Ongoing personal experiences in life shape not just brain function, but brain architecture. What's most important to an animal is usually reflected in the size of various parts of the brain. A rat's life depends on a keen sense of smell; a primate depends much more on sight, so the olfactory bulb is proportionately larger in the rat, and the visual area is much larger in the primate. If a woman is persistently more verbal than a man, it would make sense that over time, there would be anatomic changes that correspond with that. Females do have a larger communication center, and girls grow up to be more talkative. In critical speech areas, women have larger gray matter volumes and greater neuron density than men.[29] Using her brain's larger speech area, my wife frequently informs me of my larger brain asshole area.

Women's superior verbal skills appear to persist into the early stages of Alzheimer's compared to men.[30] The inescapable conclusion is that compared to females, males as a group have more difficulty developing complex communication brain infrastructure. Any factors, such as environmental toxins that interfere with that developing infrastructure, have a greater consequence to males than females.

There is at least one notable exception to this. Male canaries are much better talkers. They sing long, complex, beautiful courtship songs, while their female counterparts only "twitter" (not via their cell phones). In a coal mine, for instance, miners would likely want to just kill the canary themselves if all it could do was monotonously twitter. Actually, noticing this sex difference in bird communication was the springboard for important later research confirming that human brains differ because of their sex. Furthermore, the region from which those courtship songs originate in the brain of a male canary shows variation in size corresponding to the season when that courtship, and therefore the complex singing, is expected to take place.

About 20% more males are conceived than females. This may be because the spermatozoa carrying the smaller Y chromosome swim faster than those carrying an X, or maybe they're just better at the back stroke. But after conception, it's pretty much all downhill for males competing with females in the longevity sweepstakes for the remainder of the life cycle. Everyone knows men live more dangerously than women, but that difference starts in the womb. Because of their increased fragility, more male fetuses will not survive, such that the larger number of actual male births is only about 5% more than females.

Pregnant women carrying baby girls generally have an easier pregnancy course than if they are carrying a boy. Most pregnancy complications, even things like gestational diabetes and placental abruption, occur more often with boy babies.[31] Boys grow faster and bigger in the womb than girls, which puts them at greater risk for nutritional deficiency.[32]

When I give lectures to audiences, including other doctors, medical students or the general public, I ask them what is their most important organ. The answers are very enlightening, often entertaining, and usually make no sense. Whatever answer a male gives in public is always a lie (we all know what their favorite organ is). But if there is a correct answer (obviously there isn't) it should be the one they no longer have—their placenta.

The placenta is THE critical organ for survival for eutherian (placental) mammals and marsupials (not the biological term for a male tied to his mother's apron strings). The health of every human on earth is more dependent on their placenta than on any other organ, because fetal organogenesis (organ formation) is completely dependent on the adequacy of placental blood flow. The placenta is the most vascular of human organs. It should be intuitive that anything that impairs the robust flow of blood to the fetus would have dire, and potentially lifelong consequences.

The four primary cell types of the placenta are different depending on the sex of the fetus. This difference may be the result of reduced maternal-fetal compatibility for males, invoking a version of "graft vs. host" immune reaction, similar to the rejection that a patient with a transplanted kidney, liver, or heart may experience. More than 140 genes in the placenta behave differently depending on the baby's gender; girls' placentas have more active gene expression promoting placental development, maintenance of pregnancy, and maternal immune tolerance.[33] Exposure to maternal disorders like asthma or pre-eclampsia are examples of adversity within the womb yielding different results for male and female fetuses. Pre-pregnancy maternal obesity increases the risk of adult obesity for a male fetus, but not for a female. Gestational diabetes in their mother increases the risk of childhood obesity for boys but not for girls. Researchers describe a "placental-brain axis" where various types of maternal stress, including exposures to environmental chemicals, are associated with placental abnormalities affecting the brains of animals, males more than females.

Just about every poor neurologic outcome from pregnancy complications is more common in baby boys: brain damage, cerebral palsy, premature birth, and stillbirth. At birth, the average boy is 4 to 6 weeks behind the average girl in overall physiological development,[34] despite the fact that infant males, on average, have larger brains than females, and autistic males have even larger brains, particularly their amygdalas. It takes a greater number of cell divisions to make a male brain.[35] Due to the vulnerability of the Y chromosome mentioned before, with each division there is an increased risk of a transcription error that can be precipitated by exposure to an environmental toxin or other type of physiological insult.

As environmental toxins are increasingly identified as disrupting and damaging fetal development, especially of the brain, and setting the stage for pregnancy complications, boys are affected more than girls. A study in animals subjected first to stress and then to an environmental toxin showed, there was a significant difference between the sexes in how many neurons were killed by the toxin.

Neurons of the male were more susceptible to the toxin than those of females.[17]

Size matters! A brain developing in a newborn ICU (NICU) compared to within a womb is at an extreme disadvantage. (More about that in Chapter 5.) Premature birth is the most common reason for a newborn to end up in a NICU. A premature birth has lifelong health consequences, especially for brain function. Prematurity interrupts critical brain developmental processes, and the earlier a baby is born, the less mature the cortex structure.

Significant prematurity can result in bleeding in the brain, leading to cerebral palsy and other learning and neurologic disabilities. Babies born more than 13 weeks prematurely have a 30 times greater risk for autism. Across the board, with prematurity, baby girls have better overall outcomes, including neurologic outcomes, compared to boys.[36] Researchers used to believe that oxygen deprivation at birth or in infancy kills brain cells, and more than one third of pre-term birth babies have abnormally small brains. However, new research has found that hypoxia doesn't kill brain cells (at least in the all-important hippocampus) but rather prevents those cells from maturing normally, impairing the brain's ability to learn, probably permanently.[37]

Many things increase a mother's chance of a premature delivery, but one of the most important and ubiquitous is air pollution. A recent study concluded that almost 20% of premature births were due to air pollution worldwide (See Chapter 5). Birth misadventures that cause oxygen deprivation to the brain of a newborn cause greater damage to a boy baby than a girl.

That boys start out as the weaker sex is reinforced by the fact that they are 60% more likely to be born premature than girls, and that disparity has only been increasing, as the rate of prematurity itself is increasing. The weeks a baby loses in the womb really do matter in the development of all organs, but especially the brain. In the next chapters I'll give more detail on how chemical toxins in the NICU environment harm brain development.

Baby girls emerge from normal pregnancy and birth, as well as from complications from either, better than boys do. With female babies, there is a more robust expression of genes responsible for placental development and the maintenance of pregnancy and the maternal immune system. Newborn boys have higher rates than newborn girls do of infection, including serious infections, such as sepsis.

The superiority of female immune systems is found across virtually all species. Females' survival advantage continues throughout the entire lifespan, but it is particularly significant in the newborn period. A superior immune system is probably also a major contributor to why the mortality rate of the COVID-19 virus is about twice as high in men as in women. It is probably why women have a lower rate of acquiring cancer and dying from cancer compared to men. But it is also likely a major contributor to why women have much higher rates of autoimmune diseases like lupus and multiple sclerosis. Mast cells are the first immune cells to be called up for duty when an infection of either viruses or bacteria begins. Female mast cells produce, store, and release more inflammatory chemicals than their male counterparts. Over 4,000 genes have been found to be more active in mast cells from females than from males.[38]

There is a strong connection between the immune system and learning and memory. Cytokines are immune proteins that have received almost as much press as Taylor Swift, because their excessive activity seems to play a role in many of the deaths from COVID-19. Mice bred to have an inability to produce a type of these cytokines, called interleukins, or the immune cells, "T-cells," are unable to learn to how to swim their way to safety compared to mice that can produce that compound. Numerous other lab animal studies show that if animals have compromised immune systems, they are less able to establish short- or long-term memory and are less social. The general superiority of women's immune systems appears to be a Trump card (sorry for that) for their brain function compared to men.[39]

In lab animals and in humans, mitochondria inside female brain cells have a greater antioxidant capacity and energy production capability, which help withstand neurotoxic environmental insults.[40] Postmortem studies of the enzyme activity in human brains (research a bit more sophisticated than what was depicted in Young Frankenstein) showed that female brains had more activity of beneficial enzymes than males.[41] Other studies show that, in contrast, males have greater production of free radicals in their mitochondria,[42] a sign of biological stress.

Microglia cells, the garbage collectors of the brain, show significant gender differences. In the male fetus, after the male hormone surge, there is a parallel surge in microglia cells in several brain regions compared to females,[43] apparently because there is more garbage to collect.

Gemfibrozil is a lipid-lowering drug used to treat very high cholesterol and triglyceride levels in people with pancreatitis and other disorders where other treatments have failed to lower blood lipids. It is also an anti-oxidant and anti-inflammatory agent. When given to animals prior to a controlled brain injury, the drug was protective against brain damage in females but had the opposite effect in males.[44]

Selenium is an essential trace element that has antioxidant properties important for brain function and also stimulates male fertility. In males, selenium distribution is preferentially directed to the gonads, providing chemical proof that men prioritize their penis over their brain—hardly a surprise to any woman reading this book. In castrated male animals (intentionally simulating a female), selenium's anti-oxidant action is increased in the brain, providing protection for neurons.[45] Don't pretend you already knew that.

Parkinson's Disease is not specifically a disorder of the intellect, but it is one of the most debilitating neurological diseases, involving loss of motor function, and later, impaired cognition. Men have about double the risk of Parkinson's than women do, and on average, an earlier onset.[46] They also have a more severe preclinical phase of the disease. Researchers postulate that estrogen has some protective effects in the disease, noting also that in women, life events that correlate with estrogen production—the number of children, age at menopause, and duration of fertile life—all correlated with later age at onset of Parkinson's.[46]

Furthermore, the symptoms of the disease differ somewhat by gender. Men more often have rigidity and rapid eye movement. Women more often have dyskinesias (involuntary, erratic movements) and depression. Once the disease reaches its clinical phase, the differences between men and women start to disappear. Evidence suggests that the increased risk for Parkinson's in males is the consequence of vulnerability to toxins that impair the functioning of the testis-related gene, *SRY*. Men also have a higher risk of amyotrophic lateral sclerosis (ALS), a progressive and fatal neuromuscular disease that seems to be increasing in prevalence.

The human female brain may be superior to the male brain, but even the female brain doesn't hold a candle to an octopus's brain. (The candle wouldn't stay lit under water anyway.) Octopuses are the most intelligent invertebrate, with nine brains: a central, donut-shaped brain, and each arm has a mind of its own, literally, which can operate independently of the other seven as well as operate under the command of the central brain. They can open jars from the outside, and if they are placed inside jars, they can open them from the inside. They can use tools, they can kill sharks, and they've been observed escaping their tanks, stealing a fish from an adjacent tank, and returning to their original tank when they think no one is watching. Let's see any human females do that. Just for the record, an octopus has three hearts and blue blood.

For a myriad of reasons—anatomic, biochemical, hormonal, and physiologic—women enjoy a neurologic advantage over men. And that advantage only grows when taking into account environmental toxins as we do in the next chapter.

Chapter Four

ENVIRONMENTAL ATTACKS ON THE BRAIN (ALLEGEDLY)

> "Lack of evidence of mail-in voting fraud is the definition of fraud."
>
> —Trump Chief of Staff Mark Meadows, not currently in straight jacket

> "It's humbling being humble."
>
> —Maurice Clarett, former Denver Broncos running back

> "I tested very positively in another sense so—this morning... Yeah. I tested positively toward negative, right? So, I tested perfectly this morning—meaning I tested negative. But that's a way of saying it—positively toward the negative."
>
> .—President, Donald J. Trump, on his coronavirus test, May 21, 2020

I'd like to thank whoever wrote Chapter 3 for agreeing to a peaceful transfer of power to Chapter 4. And now that you are in Chapter 4, you can't sue me for anything that was written in Chapter 3, because I'm protected by the statue of limitations.

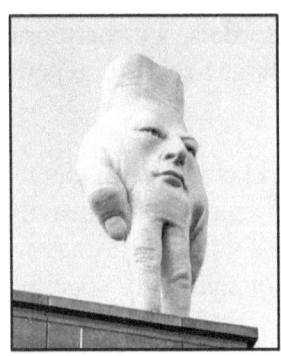

Statue of Limitations,

Provo, Utah

"There's been a staggering rise in neurodevelopmental disorders in the United States and globally," said National Toxicology Program (NTP) Toxicologist Mamta Behl, PhD, during her keynote talk at the February 2020 symposium sponsored by the National Institute of Environmental Health Sciences, entitled "Interactions Between the Brain and the Environment."

In the U.S. in 1976, the incidence of children diagnosed with learning disabilities was 1 in 30. By 2013, that had increased to 1 in 6. In 1988, Autism was diagnosed in 1 in 1,000 children. By 2013 it was 1 in 45. One in 18 children was diagnosed with ADHD in 1996. By 2012, that was 1 in 10, with more than twice as many boys diagnosed as girls.[1] Similar increases have occurred in the incidence of tic, obsessive-compulsive, and emotional disorders.

Following the same pattern of learning disabilities, by 2011, one in six children was diagnosed with some kind of neurodevelopment disorder.[2] Some observers are trying to convince themselves and everyone else that this rise reflects more aggressive diagnostic efforts and relaxing diagnostic criteria rather than any actual rise in the prevalence of these disorders. Other studies have concluded that this explanation only accounts for a modest portion of cases. This issue will be dealt with in more detail in Chapter 8. But one thing is indisputable. Boys are more often diagnosed with all these disorders than girls by a wide margin, from a ratio of 4.5 to 1 for ADHD to 2 to 1 for learning delays.[3]

Genetic changes are often invoked as an etiological explanation for this broad-based increase. This is not likely, however, because genetic-based changes occur slowly, not nearly as rapidly as the rate of increase of these disorders. Furthermore, inheritance patterns are not consistent with sex-related genetic "evolving" as a likely explanation.

Autism, which is one of the most severe developmental disorders with one of the highest rates of increase, is heavily dominated by males. Eighty percent of patients with autism have a normal genetic profile.[4] The other 20% do not share any specific, consistent, genetic abnormalities.[5,6]

Some have pointed to a higher rate of neurodevelopment disorders in siblings as being supportive of genetic responsibility for the male preponderance. But siblings also tend to be subjected to the same environmental exposures, clouding the issue. Furthermore, if genes were primarily responsible, that would likely involve sex-related genes on the X chromosome. Any affected female would have to receive the abnormal X gene from her father, but that pattern is not seen.

Almost by default, environmental exposures are the only reasonable explanation for the increase in disorders and for the male dominance.[7] So if, "It's the environment, stupid," what is it in the environment that might explain this?

Deep in the heart of the Yasuni National Park in the Ecuadorean Amazon jungle (the only place on earth where there is only one Starbucks) live between 200 to 400 Waorani tribesmen. They are "uncontacted"—living in complete isolation from the outside world, ironically, much like we all were during the coronavirus pandemic. Despite their isolation, the Waorani became world famous when, in 1956, not exactly interested in learning about Jesus, they speared to death five missionaries that had landed their plane in Waorani territory. The Ecuadorean government responded by making it illegal for outsiders to go in after them for any reason, including providing "aid," promoting religious conversion, or selling Girl Scout cookies. They are "forest people," whose feet are deformed from a lifetime of climbing trees, and they are as isolated from modern civilization as any human beings on earth. They hunt with blow darts, wear little to no clothing, and dangle dead monkeys around their necks for adornment. Even though they live in the Amazon jungle, they don't get any packages delivered by Amazon. But even they cannot live without being harmed by the mass chemical contamination of the entire globe. If we were allowed to test them, even the blood of Waorani tribesmen would almost certainly show contamination with hundreds, perhaps even thousands of the chemicals that have come to permeate the entire world in the 21st century.

From the hair of polar bears to the chromosomes that lie in the nucleus of your newborn baby's brain cells, virtually every living thing on earth is literally being bathed in harmful chemicals and heavy metals. Taking advantage of this disturbing reality has even found application in the controversial search for energy in underwater formations of methane hydrates. The age of hydrates and sediments that cover them, and therefore the origin of the hydrates, can be determined in part by whether they have traces of the legacy pesticide dichlorodiphenyltrichloroethane (DDT), which was first used in 1945. Because of its persistence in the environment and continued presence in dairy products, meat, and fish, virtually all of us still have DDT in our bodies.[9] When ingested, persistent organic pollutants such as DDT take up semi-permanent residence in the fat tissue of living organisms, making human fat a welcome mat for DDT.

In the late 1970s, chemical and oil companies began to fear that growing public awareness of the toxicity of their manufactured chemicals would start to hurt their business, so naturally, they responded with a massive public relations (PR) campaign, apologizing for any harm they may have done.... Just kidding, of course. They responded with a massive PR and advertising campaign rather than an apology or re-evaluation of the safety of their products. For instance, Monsanto started running print ads showing a young child with a puppy above the slogan, "Without chemicals, life would be impossible." Actually, without their chemicals, the only thing that would be impossible is their profits. Your life, on the other hand would be just fine, perhaps a bit more inconvenient, but otherwise fine and much healthier.

The term "Chemosphere" currently refers to a famous, futuristic, octagon-shaped house in Los Angeles designed by architect John Lautner. The name more appropriately could be applied to 21st Century Earth—the Chemosphere—because our planet is a giant sphere, now drenched in a toxic chemical bath. Multiple studies have confirmed universal contamination of the global environment and virtually all living things with a dizzying array of manmade compounds. Virtually none of these chemicals improve or augment natural biologic systems, and many are toxic to life forms of all types, including humans, especially the brains of humans.

Through the air you breathe, the water you drink, the food you eat, the couch you sit on, and the cell phone you can't put down long enough to read this book (or on which you read this book), life in modern civilization exposes all of us to an almost endless list of chemical toxins. The United States manufactures or imports 42 billion pounds of chemicals every day, only half of which are used to hold Donald Trump's hair in place. The term "xenobiotics" refers to chemicals found in an organism but not produced by that organism—a foreign invader, if you will. Most of these industrial chemicals are xenobiotics, many of which are neurotoxins. Common fruits and vegetables can contain residues of as many as 60 different pesticides. In the average indoor air in homes in the United States float 400 different chemicals.[10]

The chemical industry wants you to think there's nothing to worry about. In-house company science of course exonerates their products, but it doesn't require more than a nanogram of skepticism to wonder about the self-serving conclusions that in-house science might provide. Routine, independent, and what should be objective science behind those assumptions either doesn't exist, because no tests were ever done, or the science is based on principles that are badly outdated and completely unable to address the risks. We are all essentially human guinea pigs in a massive toxicology experiment that we didn't consent to, that has no scientific design or constraints, and that is conducted by people who have little to no concern about how the experiment will affect your health and your life. And it's an experiment that has been going on for more than 140 years.

Since at least the Industrial Revolution, officials of virtually every major industry and of every level of government, including public health officials, i.e., "the establishment," have demonstrated a commitment to downplay risks to the public of industrial toxins and contaminants.

The Poison Squad, a fascinating book by Deborah Blum and a PBS documentary, details the heroic effort by Dr. Harvey Wiley at the turn of the 20th Century to rid American kitchens and dinner tables from countless toxic chemicals, preservatives, fillers, and fraudulent ingredients added by large corporations to their processed products. For years, the official narrative, if there was one at all, was that it was all safe for human consumption. In the era before consumer protection laws, Wiley launched a decades-long crusade to expose the careless, and in many cases deliberate contamination of America's food supply with sulfur dioxide, plaster of paris, boric acid, salicylic acid, copper sulfate, cocaine, morphine, cotton seed, sodium benzoate, formaldehyde, and saw dust, among many others. His work was instrumental in developing the first consumer protection laws, and he is regarded as the Father of the U.S. Food and Drug Administration (FDA). He ultimately resigned from his leadership role in government, frustrated by the stonewalling of food corporations and their heavy lobbying influence over federal and state government bureaucracy.

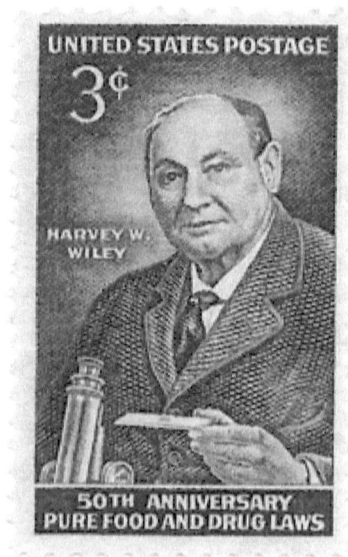

"Radium Girls" is a name given to young female factory workers whose job it was to paint watch dials with radium-based luminous paint in the early part of the 20th century. They were told the paint was harmless and were instructed to use their lips or tongue to give their brushes a fine tip before each dip into the paint because using rags or water took longer and used more raw materials. The company executives and their "scientists" continued to insist on the "lip, dip, paint" method long after they knew the radium paint was poisonous. Many workers died and/or suffered hideous bone, tissue, and skin deformities and diseases, consequences of the radiation that penetrated their lips and mouths. One watch-painting company appealed its lost lawsuits eight times before issuing its employees protective gear, and only then withdrew the requirement of employees to point the brushes with their lips. As late as the 1970s, radium was still being used on watch dials. I had no idea that it was radium that caused the dial on my first watch as a teenager to glow in the dark. I just thought that's what watches were supposed to do. (Current phosphorescent watches use paint that includes no radium and that absorbs and re-emits light.) This appalling example of corporate indifference to workers' health and safety has been referenced and featured in short and longer fiction, poetry, historical fiction, as well as historical narratives, documentaries, a play, and a feature film.

A similar dynamic played out with many of the neurotoxins detailed in this and the next chapter. Whatever neurotoxin you might name—lead, mercury, arsenic, fluoride, cigarette smoke, radiation, pesticides, Teflon, cell phones—invariably government authorities and powerful businesses spent decades protecting the businesses responsible for the contamination, rather than the public from the contamination. And in many cases, this continues today.

Furthermore, in many years of observing local and national environmental events, including oil spills, wildfires, floods, industrial disasters, military mishaps, chemical explosions, and nuclear accidents, public health officials' default priority is to downplay the risks, presumably to avoid panic, rather than prioritize public health protection. We saw the Environmental Protection Agency (EPA) absurdly declare ground zero "safe" after the 9/11 attack on the World Trade Center. The human health hazard of the Deepwater Horizon oil spill was initially dismissed. The lead contamination of the water supply of Flint, Michigan, was swept under the rug for months. The Three Mile Island, Chernobyl, and Fukushima nuclear accidents were all smoothed over with layers of denial, obfuscation, and propaganda that served to protect those responsible instead of the public.

The Erin Brockovich saga, Love Canal, the Camp Lejeune water contamination disaster, and countless others have followed the same pattern. I've seen local health officials downplay the risks of oil spills in my home town of Salt Lake City, and have consulted with exposed communities throughout the Western United States experiencing similar events. In my role as board chairman of Doctors and Scientists Against Wood Smoke Pollution, I see a steady stream of people being harmed by wood smoke from neighbors and restaurants. Health officials usually inexplicably dismiss the hazard, and nationwide little to nothing is done about it.

In 2021 an alarming study about heavy metals in baby food was released in a congressional report. An article about the study begins, "A House report finding that top baby food products contain heavy metals has sparked panic among parents—and a lawsuit. But experts advise parents to "stay calm." Why? Why do experts want parents to stay calm? In fact, if they are really "experts," staying calm is definitely not the advice they should be offering. Yes, there is no reason for parents to light their hair on fire, but only because that wouldn't help. But there is every reason for parents to stop feeding their infants these manufactured foods, and where possible, start making their own baby food. Moreover, the message for everyone, not just parents, is that we must demand from our government strong and effective oversight of our agricultural system, and specifically begin an investigation into why our food supply is so thoroughly contaminated with heavy metals and other toxins. (More about that in Chapter 9.)

WWI became the first large-scale demonstration of the power and horror of chemicals to disable, maim, and kill soldiers. The use of tear gas, mustard gas, phosgene, and chlorine led to the labeling of WWI as "the chemists' war." In response, the 1925 Geneva Protocol for the Prohibition of the Use of Asphyxiating, Poisonous, or Other Gases, and Bacteriological Methods of Warfare, was adopted by the major nations of the world. WWI was also referred to as the "war to end all wars," in part because of the horror that chemical warfare wrought upon the troops.

But while the use of chemicals was finally being regulated in war, ironically and simultaneously, a virtual free-for-all was unleashed in the use of chemicals and deadly substances in consumer goods and countless civilian applications. DDT was indiscriminately sprayed all over American cities, including residential neighborhoods, and we all started inhaling it, swallowing it, and absorbing it through our skin. Teflon was laminated onto cookware, and we all started eating it with our scrambled eggs. Polychlorinated biphenyls (PCBs) were dumped into our rivers, and we all started drinking them. Radiation was launched into the atmosphere, falling down upon us whenever it rained, lodging in our thyroids, bones, and soft tissues. Radium was included in cosmetics and creams and was the featured ingredient in Radithor, "A Certified Radium Drink," It was added to sprays for use as a bug killer, furniture polish, and disinfectant. Lead became almost ubiquitous in drinking water, paint, and gasoline, and arsenic was added to cosmetics and was the "active ingredient" in the medical tonic, "Fowler's Solution." Chloroform was added to liniments. Asbestos was added to toothpaste. The most toxic and deadly neurotoxin that we know of, mercury, was a common ingredient added to teething powders for babies, diaper rash creams, and laxatives for adults. If I skinned my left knee on the asphalt playground at William Penn Elementary in the 1950s, having been shoved there by Johnny, who clearly deserved to go to prison in the third grade, the teacher or school nurse would put Mercurochrome (an antiseptic containing mercury) on the abrasion so it wouldn't get infected. That's like using a weed whacker to clean your kitchen floor, doing more harm than good and not being terribly effective. By the way, Mercurochrome is the reason my left knee is so much dumber than my right.

Using toxic chemicals as weapons for war had been banned, but businesses were subjecting civilians at home to an all-out toxic hemical attack. Little concern about the consequences of these toxins was raised by the public, the government, health experts of the time, and certainly not the companies that manufactured them. Whatever concern was raised only targeted one toxin at a time. But no one started thinking about the end result of the cumulative exposure of all those biologic poisons.

It was once thought that the placenta provided a protective shield for intrauterine fetal development, but that idea has become an anachronism. For 50 years or more, doctors have advised pregnant women not to smoke or drink alcohol, because the chemicals could cross the placenta and harm the baby's development. Many of us have cringed watching videos of ultrasounds of unborn babies and how they physically respond almost immediately to a pregnant mother's smoking. If we had time-lapse ultrasounds of how babies in utero respond to many other environmental toxins we would be just as stunned. For nearly 40 years, doctors have advised pregnant women to avoid taking any non-essential medication for the same reason. Why have we not thought about the possibility of other chemicals, those not manufactured by the pharmaceutical industry, the tobacco industry, or the alcohol industry, also crossing the placenta? Why have we not considered that the chemicals in air pollution, personal care products, our clothes, or the food we eat could interfere with fetal development?

In 2005 and again in 2009, the Environmental Working Group commissioned five laboratories to examine the umbilical cord blood of 10 babies; they found more than 200 chemicals in the blood of each newborn.[11] In fact, 200 is undoubtedly a gross undercount, because the researchers only tested for a few hundred chemicals. Of the ones found in umbilical cord blood, 158 were determined to be neurotoxic based on other studies. More research done specifically on the blood of pregnant mothers showed the same disturbing result. Virtually all pregnant women are walking chemical repositories. Tracking 163 chemicals, 99% of pregnant women tested positive for at least 43 different chemicals.[12]

The Great Brain Robbery –Brian Moench

Back in 1980, a government scientist concluded that human breast milk was so contaminated with industrial toxins and pesticides that if it were regulated by the U.S. Department of Agriculture (USDA) it would be banned. As unnerving as this information is, it really should not be a surprise. The average human in a developed country is now exposed to over 140,000 industrial chemicals, about 100 times more than just two generations ago.[13] Even if only a fraction of those 140,000 are in breast milk, the most essential of human food, that should be terrifying to us all.

A website called ChemicalSafetyFacts.org disputes much of what I have just written. They have an article titled, "Debunking the Myths: Are there really 84,000 chemicals?" Yes, there are actually many more. They claim there are only 8,707 chemicals used in commerce today, and with a zippy, hipster video, they declare that not only is there nothing to worry about, you'd be a naked, hopeless, blithering idiot without them, i.e. a college student.[14] Well, worry anyway, even if you're fine being naked, blithering, and an idiot.

Even if the website were correct, the number of chemicals in commerce today is hardly the number of chemicals you are still exposed to, because so many of the worst of them don't break down for decades or longer, something they conveniently left out of their Pollyanna video. And by the way, the site is run by the American Chemistry Council, the trade organization of the chemical industry. I rest my case.

> My flesh-eating attorney has just informed me that the words "allegedly," "forthwith," "defacto," and "res judicata" need to be inserted at the beginning of every sentence in the previous 4,000 paragraphs.

It is hardly a surprise that pregnant mothers would have at least a few hundred chemicals in their blood stream and that some of them, maybe even most of them, will cross the placenta and contaminate the developing brain of their babies in utero. It defies common sense that this would not have clinical significance.

In March 2014, prominent researchers from the Mount Sinai School of Medicine in New York and the University of Southern Denmark issued a warning that "a global, silent pandemic of neurodevelopmental toxicity" was sweeping over developed and undeveloped countries alike. They cited strong evidence that "children worldwide are being exposed to unrecognized toxic chemicals that are silently eroding intelligence, disrupting behaviors, truncating future achievements and damaging societies."[15] It was a follow-up to a similar warning they had released in 2006. They identified eleven different environmental exposures, common throughout the world, as toxic to the brain development of children, virtually all with permanent consequences. The developmental disorders include autism, ADHD, dyslexia, and other cognitive impairments.

The toxins and pollutants, all related to consumer goods and industrial activity, include lead, methylmercury, PCBs, arsenic, toluene, manganese, fluoride, organochlorine and organophosphate pesticides, tetrachloroethylene (a solvent), and the polybrominated diphenyl ethers (flame retardants). The authors also postulated that "even more neurotoxicants remain undiscovered."

These brain toxins are found in the clothing you wear, the air you breathe, the food you eat, the couch you became a potato on, and the soil your kids play in (that is if any kids playing outside or in the soil is something other than a relic of the past). This short list of chemicals and compounds is just a fraction of the real-world culprits. Rest assured, these researchers only scratched the surface of the problem. The number of chemicals that are toxic to the brain, interfering with the delicate process of organizing fetal brain architecture, is orders of magnitude greater than these eleven, and other experts add to this list components of typical air pollution—polycyclic aromatic hydrocarbons (PAHs), fine particulate matter, nitrogen oxides,[16] glyphosate (the main ingredient in the herbicide Roundup), radiation, perchlorate, and aluminum adjuvants (often used in vaccines).[17]

It is a popular misconception, fed in part by weak government regulations, that toxins produce an all-or-nothing effect.

Levels above "safe" doses are acknowledged to be harmful, but below "safe" levels are misinterpreted as harmless. But that's not how the body works, especially the developing brain.

Brain-damaging chemicals can provoke the entire spectrum of outcomes, from imperceptible changes to severe neurologic handicaps. Furthermore, the absence of cognitive or behavioral problems in childhood is not necessarily evidence that an early exposure to a neurotoxin had no adverse effect on brain development. Studies in both animals and humans have demonstrated that some substances cause damage to the brain that is manifested only in a delayed onset of learning problems, attention deficits, and changes in emotional regulation, which can have long-term consequences but don't emerge until teenage and early adult years.

Of the hundreds or even thousands of exogenous chemicals that pregnant mothers are exposed to, and that cross the placenta during embryonic and fetal development, many of those undoubtedly reach the brain during critical windows of brain formation. None of them enhance the natural process of brain growth and maturation, and many of them are known to be outright toxic to neurons and brain tissue. The immature brain of an embryo, fetus, or infant is at risk for significant and permanent damage from exposure to chemicals, such as pesticides, at levels that may have no detectable impact on adults. Public policies, which too often focus on adults, fail to protect developing brains during pregnancy and early infancy.

After investigating this research for a couple of years, I noticed a consistent pattern beginning to emerge for most of the neurotoxins studied. They had a greater impact on males than females. If this is part of a battle of the sexes, no one knew it was even being fought, and the research is telling a very disturbing story about the outcome. Men, you're losing this battle.

The remainder of this chapter and the next is a breakdown of the most well studied of the most prevalent environmental neurotoxins.

LEAD

In the toxic substances Hall of Shame, lead has achieved a level of infamy almost unequaled by anything except perhaps radioactivity. All of us have some lead in our bodies, the result of living in an industrial world with a sinister lead industry that for decades successfully fought off attempts to curtail products it knew were deadly and toxic. All of us have had our cognitive capability compromised by the lead to which we were exposed. We are all little less than who we could have been.

Lead's toxicity extends far beyond the brain, its effects can be devasting to all major organ systems. It is highly toxic to the kidneys and cardiovascular system and to pregnancy viability. Given the theme of this book, we will focus only its neurotoxicity.

There is no "normal" or "natural" blood level of lead, and it serves no physiological purpose. The CDC and medical organizations like the American Academy of Pediatrics have officially stated that no amount of lead exposure can be considered safe; even very small amounts are neurotoxic.[18] A recent report from UNICEF says that one in three children worldwide have toxic levels of lead in their bodies, high enough to trigger government interventions.[19] Few of those interventions are actually happening.

Lead has become the most widely recognized environmental neurotoxin in human history. The average American child growing up before the 1980s lost at least 6 IQ points from leaded gasoline and paint.[20] That's the difference between being a Republican or a Democrat (I'll let you draw your own conclusion on who has the upper hand of that IQ disparity.) In the aggregate, that is an astounding societal loss. By shifting the bell curve, that degree of IQ loss decreased the percentage of the population qualifying as "intellectually gifted" by about 40% and increased the population of the "mentally challenged" by a similar amount.

Lead was a known neurologic poison well before it was added to gasoline in 1923. Lead, like most other heavy metals, is not combustible, does not degrade, and cannot be destroyed. Every ounce of lead that has been produced and refined from the original ore and added to products like paint and gasoline is still somewhere in the environment, in corroded pipes, inside homes in deteriorating paint, suspended in the air along freeways, on road surfaces, and embedded in the tires of your car. Much of it has moved, has become recycled or has been distributed differently from where it was 50 years ago, but it is all still somewhere, and much of it is mobile enough in the environment to continue exposing us. Thousands of pounds of vaporized lead escape every year out the smokestack of the Rio Tinto copper smelter about 20 miles from my home. It steadily accumulates in the environment of Salt Lake City, and some of it undoubtedly makes it all the way to Denver, 520 miles away.

Years ago, I bought a truck load of crumbled tires (painted green to symbolize that they were "eco-friendly" I suppose) to cover the playground in my backyard, underneath the swing set, climbing poles, and monkey bars. I was so proud of myself for finding a good way to recycle and keep a few tires out of landfills. Years later, I realized the playground I had so proudly constructed for my granddaughter was probably full of lead because lead is embedded in vehicle tires from all the tail pipe emissions from the era of leaded gasoline of decades ago. There are similar concerns regarding many artificial turfs that have been shown to be sources of lead dust, putting young football and soccer athletes at risk. People who might want to raise a garden in an urban environment or on property next to a heavily trafficked road should have their soil tested for lead before they try to grow a vegetable garden. There is still a little bit of lead in many paints, water pipes, ceramics, kitchen dishes, crystal, herbal and cosmetic products, and children's toys.

Even with everything we know now about lead's extreme neurotoxicity, inexplicably and indefensibly, it is still found in aviation fuel for small airplanes and helicopters, known as "avgas." Approximately 150,000 piston-engine aircraft across the nation are allowed to use it. For more than two decades, EPA has rebuffed petitions from multiple environmental and public health advocacy groups to force the elimination of avgas. A 2011 study from Duke University showed elevated levels of lead in the blood of those living up to one kilometer away from these small aircraft airports.[21] The EPA estimates that 16 million Americans live close to one of

22,000 airports where leaded avgas is routinely used, and three million children go to schools near these airports.[22]

There is a strong correlation between levels of heavy metals (lead, mercury, and manganese) in the blood, plasma, and urine of adolescents and aggressive behavior.[37]

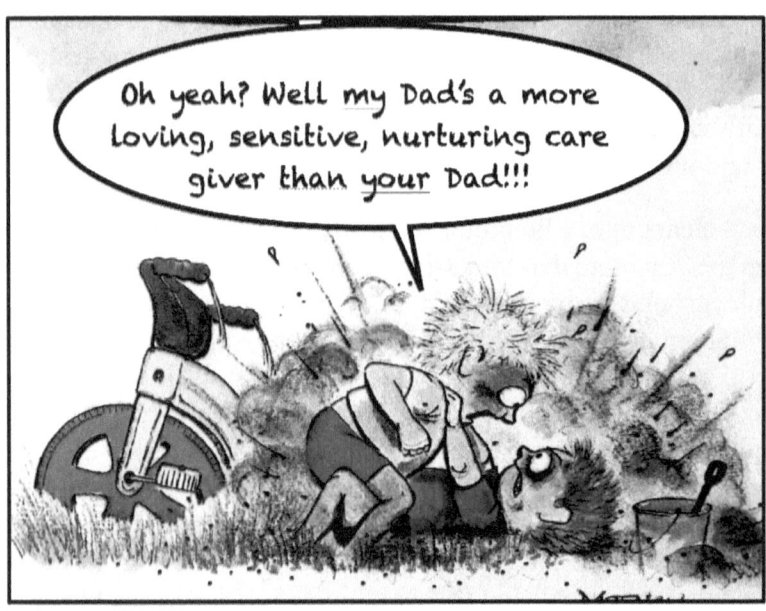

Other research shows a strong correlation between atmospheric lead levels and violent crime rates (but not necessarily white-collar crime). A study published in Environmental Research, which used data spanning more than fifty years, reported a "very strong association" between lead levels in children and crime rates twenty years later when they became young adults. The decline in U.S. crime rates, which began in the early 1990s, fits the pattern with the reduction of leaded gasoline in the early 1970s. Other countries that followed suit saw similar declines, also delayed by twenty years.

A Pittsburgh University study showed that juvenile delinquents averaged lead levels four times higher than adolescents with no history of trouble with the law. Some health authorities believe the data suggests that 90% of the international drop in crime over the last 20 years can be attributed to reducing lead exposure.[23]

Prenatal lead exposure is also associated with antisocial behavior, including aggressive, violent criminal activity and arrests for this behavior as adults.[24]

Ninety percent of the ten billion rounds of ammunition sold in this country to the military, police, and the public is lead ammunition.[25] A little bit of lead is vaporized every time lead ammunition is shot at any target. Frequent shooters are exposed to enough volatilized lead dust and lead fragments that their own health, especially their mental health and judgement, can be the most important casualty of their gun fascination. Even in a well-ventilated gun range, lead dust drifts onto shooters' hands, arms, and clothing and stays suspended in the air long enough to be inhaled. The chronic baseline blood levels of shooters are about 67% higher than the average non shooter. When customers and employees of shooting ranges go home, they can carry enough lead dust with them to contaminate their households and harm their family members.[26]

As suggested by the association between lead and crime rates, the neurotoxicity of lead causes poor judgement, impaired executive functioning, and aggressive, antisocial attitudes. Realizing this prompts me, and it should prompt others, to wonder about the role that lead exposure may be playing in the extremely aggressive, anti-government, anti-social behavior of white supremacists, right-wing militias, and the gun-fanatic faction among conservatives.

Some of this violent behavoir has been shockingly imbecilic. Thirteen members of one of these self-proclaimed militias were arrested for plotting to kidnap and execute the governor of Michigan. That was merely a small opening act for what happened on Jan. 6, 2021, when the nation's Capitol Building was overrun by thousands of maniacal Trump supporters with a variety of weapons attempting a violent overthrow of the government.

Gun fanatics are the people most likely to go shooting for target practice, either for fun or something more sinister. Target shooting and gun play exposes them to more lead, which would only make their irrationality and aggression worse, leading to a malevolent, dangerous, self-reinforcing feedback loop. The connection between lead and poor judgement, violence, and criminality should provoke a demand for legislation requiring testing for blood lead levels as a companion to mandatory background checks and waiting periods for purchasing firearms. Scrutinizing lead exposure is certainly not the only answer to controlling criminality and gun violence, but given the magnitude and complexity of the problem, there is no reason to not add it to the basket of needed reforms.

All of us, no matter how old or young we are, how clean our air and water is, no matter where we grew up, have been harmed and are still being harmed by the lead carelessly or deliberately released into our environment. Blood lead levels far below what is officially considered toxic have been shown to harm the brain development of children.[27]

Children are more vulnerable than adults to the neurotoxicity from lead, and they absorb a higher percentage of the lead that is swallowed. The microvasculature of a child's developing brain, specifically, the immaturity of the BBB (see Chapter 2), is exploited[28] by lead exposure and is uniquely susceptible to high-level lead toxicity. The end result can be cerebellar hemorrhage, further permeability of the BBB, and blood vessel–related brain swelling.

Lead also affects many of the biological functions of nerve cells themselves, interfering with critical enzymes and chemicals that act as neurotransmitters, displacing calcium movement in and out of cells and disrupting the protective myelin coating nerve axons. Occupational lead exposure is associated with brain atrophy, permanent white-matter lesions, and overall small brain volumes.

Lead has a half-life in the blood of 35 days, meaning that 35 days after an exposure, the blood level has decreased by 50%. But lead mimics calcium and follows the same biological migration pathways, steadily accumulating in bones and teeth. If you want to know someone's acute lead exposure, you would measure it in the blood. However, the record of what you were exposed to in the past, including the distant past, is kept in the bones and teeth. Baby teeth begin forming in utero, and the amount of lead exposure a baby may have experienced before birth, at the most critical neurodevelopmental stage, is recorded in those baby teeth.[29]

Men generally have higher blood levels of lead than women do. But during pregnancy and lactation, lead, like calcium, is mobilized from bones because of the increased bone turnover, and that can release lead into the blood and the breast milk. However, in most cases, breast milk contains less lead than formula. Calcium supplements can decrease blood lead levels in pregnant and lactating females.

In the fall of 2023, the CDC became aware of nlarly 500 cases of lead poisoning in children. Bear in mind in order to have symptoms of poisoning, the levels of exposure would have to be significant, and number of children that suffered some degree of brain damge without obvious symptoms would have been much greater. The culprit turned out to be pouches of infants' cinnamon applesauce sold at dollar stores and other outlets under the brand names, WanaBana, Schnucks and Weis. Children in 44 states ate the toxic applesause.

The lead was likely added intentionally either to give the cinnamon a brighter color, or add weight to bulk containers of the spice that were usually sold by weight. In either case the moral depravity of such a business decision is incomprehensible. Food safety experts note that deliberate contamination has long been known to be a problem with spices that have a reddish hue and are sold by weight. In this case the cinnamon originated in Sri Lanka and shipped to Ecuador where it was likely mixed with lead chromate. After changing hands a few more times, the leaded cinnamon was sold by a company with a sinisterly ironic name, Negasmart, to Austrofood who then manufactured the applesauce pouches in Ecuador.

A New York Times investigation from 2024 found that the contaminated applesauce "sailed through" multiple check points set up by the FDA, and that American inspectors had not visited Austrofood in five years. Ecuador didn't have the goverrnment funding to inspect the involved ingredients either.

Private safety auditors hired by American importers thereotically ensure product safety. But you can guess how well that works. A private company audit of Austrofood gave it an A+ rating while American parents were unknowingly poisoning their own children.

In an example of the nation's misplaced priorites, FDA policies on lead in food consumed daily by children are less rigorous than government standards that apply to the cribs they sleep in. For years studies of lead levels in baby foods have revealed high enough levels for the FDA to take action and in 2023 the agency proposed maximum limit standards. But the draft guidance was not finalized but would not have been mandatory even if it had.

The FDA however is not the real culprit because they have limited authority to enact standards like that. The FDA is only able to inspect about 1% of international food manufacturers. The food industry is not legally bound to test either its ingredients or its final products for contamination. The real culprit is Congress, and in case you haven't met Congress lately, don't expect them to solve any problem no matter how much damaging is being done to children. In 2022, the F.D.A. requested authorization to set limits on heavy-metals in baby food, and to require baby-food makers to test for them. Two years later Congress has done nothing on the issue. As of late 2023, only two "blue" states, New York and California, have acted to protect the safety of baby food beyond the limited action of the FDA. More about the failure to ensure the nation's infants are consuming non-toxic baby food is found in Chapter 9.

> There's a certain political party that won't spend money to provide food to kids in poverty, that want to kick poor families off Medicaid, defund schools, and role back child labor laws. But if you're an embryo in a deep freeze they'll do anything to protect you...until the day you're born. Then you're on your own.

During the 2014 scandal and tragedy at Flint, Michigan, where lead was allowed to contaminate the drinking water of over 100,000 mostly poor African Americans, the entire country was newly awakened to the brain-damaging effects of lead exposure, especially to children. But lost in the coverage of that disaster was the information on how much more boys are impacted than girls.

One of the earliest studies on children's lead exposure measured lead levels in lost baby teeth and found that IQ deficits were much greater in boys than girls.[30] Testing children three to six years old, researchers found that boys had much greater loss of cognitive abilities, specifically, executive functioning and reading readiness, compared to girls for the same amount of lead exposure.[31]

Heavy metals, such as lead and mercury, easily cross the placenta by passive diffusion and contaminate the fetus. Lead can be detected in the fetal brain at 12 weeks after conception. Lead increases the risk of many common pregnancy complications that independently increase the risk of poor fetal brain development. Maternal lead levels are inversely proportional to the risk of low birth weight and length, premature birth, and head circumference.[32]

Several studies have found that prenatal exposure to lead impairs neurodevelopment more in boys than in girls.[33] The discrepancy in cognition persisted at least as far out as adolescence.[34] The lead-related antisocial, aggressive behavior discrepancy between males and females was also found to persist into adulthood.

Childhood lead exposure is associated with volume loss of gray matter, in particular in the frontal cortex, measured by MRI scans years later in adulthood. That anatomic aberrancy correlates with impulsive, aggressive behavior. The volume loss is greater in men than women for the same amount of lead exposure.[35]

Lead exposure causes an increase in levels of the stress hormone cortisol in males but not in females. The preponderance of animal studies also shows that males are affected more than females by lead exposure.[36] There are at least 30 lead-responsive genes whose expression can be altered in opposite directions depending on a person's sex. A portion of these genes have a role in creating susceptibility to depression, setting up females for a greater risk of depression from lead exposure. This is the only aspect of brain function where lead has a greater impact in women than men, but it is consistent with females' overall increased vulnerability to depression.

One take home message should not be overlooked. Infants should be routinely screened for blood lead levels. The only reason the lead contaminated applesauce scandal was exposed was a routine blood lead screening of two children from one family in North Carolina. Blood lead testing is required for children on Medicaid, but it is optional for all other parents. Elevated blood lead cannot be identified in children who are not tested, and the damage is irreversible, with lifelong consequences.

MERCURY

Humans have been burning coal since the Roman Empire. In the 1300s, the Hopi Indians living in the American Southwest burned coal for cooking food and heating their homes. The American coal industry began in Virginia in the 1700s and then moved to Pennsylvania on a commercial scale in the early 1800s, where coal with a higher carbon content (anthracite) was discovered. Nothing was more integral to the Industrial Revolution than coal combustion. The first coal-fired power plant, the Edison Electric Light Station, was built in London in 1882. Twenty percent of electricity generation in the U.S. still comes from coal combustion as of 2022.

Mercury is the most potent of all the neurotoxin contaminants released from coal combustion. Numerous other industrial processes, in particular, medical waste incinerators, chlor-alkali plants (they produce chlorine and caustic soda), cement plants, and countless small-scale, often illegal gold-mining operations in developing countries also emit mercury into the global environment.

Like lead, mercury has no beneficial biological function. In fact, any mercury atom that ends up in the body can be toxic to a wide variety of cells. Mercury is between 10 and 1,000 times more potent in its toxicity than lead.

The Great Brain Robbery –Brian Moench

A distinguished group of 23 mercury scientists stated in a letter to President Obama in 2011: "Mercury is such a potent toxin because it bonds very strongly to functionally important sites of proteins including enzymes, antibodies and nerve growth-cones that keep [brain] cells alive, 'intelligent,' and safe. Target enzymes, organs, or metabolic pathways vulnerable to mercury poisoning may change from cell to cell, person to person, and in the same individual over time." Mercury inhibits the action of neurotransmitters, such as acetylcholine, serotonin, dopamine, glutamate, and norepinephrine,[1] and can literally make the axons of neurons shrivel up.

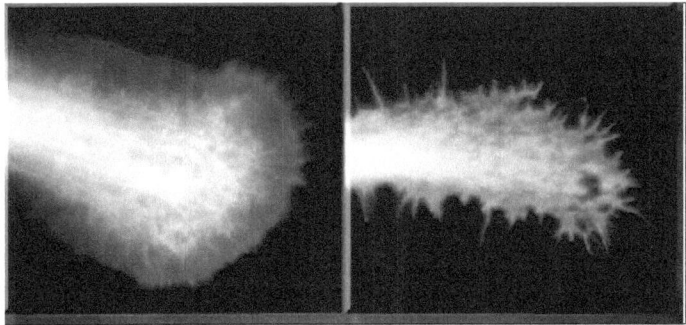

This is an electronic microscopic view of a nerve growth cone from a nerve in a petri dish. On the left is the before picture, on the right is the same nerve after researchers at the University of Calgary added a tiny amount of mercury to the petri dish. The microtubular structures disintegrated within 30 minutes after exposure. Other neurotoxins, lead, aluminum, cadmium, and manganese, added at the same concentration, did not have this effect, providing visual evidence of the unique potency of mercury neurotoxicity.

Methylmercury is the organic form of mercury, because it contains a methyl group that includes a carbon atom. In this context, the term "organic" means that the element carbon is part of the compound, not that it is otherwise uncontaminated, as in "organic produce." Humans are exposed to methylmercury when they eat fish, and it is considered the most toxic form of mercury. The USDA website says, "At high exposure levels methylmercury can be toxic to people." That statement is a disservice to the public, and can only be explained as a concession to the tuna and coal industries.

All medical and public health groups have agreed for many years that there is no safe level of exposure to lead. So how can there be a safe level of mercury exposure for infants or anyone else when mercury is orders of magnitude more neurotoxic than lead? Pregnant women shouldn't eat tuna fish, period.

In 2004, the EPA estimated that one in six women of child-bearing age has enough mercury in her blood to impair the brain development of her child.[3] Other researchers estimated that the real number was twice that.

We know that for many reasons, renewable energy must replace coal combustion, and reducing mercury contamination of our air and water is just one of those reasons. But do you also need to worry about mercury in your Coke, Sprite, or Pepsi? With a name like Dr. Pepper, that's got to be just what the doctor ordered, right? Mercury is found in vegetable oil and high fructose corn syrup (HFCS), a nearly ubiquitous sweetener and ingredient in countless processed foods,[4] especially sweetened beverages. The chlorine used to bleach wheat flour may contain as much a 1 ppm (part per million) inorganic mercury.

On average, Americans get about 10% of their calories from HFCS, consuming about 36 pounds of it per year. It could be the worst 36 pounds in their annual diet. Mercury contaminates HFCS through an industrial substance called caustic soda, used to break down corn to produce syrup. Although supposedly, this process is being phased out in the U.S., it is not being phased out in other parts of the world. No government agency really knows how much mercury is in most HFCS. Probably because it would be inconvenient to find out and would be a black eye for industrial agriculture, the U.S. government refuses to bother testing for it. I guess their motto is, "What you don't know, you don't need to know, and we're not going to let you know—sue us."

Dr. Renee Dufault retired early from the FDA in 2008 after having been blocked by the FDA from publishing research about mercury in HFCS. She published data indicating that half of HFCS samples they tested had detectable levels of mercury, and other researchers found a third of supermarket processed food and beverages had mercury in them. Canadian researchers found similar results. Dr. Dufault then showed that a diet with reduced processed food was associated with less mercury in the blood. The Smithsonian Institute was impressed enough with Dr. Dufault's research that they invited her to present her findings to them.[5]

In order to get beyond the FDA's roadblock and get her research published, she had to resign as an employee of the Public Health Service. That also freed her up to write a book, *Unsafe at Any Meal: What the FDA Does Not Want You to Know About the Food You Eat*. What she came to realize was that the mercury in HFCS was more than an unavoidable contaminant in processed food; it was at least indirectly intentional and served a purpose. By acting as a preservative, the same reason mercury was added to vaccines, mercury would suppress mold and bacterial growth and prolong the shelf life of processed food. Bread manufacturers would even boast that adding HFCS would increase shelf life. Furthermore, chlorine—the same chlorine used to disinfect swimming pools, and that is used as a potent, toxic disinfectant, like whatever disinfectant Donald Trump suggested could be injected to "clean the lungs" of people infected with COVID—is also used to bleach flour to make white bread. That chlorine is most often made from a process that contaminates it with mercury.

Hydrogen chloride and sodium hydroxide are two common food preservatives that are also contaminated with mercury because of the process used to manufacture them. The bottom line is, there are multiple reasons why many processed foods contain the deadliest known neurotoxin. Rather than protecting consumers, to anyone but the most biased observers, the FDA seems to be running interference for "Big Agriculture" corporations, and the Corn Refiners Association (CRA) in particular.

After their mercury problem was publicly exposed, the CRA issued a hostile response, casting aspersions on the "relevance and accuracy" of Dr. Dufault's test results. Then they released a tepid and evasive statement from a hired-gun scientist, Dennis J. Paustenbach: "To imply that there is a safety concern to consumers based on the findings presented, is both incorrect and irresponsible."[6]

The Environmental Working Group described Paustenbach this way: "Dr. Paustenbach has spent virtually his entire career as a paid expert for polluting corporations arguing for weaker health protections for workers and the public from some of the most notorious toxic substances ever known."[6] Paustenbach had worked to defend Pacific Gas and Electric's chromium-6 pollution in the case made famous by the movie, *Erin Brockovich*, starring Julie Roberts. Despite these highly publicized studies of mercury contaminating our food, the FDA did no follow-up investigations, demonstrating their subservience to corporate influence.

Dental amalgams with mercury are a known route of human exposure to the toxic metal. Boys retain and accumulate significantly more mercury than girls from a similar dental-route exposure. In children that had certain gene variants, the toxicity caused by mercury was much greater in boys than girls.[7]

Some of the most toxic elements in the periodic table have been used in multiple applications as preservatives: mercury, silver, copper, arsenic, and the halogens (chemical elements that form a salt when reacting with metal), like chlorine, fluorine, and iodine. But the chemical reaction that affords heavy metals efficacy as antibacterials, i.e., inhibiting key enzymes and denaturing proteins, is not selective to microbes. They can bioaccumulate in human cells as well, and with toxic effects.

Thimerosal has been used as an antimicrobial preservative since the 1930s. About 50% of thimerosal is metabolized into ethyl mercury, which is more quickly eliminated by the body than methylmercury, and is therefore presumed to be less dangerous. But less dangerous doesn't mean not dangerous. Ethyl mercury moves freely throughout the body, including crossing the BBB.[8] Research suggests that ethyl mercury impairs the functioning of the BBB just like methylmercury.[9]

Over many decades, evidence accumulated that thimerosal is not terribly effective as an antimicrobial, and it's potency as neurotoxin was increasingly obvious. Little attention was paid to either liability, however, until the 1980s, when the USDA admitted that topical products with thimerosal failed on both counts. Simultaneously, and with dubious justification, thimerosal wasgiven a second career to be used in vaccines for children and pregnant women.

At least one study found that inorganic levels of mercury in the brain are much higher with ethyl mercury compared to methylmercury.[10] Ethyl mercury has been shown to be toxic to nerve cells (astrocytes), in particular, damaging the DNA and energy production (mitochondria) of the cells.[11] Other laboratory studies (i.e., in petri dishes) show that ethyl mercury and methylmercury are equally toxic to nerve, cardiovascular, and immune cells.[12]

Thimerosal is central to the hornets' nest controversy about whether vaccines cause autism. Because of public alarm about the possible connection, in July 1999, without admission of any errors in judgement or past mistakes, Public Health Service agencies, the American Academy of Pediatrics, and vaccine manufacturers agreed that thimerosal should be reduced or eliminated in vaccines as a precautionary measure. In 2001, thimerosal was removed from all childhood vaccines in the United States except flu vaccines. That thimerosal is still in flu vaccines is a more important consideration than it may have seemed at first, given that flu vaccines have to be given annually, and recall that, like most other heavy metals, mercury does not dissolve or degrade. That concern became magnified beginning in 2002 because the CDC began recommending that infants and pregnant women receive the flu vaccine.

But removing thimerosal from the other vaccines raises an obvious question—if flu vaccines are safe with thimerosal, why remove it from others? And if it was an appropriate precaution to remove it from the others, why was it left in flu vaccines? You can forgive the public for wondering if it was Groucho Marx making these decisions.

Public health experts are justified in defending the integrity and safety of vaccines. As preventive medicine, vaccines have contributed greatly to public health and safety perhaps more than any other medical intervention. Vaccine eradication of such hideous diseases as small pox and polio, and near eradication of other often devastating diseases like measles and rubella has been forgotten by far too many people, especially those young enough to have never seen or experienced those diseases.

With the country awash in ludicrous conspiracy theories, the last thing we need is absurd claims about dangers that don't exist, especially when vaccines will be the key to ending future devastating epidemics like COVID. As this book is being updated, there is a tragic and completely preventable outbreak of measles in Florida that only happened because of the political opportunism of its governor, Ron Desantis, and his idiotic appointee as Surgeon General, Joseph Ladapo. The idea that herd immunity is preferable to vaccines for these deadly diseases is nothing but herd stupidity.

However, many health experts have not been entirely honest with the public, either. By defending vaccines in all their forms, with all their schedules, at all costs, they seem to have been willing to overlook some serious, legitimate concerns, and in my view that has backfired in fighting against the fanatical anti-vaccine movement. What may make sense from the perspective of a broad public health campaign may not make anywhere near as much sense at the level of many individual patients. If, in fact, it is true that vaccines never did cause autism, it is also true that giving an infant multiple vaccines with a proven neurotoxin, for which there is no safe level, is impossible to defend.

Countries such as Sweden and Denmark reduced the amount of thimerosal in vaccines many years before the United States acted. Other countries, including Japan, Austria, the UK, and even Russia (hardly at the cutting edge of medical advances) eliminated it entirely nearly a decade before the United States did. On the CDC website is a page that addresses thimerosal in vaccines.[13] The CDC points to epidemiological studies that showed autism rates continued to increase in those countries for at least seven more years, as proof that thimerosal doesn't cause autism. Great! But it also goes beyond that, claiming, "The evidence is clear: thimerosal is not a toxin in vaccines, but merely a preservative, preventing contamination." Not causing autism and "not a toxin" are not the same thing at all. Autism is hardly the only possible manifestation of harm from thimerosal.

The CDC cites very little evidence to justify giving mercury in vaccines essentially a clean bill of health. The few epidemiological studies cited as evidence that ethyl mercury in vaccines does not cause more subtle, non-autism neuropsychological harm are not very convincing. In fact, those studies cannot be considered terribly useful. One was retrospective and had no reliable way of proving the studied groups' levels of exposure to vaccine-related mercury.[14] Another tried to determine if there was a difference in the results of eleven standardized tests for memory and learning, attention, executive functions, visuospatial functions, language, and motor skills, ten years after vaccination in two groups of children. The only difference between the two groups was different doses of thimerosal. That is not a real, unexposed control group and cannot be considered an exoneration of thimerosal. Even in that study, girls given the higher dose of thimerosal performed more poorly in two of the eleven tests.[15]

What if instead of autism, we determined that the mercury in childhood vaccines indeed acted exactly as the neurotoxin it is known to be and decreased the IQs of children by 2 points? 3 points? 5 points? Can anyone still defend having used it? How many IQ points can we justify sacrificing to suppress a certain disease? One point to suppress a season of influenza? Ten points to eradicate small pox forever? Can we say that we did right by the millions of children whose intellect suffered just enough that their career options became more limited, but they didn't become autistic? If those numbers seem small individually, in the aggregate, across an entire nation, a small loss of cognitive ability can have broad, national and societal consequences for economic growth, scientific innovation, and technological progress.

The letter that mercury experts sent to President Obama, referred to before, also stated, "Exposure to mercury in any form places a heavy burden on the biochemical machinery within cells of all living organisms." By 6 months of age, infants receiving three doses of the diphtheria/tetanus/pertussis vaccine, three doses of the H-flu vaccine, and three doses of the hepatitis B vaccine would have received 187.5 micrograms of mercury.[16] For infants at critical stages of brain development, that cannot be brushed off as an insignificant. If it were lead in vaccines instead of mercury, there would be even more public outcry, and as we have mentioned, mercury is orders of magnitude more toxic to the brain than lead. Thimerosal should never have been an ingredient in any vaccines, let alone children's vaccines. There are other alternatives for preservatives, none of which include the most potent neurotoxin known.

Other epidemiologic studies in infants have found an increased incidence of impaired neurodevelopment in association with thimerosal exposure in male children compared to female children, even when the males were exposed to a lower dose than the females.[17]

Mercury is not just a full-service disaster for the brain development of children; it's making our native fish population stupid as well. I assume that affects their ability to compete with Russian fish in chess tournaments. If you are reasonably well informed, you are likely aware that large fish, such as tuna and halibut, have high enough levels of mercury in their flesh that people should eat very little, if any of these fish. A tuna fish can have concentrations of mercury a million times higher in its flesh, than exists in the ocean they swim in. But the problem is worse than just large fish. In 2009, the U.S. Geological Survey tested fish from 291 streams across the country for mercury. They found mercury in every single fish tested, and 25% exceeded the lax guidelines from the EPA. There is no reason to think that fish are any less contaminated now, meaning they are not safe for anyone to eat on a regular basis, especially children or pregnant mothers.

The waters of the Great Salt Lake have the highest concentration of mercury of any inland body of water in the United States. The ducks and other waterfowl that nest along the wetlands of its shores are heavily contaminated with mercury to the point where they have triggered the only advisories in the nation against human consumption of water fowl. Fortunately, when I learned about these warnings, I didn't have to alter my culinary preferences, given that I drank very few duck smoothies. I always thought ducks tasted just like the mud they wade in, and even my mom's gravy couldn't rehabilitate them (see Prologue). However, a top-notch surgeon I worked with was an avid duck hunter who spent many weekends in the wetlands of the Great Salt Lake. For years, before he realized how contaminated the ducks were, he ate much of what he shot. I saw him several times after he retired, and he lamented what the mercury had done to him—slowed his movements, his speech, and his cognition, long before what aging should have done.

Florida has had a growing problem with an invasion of Burmese pythons overrunning the Everglades. The Florida Fish and Wildlife Conservation Commission wants the public's help in culling the population. So, in an effort to make hunting them more attractive, they want people to eat the python meat, because, stop me if you've heard this comparison before, it tastes like chicken— "Chicken of the Glades." The only problem is that the pythons are heavily contaminated with mercury, about eight times more than the limit set by the EPA (which you can count on as being too lax). So, in case you were worried that the meme "Florida Man" is at risk for running out of new material, this new state campaign solves that problem as well. If enough Florida men eat these pythons, Florida's perch at the top of the stupidity pyramid will be secure for generations.

Like with lead, most research has shown that boys are more susceptible to the neurotoxic effects of mercury than girls.[18] Among many other reasons, females have a better armament of antioxidant defenses.[19] Researchers at Harvard University recently found that mercury in the red blood cells taken from the cord blood of newborns suppresses the gene *PON1* in boys but not girls.[20] The amount of gene suppression correlated with impaired cognition in boys during childhood but not in girls. This particular gene is also an important contributor to a person's ability to break down pesticide residues.

In laboratory animals, methylmercury exposure shortly after birth caused more brain damage in males than in females, specifically demonstrating more inhibition of cell division.[21] Males are consistently found to be more vulnerable to neurotoxicity from thimerosal. A study in lab animals showed that in determining a lethal dose, females are able to tolerate three times as much thimerosal as males.[22]

Male fetuses' exposure to methylmercury causes more severe alterations in nerve-cell migration and nerve extensions than occurs with a similar exposure in female fetuses.[23] Genetic sex differences probably account for higher systemic accumulation of mercury in boys compared to girls.[24] Upon exposure to methylmercury, the profile of changes in expression of multiple genes is different in the two sexes.

One mechanism of brain toxicity triggered by thimerosal appears to be localized hypothyroidism. Adequate thyroid hormone is critical to normal brain development. Supporting that concept is the elevation of thyroid-stimulating hormone in male but not female rats exposed to thimerosal.[25] In evaluating the differences in the ability of aged laboratory animals to eliminate heavy metals like mercury based on their sex, researchers found that female animals had a distinct advantage over males.

Multi-dose flu vaccine bottles still contain thimerosal as a preservative. Parents can request a vaccine from an individual bottle that does not contain the compound, as we have done with our granddaughter. We should all hope that future vaccines do not contain thimerosal for adults or children.

> No child labor was used in the writing, research, formatting, vetting, or proof reading of this book…just a bunch of really childish, immature adults who have nothing better to do.

ARSENIC: THE POISON OF KINGS

The poisonous properties of arsenic were known as early as the 4th century B.C. by such prominent scholars as Hippocrates, Theophrastus, Pliny the Elder, and the Greek physician Pedanius Dioscorides. It is known in history as the "Poison of Kings" and the "King of Poisons," because it was the preferred weapon of anonymously assassinating kings, emperors, and aristocracy. It has no smell or taste, and an amount the size of a pea could be fatal and easily dissolved into food or drink. Nero, before his fiddling recital during the burning of Rome, used it to murder his stepbrother, Britannicus, who invented the encyclopedia (not really), paving the way for him to become one of Rome's most notorious emperors.

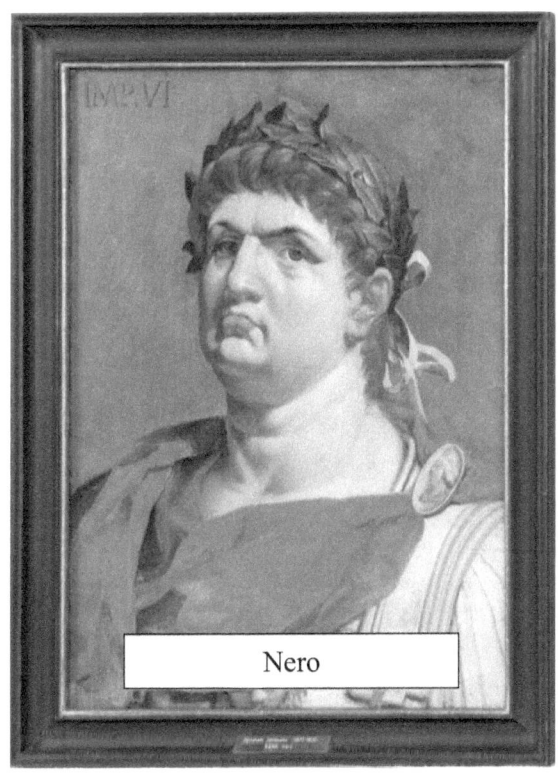

Nero

The European Renaissance not only elevated art, science, government, and culture, but also, ironically, the art of murder. Professional arsenic assassins did a booming business among the elites, work that would have garnered the admiration of today's most cuthrot assassin, Voldemort Putin himself.

But arsenic's reputation was actually bipolar. Arsenic was used as a cure for a wide array of medical disorders, for example, ulcers, as early as 2,000 B.C. In the eighteenth century, it was the primary ingredient in the popular Fowlers Solution, a snake oil marketed as an all-purpose tonic, good for whatever ailed a person, much like Geritol of the 1950s or whatever Gwyneth Paltrow is selling this weekend in her *GOOP* lifestyle catalogue.

Arsenic has the distinction of being the principal compound in the first antimicrobial ever produced, used in the treatment of syphilis, for which it was named the "Savior of Syphilis." It remained the treatment of choice until the advent of penicillin 40 years later. Some women in India still take arsenic during the first trimester of pregnancy due to a very unfortunate cultural superstition that it increases the chance of having a boy. Unfortunately, it only increases the chance of having a mentally impaired baby, ironically, even more so if the baby is a boy.

In Japan, over four months in 1955, contaminated milk powder caused a mass arsenic poisoning of bottle-fed infants. Of about 13,000 infants exposed, more than 100 of them died. Studies of survivors, years later in adolescence, found they had suffered from IQ loss, including being ten times more likely to have IQs below 85 compared to controls. Fifty years after exposure, some of the survivors were examined and were found to have higher risk of intellectual disability, schizophrenia, and depression.[38]

As late as the early 2000s, arsenic was used as a principal ingredient in pesticides for both agriculture and wood preservation. Like most other heavy metals, it does not break down and is not destroyed in the environment. Arsenic is also present naturally as a ubiquitous environmental contaminant found commonly in soil and water. It is highly toxic in its inorganic form. Arsenic-contaminated drinking and irrigation water and food preparation are the largest sources of exposure for most people. The metal is harmful to almost every major organ in the body, especially the brain.

Over 100 million people drink water that has unacceptable levels of arsenic, a particular problem in the Western United States. The legal limit in public water is 10 parts per billion (ppb), and 5 ppb is common in many parts of the country. A study by Columbia University evaluated 272 third-to-fifth graders in Maine who lived in homes whose drinking water had levels of arsenic above 5 ppb. The study found an average loss of 5-6 IQ points among these Maine children related to the arsenic from their well water.[26] That would be a devastating loss for any child.

Arsenic was added to chicken, turkey, and pig feed beginning in the 1940s via the animal drug Roxarsone, which is converted to inorganic arsenic. It was believed that Roxarsone enhanced muscle growth, prevented disease, and made the meat pinker. Roxarsone is no longer approved by the FDA, but it is still in use in other countries. The breakdown of Roxarsone-type compounds in animals creates metabolites that are significantly more toxic than the initial additives.[27]

Arsenic is a common contaminant of just about every type of rice—white, brown, wild, organic—because the grain absorbs it as a residue from pesticides and from the soil itself. Brown rice has even more arsenic than white rice. Arsenic is also common in apple juice because it is absorbed by apples from the soil, as well as the fact that two thirds of apple juice comes from China, which has no regulations on the use of pesticides. Between 60-90% of the arsenic ingested is eventually taken up by the bloodstream.[28]

All forms of arsenic accumulate in the brain. It can cross the placenta and the BBB and interfere directly with intrauterine brain development. It can kill fetal brain cells[29] and provoke neurologic birth defects, such as neural tube malformations. In studies of children in countries all over the world, chronic exposure to arsenic is associated with a profile of neurologic damage similar to lead exposure.[30] Gender differences in neurological deficits have not been well studied, but one study of 602 children compared cognitive performance tests to arsenic urinary levels and found an inverse correlation in boys but not girls.[31] Arsenic was also found to affect male lab animals more than it affected female lab animals.[32]

Impaired brain function is not the only health consequences of arsenic exposure. Devastating birth defects—neural tube deficits, anencephaly (missing a brain) and encephalocele (brain herniation through a skull defect)—occur more frequently among pregnant mothers exposed to arsenic.[33] Symptoms of lung disease and impaired lung function have also been found to be the result of early-life arsenic exposure.[34] Early-life exposure causes a six times greater chance of premature death in young adults, primarily related to increased risk of lung cancer.[35]

Children in Matlab, Bangladesh, were exposed to high concentrations of arsenic in drinking water as infants. When examined years later as teenagers and young adults, symptoms of respiratory disease related to their arsenic exposure had largely disappeared in females but had persisted in males.[36] These studies found evidence for a difference between the sexes on how arsenic is metabolized, providing a possible explanation for the greater toxicity of arsenic in males on the brain and lungs.[37]

Specific recommendations for baby foods to avoid because of arsenic contamination are found in Chapter 9.

MANGANESE

If you fly over Texas, Colorado, Wyoming, Utah, the Midwest, and many other parts of the country from 30,000 feet in the air, it looks like the earth has become stricken with small pox. In fact, in many ways, it is being attacked by an ugly, if not deadly disease. Between 13,000 and 17,000 new oil and gas wells are drilled in the U.S. every year. Around one million wells are active. Over 18 million Americans live within a mile of a fracking site, and that number constantly growing.[38]

Most drilling for oil and natural gas is now done by fracking, the nickname for the process that requires injecting a slurry of water, chemicals (many of them toxic), and sand under high pressure to release oil and gas trapped in tight shale formations. Fracking is considered a climate villain by anyone concerned about the climate crisis, which, of course, should be everyone. But the fracking industry enjoys powerful political clout, even in liberal states like California, whose wildfires have become the signature of America's climate-related environmental destruction.

Fracking operations are pollution nightmares. Much of the air pollution related to fracking will be dealt with in the next chapter. But arsenic and manganese are both prominent contaminants of the water that flows back from fracking wells. Depending on how this water is used or disposed of, the "produced water" (a terrific euphemism for toxic water) can eventually contaminate streams,

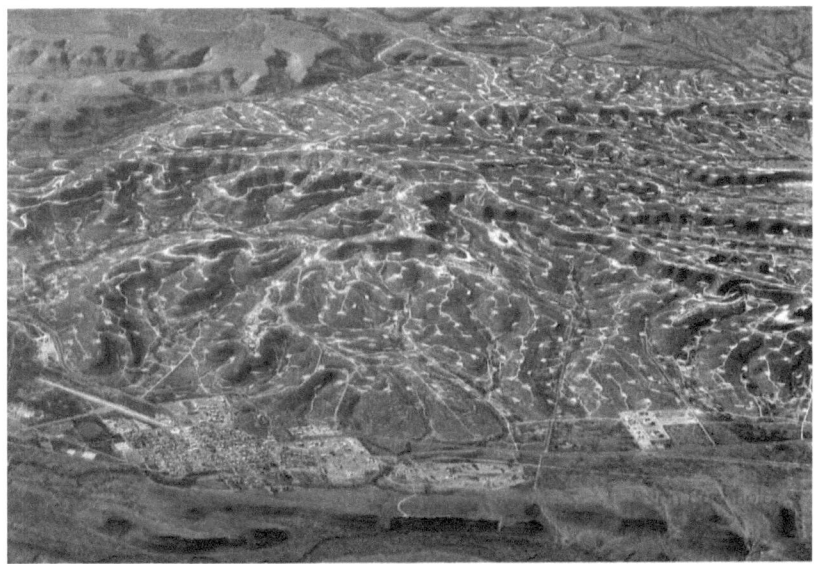

Aerial view of the Permian Basin fracking field that spans Texas and New Mexico

aquifers, and other sources of drinking water. With neurotoxicity quantitatively and qualitatively similar to arsenic, manganese is damaging to the brain by itself, but when accompanied by arsenic, as it often is, it is particularly so. In both animal and human studies, simultaneous exposure to arsenic and manganese can augment each other in harming the intellectual development of newborns.[39] Both arsenic and manganese appear to be toxic at levels in drinking water well below the EPA's standard for clean water.

If there is any difference in how manganese affects boys and girls it's that it reduces socialization in girls, and increases emotional disturbances in boys.[40]

ALUMINUM

Aluminum is the third most common natural element on earth after oxygen and silicon. The earth's oxygen reservoir exists primarily in the form of a molecule consisting of two atoms close together, O_2, and the earth's silicon deposits exist primarily in the various body parts of the Kardashian sisters. Aluminum represents about 8% of the earth's crust and is easily taken up from soil by grains, vegetables, and seaweed. It reaches humans through bioaccumulation in the food chain.

Aluminum is also used in antacids, deodorants, makeup, sunscreen, aspirin, beverage cans, and as a food additive. Human exposure to aluminum is increasing to the point where some have described us as living in the "Aluminum Age."

As with lead, aluminum has no beneficial role in human physiology. Aluminum not only bioaccumulates in the food chain, but once consumed, it bioaccumulates in particular organs, including the brain. Its presence in brain tissue at any level is detrimental, and it is not evenly distributed, leaving some areas of the brain more vulnerable than others to toxicity. The consequences include abnormal blood flow to the brain.[41] Compared to healthy controls, in patients with Alzheimer's, multiple sclerosis, and autism, brain concentrations of aluminum are elevated.[42]

Neurotoxicity of aluminum has been demonstrated in the laboratory, in tissue and cell culture experiments, in live animals, and in humans.[43] Individual neurons slowly and steadily accumulate aluminum, which in turn, increases their energy demand, while their energy supply is relatively fixed. When energy demand exceeds supply, the viability of the cell is jeopardized.[44] The progressive increase in aluminum within the cell corresponds to a pathologic continuum going from neuronal dysfunction to degeneration to apoptosis (programmed death that is part of the normal life cycle of cells and organisms), and ultimately, to a worse, sudden, and violent death, i.e., "necrosis," that can cause collateral damage to nearby cells and brain tissue, like the explosion of a microscopic hand grenade. The toxicity of aluminum, mercury, lead, and arsenic occur through similar biologic pathways, which can be thought of as committing murder of neurons.

Aluminum is particularly potent at increasing brain inflammation, activating microglia (reminder—that's the brain's garbage collection service), and the amyloid precursor proteins associated with Alzheimer's.

Children with ADHD and learning disabilities have higher levels of aluminum in their blood.[45] Aluminum concentration is 10 to 20 times higher in cow's milk–based infant formulas and 100 times higher in soy-based formulas compared to breast milk.[46] Animal studies indicate that aluminum in maternal breast milk ends up in the brains of infants and remains in the brain for their lifetime.[47]

Hair is a much more utilitarian tissue than most people realize. It serves a purpose beyond improving one's aesthetics or providing a reason to buy shampoo. I've been in mourning ever since the hair on my forehead lost its will to live. Hair is a unique tissue containing protein we call "hard keratin," which has high levels of cysteine residue that binds heavy metals and helps eliminate them from the critical organs of the body. Children between the ages of 3 and 9 have three times higher levels of aluminum in their hair than adults.[48] As early as 1996, the American Academy of Pediatrics warned against possible aluminum neurotoxicity in children from multiple exogenous sources,[49] despite the fact that only 0.1% of orally ingested aluminum is absorbed from the GI tract.

Aluminum is the most often used adjuvant (a compound that increases immune response, and therefore effectiveness) for vaccines, in the form of aluminum hydroxide, aluminum phosphate, and aluminum sulfate. It is assumed to be safe by the pharmaceutical industry and by government agencies such as the FDA. But it is still controversial because of its well-established biological and nervous-system toxicity.[50]

A research paper from 2015 begins, "Use of highly pure antigens to improve vaccine safety has led to reduced vaccine immunogenicity and efficacy. This has led to the need to use adjuvants to improve vaccine immunogenicity."[51] That means that the attempt to increase vaccine safety has come at the cost of reduced effectiveness. Aluminum adjuvants are used to increase effectiveness, but here is at least some acknowledgement that effectiveness comes at a price. The paper goes on, "Unfortunately, adjuvant research has lagged behind other vaccine areas, such as antigen discovery, with the consequence that only a very limited number of adjuvants based on aluminum salts, [or]monophosphoryl lipid A, and oil emulsions are currently approved for human use."

Aluminum particles injected as part of a vaccine eventually get picked up by the lymph system and appear in lymph nodes, the spleen, and most worrisome, are actively transported to the brain, in what's been described as a Trojan horse process.[52]

Not surprisingly, some studies have also shown increased aluminum levels in the hair and urine of autistic children compared with healthy controls.[53] Multiple exposures from aluminum adjuvants, organophosphate pesticides, lead, and mercury can trigger an exaggerated immune response, which leads to systemic inflammation that can carry with it damage to the brain.[54] Yet the cumulative impact of multiple, simultaneous toxic exposures is completely ignored in the government's regulatory structure. From the moment of conception on, every day for the rest of a person's life, they are exposed to at least one neurotoxin, and often several.

The number of childhood vaccines considered necessary by public health officials has increased from 10 in the 1980s to 32 currently. Eighteen of those typically use aluminum adjuvants. With a standard vaccine program in the U.S. in the first six months of life, babies are scheduled to receive between 14.7 and 49 times more aluminum than the FDA's daily safety threshold.[55] If some of those vaccines are also an annual flu vaccine, then you can add thimerosal to the possible neurotoxic mix, as addressed previously.

I'm going to repeat what I wrote in the section on mercury. This is not to be interpreted as an anti-vaxxer rant. It is not. But that doesn't mean that tunnel vision of public health officials isn't causing them to overlook some of the possible consequences of the program. Some of the concerns of the safety of vaccines are legitimate, and perhaps more concerning is the recommended schedule of childhood vaccinations, and whether safer preservatives or adjuvants are possible.

Soon after birth, most children are given a Hepatitis B vaccine that contains 250 micrograms (mcgs—i.e., one millionth of a gram) of aluminum. Yet the FDA guidelines for a one-time exposure for an 8-pound baby is only 18.16 mcg. During well-baby checkups at 2, 4, and 6 months of age, the typical child gets several more vaccines at each visit. Many children end up getting up to eight vaccines in a single visit, and that can be more than 1,000 mcg of aluminum.

Furthermore, placebos used in clinical trials to help determine safety of vaccines often contain as much or greater amounts of aluminum than the trial vaccine.[55] Any methodology that takes for granted the safety of aluminum is flawed. It is easy to see that adverse reactions to the aluminum adjuvant itself would be obscured. Aluminum adjuvants alone, in amounts "equivalent to human exposure," induced behavioral abnormalities in female mice.[56]

The U.S. military was concerned that our troops could be exposed to anthrax during the first Gulf War. Normally the anthrax vaccine involves five doses given over 18 months.[57] Under the pressure of the war, in a calculated risk, that schedule was accelerated, and military personnel had to be given numerous vaccinations over a short time frame. A study in lab animals of aluminum hydroxide exposure at levels comparable to what was administered to the military personnel via those vaccines found significant motor neuron degeneration and memory deficits.[58]

There are several alternatives to aluminum for adjuvants. Calcium phosphate was used in France as an adjuvant for diphtheria, pertussis, and tetanus vaccines beginning several decades ago. It is already naturally present in the body and may be as effective as, and safer than, aluminum.[59]

Aluminum as an occupational exposure has been linked to elevated concentrations in the brain and neurological diseases such as Alzheimer's. A recent autopsy study of people over 70 years old found that in 70% of the patients, at least one part of their brain had an elevated concentration of aluminum.[60] A meta-analysis of studies, which included 10,567 patients, found that increased aluminum exposure increased the risk of Alzheimer's by over 70%.[61] Several studies have shown a strong positive association between rates of Alzheimer's and the concentrations of aluminum in drinking water in multiple countries.[62] Furthermore, lowering the body burden of aluminum resulted in some improvement in cognitive performance in patients with moderate to severe Alzheimer's.[63]

Aluminum is one toxin for which there is not much research to indicate a significant gender disparity in negative impacts. Avoiding aluminum is important for everyone from newborns to the elderly. The proverbial "tin foil hat" brigade (made of aluminum foil, of course) already demonstrates severely compromised cognitive skills. They should definitely switch from aluminum to something less neurotoxic, like PBS instead of Fox News.

But aluminum is hard to avoid entirely, given its widespread use in food processing, in containers for prepared and cooked foods, and in cosmetics. One study found that cooking red meat in aluminum foil can double or quadruple the amount of aluminum contaminating the meat. Aluminum is practically a routine ingredient in anti-perspirants and is common in toothpastes. It is wise to stick to products that don't use it. It is also prudent to avoid cooking, preparing, or storing food, in particular salted and acidic foods, in uncoated aluminum containers, pots, or foil. Aluminum can leach from rock and soil to enter any water source, so it is another reason for getting a water purification system that will eliminate it and other heavy metals from your drinking water.

CADMIUM

Treat yourself to your favorite meal before reading this section, because you may want that to be your "last supper." If you have ever heard the aphorism, "You are what you eat," the practice of dumping sewage over pasture and farmland as cheap fertilizer should give that phrase entirely new meaning.

Among neurotoxic heavy metals that we are commonly exposed to, cadmium is a second-tier player that comes off the bench when the first string needs a rest. It is rated by the Agency for Toxic Substance and Disease Registry (ATDSR) as the seventh most toxic heavy metal, keeping it firmly in the Hall of Shame of environmental toxins. There are numerous occupations that place workers at risk for significant exposure, but the most common pathway for the general population is food consumption and cigarette smoking.

The accumulation of cadmium in soil and eventual absorption by crops make it a common contaminant of food, often from the practice of spreading sewage or industrial waste on farmland. Nearly half of municipal sewage sludge ends up applied to land, often farmland. The practice pollutes water supplies and exposes us to numerous harmful chemicals in addition to heavy metals, and cadmium is only one of them. Wastewater plants treat municipal sewage and industrial and factory waste to reduce pathogens, bacteria, and odors, and all this is converted into a fertilizer, euphemistically called "biosolids." The nitrogen in human waste can reduce the use of artificial fertilizer. But sewage treatment plants were never designed or intended to produce fertilizer.

Thinking about having your comfort food grown in sewage likely brings you anything but comfort. It may make you commit to never eat again. It takes no imagination to think that what gets sent into a public sewer system is a witch's brew of the 140,000 industrial chemicals mentioned earlier and everything else you don't ever want to be exposed to. PCBs, dioxins, flame retardants, pesticides, and pharmaceuticals are all found in sewage sludge. Heavy metals, many of the hormones, pharmaceuticals, chemicals, and pathogens in the sludge are not neutralized, killed or broken down during the composting, pasteurization, centrifuge, or air drying used in waste treatment. Farmers who apply sewage sludge to their land have no idea what's in it. There is no testing required of the crops themselves for chemical and heavy metal content, and there are no labels required on produce grown with sewage sludge, despite the fact that numerous food crops can absorb these toxins.

In theory, the EPA establishes safety limits for biosolids, but only for ten heavy metals, and it only tests anywhere from once per month to once per year. But as with so many other safety thresholds, those limitations in sewage sludge are grossly (pun definitely intended) inadequate. Some of those heavy metal safety thresholds are 100 times greater than what is allowed in other countries.[64] The EPA only looks at one metal alone and in isolation, not the cumulative total of toxins. That makes as much sense as playing a football game with only one player. Moreover, year after year, the soil contamination steadily increases, and so does the contamination of crops raised on those fields.

Water recycled from sewage treatment plants is often turned back into waterways, streams, and rivers, but it is also used to water crops. While the treatment may break down some chemicals and some pathogens, it certainly doesn't remove all of them, and it may not adequately remove even the toxic, drug-resistant bacteria, e-coli and salmonella. Contaminated water may be the cause of numerous outbreaks of contaminated fruits and vegetables shipped to consumers in recent years.[65]

While I raise this issue in discussing cadmium, this toxic heavy metal is just one drop in a proverbial bucket of contaminants being absorbed by the plants and livestock that make it to your dinner table. A study of grocery store food items from 2014 to 2016 found cadmium present in 65% of almost 3,000 food items tested.

Because it is excreted only very slowly from the body, cadmium has a long biological half-life, 20 to 30 years. In addition to causing liver and kidney damage, osteoporosis, diabetes, endocrine disruption, and reproductive disorders, it is a potent neurotoxin and contributes to the neurodegenerative diseases Alzheimer's, Parkinson's, ALS, and multiple sclerosis. Several years ago, like with aluminum, studies found that IQs were inversely proportional to concentrations of cadmium in the hair of children.[66] Learning disabilities and special education utilization are three times more common among children who are in the highest 25% in the amount of cadmium excreted in their urine.[67] This association with cadmium was found at exposure levels common among American children, levels previously thought to be benign.

A common denominator for these pathologies related to cadmium is inhibition of DNA repair mechanisms. Cadmium can penetrate directly into peripheral nerves and brain cells. It can cause olfactory dysfunction, peripheral neuropathy, neurologic damage, impaired cognition, learning disabilities, loss of movement and coordination, and aberrant behavior in both in adults and children.[68] The mechanism of brain damage provoked by cadmium involves oxidative stress, damage to the brain's network of microscopic blood vessels, and alterations in the expression of genes.[69]

HOW FLAME RETARDANTS BECAME BRAIN RETARDANTS

If we were to give out awards for the most worthless, yet toxic products that humans have ever produced without any compensatory benefit, polybrominated diphenyl ethers (PBDEs), i.e., flame retardants, might be the winner. At least lead has a few beneficial properties, like durability and malleability, depending on the application. Cigarettes at least gave people a nicotine buzz, and some smokers think smoking makes them look debonair and rebellious, until it makes their teeth fall out. With nuclear radiation, at least you may think you look cool glowing in the dark. But with PBDEs, even the supposed benefits were all a fraud.

The story of flame retardants is emblematic of the devastating consequences of the corporate profit imperative and the abject failure of government oversight. North American residents' contamination with flame retardants is between 10 and 100 times higher than the contamination in people from other parts of the world.[1]

Big Tobacco has made billions by destroying hundreds of millions of lives. The more lives destroyed, the more money they make. But they managed to accomplish that feat in ways beyond getting people addicted to cigarettes. Big Tobacco, in fact, figured out a way to cause massive harm to the health even of people who didn't smoke, by engineering a campaign to soak many of our household items, especially furniture and electronic appliances, in toxic, flame-retardant chemicals, in a highly successful strategy to divert attention from the fire danger inherent in smoking.

The Pulitzer Prize winning, six-part series from the Chicago Tribune, *Playing with Fire*,[2] and the book and documentary,

Merchants of Doubt, reveal Big Tobacco's central role in exposing everyone, including non-smokers, to deadly chemicals.

Decades ago, cigarettes first became the object of public condemnation, ironically not so much for smoking-related diseases, but for their role in killing people by sparking home fires. Placed firmly in the hot seat, pun definitely intended, tobacco executives decided that pursuing the most obvious solution, creating a "fire-safe" cigarette—one less likely to start a blaze—might hurt their appeal to consumers, and consequently, their profits. So, the industry decided it couldn't or wouldn't make a fire-safe cigarette, and instead shifted attention to the couches and chairs that were going up in flames. They made it the furniture's fault. That makes as much sense as blaming the existence of forests for forest fires, something that legislators in my home state of Utah have actually done.

State and federal lawmakers had tried unsuccessfully since the 1920s to enact laws requiring fire-safe cigarettes. They were joined by advocates for burn victims and firefighters pushing for changes to cigarettes. So Big Tobacco changed the playing field entirely by launching an aggressive and cunning campaign to get firefighting organizations to adopt tobacco's cause as their own. The industry poured millions of dollars into the effort, hiring consulting groups to court fire safety groups and doling out grants to them. One executive of the Tobacco Institute boasted, "Many of our former adversaries in the fire service defend us, support us and carry forth our federal legislation as their own."

Ultimately, regulators in the pivotal state of California succumbed to the Big Tobacco strategy of "let's make everything but the cigarette fireproof." In 1975, the state of California passed a law that required polyurethane foam to resist an open flame, launching one of the biggest mistakes in public policy in the history of the U.S. Almost all furniture manufacturers found it too difficult to comply with different standards for different states, so by default, California's ill-advised flame-resistant standard became the de facto standard of the entire nation.

The Great Brain Robbery –Brian Moench

Hiring a former fire marshal lobbyist, the three companies that made flame retardants, Albemarle, Chemtura, and Israeli Chemicals, eventually succeeded in a campaign to create worldwide standards requiring that plastic casings of electronics resist a candle flame and posted internet videos comparing the flammability of computer monitors with and without flame retardants.

Achieving scientific consensus on any issue or controversy is usually a slow process, coming only after extensive peer-reviewed studies and eventually requiring the buy-in of the majority of the world's relevant scientific experts. Changing public policy based on that scientific consensus is a subsequent and equally slow process, often dragging out for decades, even after consensus among the real experts is reached. Ever since the age of the dinosaurs, in every law ever passed by Congress, corporate lobbyists always have a dominant say in the outcome, and sometimes the only say. Most laws involving environmental protection have followed this painstaking and regrettable scenario.

But even this inadequate template was turned inside out for flame retardants. Despite the fact that independent testing showed flame retardants didn't work (the chemicals did virtually nothing to prevent fires in foam-covered furniture or appliances), the foundation was laid for an entire industry to be created to keep us safe by drenching us and everything we touch in toxic chemical additives. Let me repeat, the scientific evidence supporting this public policy was nonexistent. Even the authors of the only two studies cited as supporting flame-retardant efficacy have publicly stated their research was misrepresented. In contrast, evidence revealing the hazards of flame retardants steadily mounted almost from the day they were introduced. Even the manufacturer-sponsored studies raised serious concern.

In 1977, a flame retardant, brominated Tris, was banned from use in children's pajamas after researchers showed that it could damage DNA in animals. But once a chemical is released to the marketplace, it is virtually impossible to remove it because of either the limited powers of the EPA, the enormous power of lobbyists, or simple apathy rather than political will.

"Despite consumer demands and even policy actions by states to phase out some of the worst flame-retardant chemicals, the chemical industry has not responded by producing safer chemicals, they're simply substituting other equally toxic chemicals," said Steve Taylor, program manager at the Environmental Health Strategy Center. So, we're stuck in a game of chemical Whac-A-Mole.[2]

Flame retardants are semi-volatile organic compounds. They are not embedded in the furniture manufacturing process but are sprayed on afterward. Therefore, they routinely escape as vapor or airborne particles that will land on surfaces or settle in dust. Friction and heat generated through normal use of a product, like furniture for example, can provoke their release. The cushions of a typical living room couch can contain up to two pounds of flame-retardant chemicals that are in the same family as banned pesticides such as DDT. Sitting or lying on the couch releases into your indoor air a plume of flame-retardant chemicals that is either inhaled or absorbed through your skin. Letting your kids jump on the couch is an excellent way to increase their tissue levels of flame retardants. Lounging on your couch is also an excellent means of contaminating yourself and your clothes. In fact, putting your couch in a storage shed and looking at pictures of it may be the only way to avoid getting contaminated by it. Most human exposure to flame retardants comes from ingesting or inhaling large amounts of contaminated household dust rather than from people's diet or what they absorb through their skin.[3]

Blood levels of flame retardants doubled in adults every two to five years between 1970 and 2004. A typical American baby is born with the highest concentrations of flame retardants of all the world's infants. A study by the Environmental Working Group revealed that toddlers average five times higher levels in their blood than their mothers do.[4]

Concentrations of flame retardants are particularly high in human breast milk. That should be alarming to any nursing mother, unless she's had a problem with her breast milk catching on fire.

To everyone else, that should be appalling. PBDEs also cross the placenta, showing up in fetal blood and liver.

Essentially worthless and persistent flame-retardant chemicals have now permeated everything on the planet, and they are largely impervious to degradation. But their lack of efficacy just scratches the surface of the absurdity and perniciousness of it all. The U.S. government allowed one generation after another of flame retardants onto the market with minimal to no assessment of the potential health risks. Many of the chemicals bioaccumulate (they are absorbed into the body at a higher rate than they are eliminated), and biomagnify (the concentration increases as you move up the food chain). Humans reside at the top of the food chain, especially a nursing infant, and that's why even small concentrations of toxic compounds distributed throughout the environment can translate into serious public health threats. Dr. Arlene Blum, U.C. Berkeley chemist and executive director of the Green Science Policy Institute, calls flame retardants the asbestos of our time.[5]

Thanks to the smoke and release of numerous toxic chemicals during a house fire, not the least of which are flame retardants, firefighters have markedly increased rates of cancer. Female firefighters in California between ages 40 and 50 have a rate of breast cancer six times higher than the national average. Firefighters have increased rates of cancers of the respiratory, digestive, and urinary systems[6] and significantly increased risk of brain cancer, leukemia, non-Hodgkin's lymphoma, and multiple myeloma.[7]

Fires release common pollution components like particulate matter, recently declared the most important environmental cause of cancer. But other, more unique toxic compounds are present in smoke from fires, some of which, ironically, are the flame retardants that were supposed to make fires less dangerous. PBDEs have been the most commonly applied flame retardants, and the greatest health concern is their association with developmental neurotoxicity.[8]

Studies in laboratory animals and humans have linked them to thyroid disruption, memory and learning problems, delayed mental and physical development, lower IQ, premature puberty, and reduced fertility. The largest study of children and flame retardants, led by Brenda Eskenazi, director of Berkeley's Center for Environmental Research and Children's Health, showed that children with higher exposures to PBDEs in utero or in infancy have impaired physical coordination and attention and have IQ deficits. Pardon the politically incorrect term, but these toxic chemicals are far more effective as brain retardants than they are as fire retardants.

Since Tris flame retardants (Tris—2,3-dibromopropyl—phosphate) were removed from children's pajamas in the 1970s, more than 3,000 peer-reviewed studies have documented the ability of similar classes of flame retardants to accumulate in humans and/or show adverse health effects.

Other specific flame retardants have been linked to the cancer rates mentioned. Firefighters have been shown to have levels of the PBDEs in their blood three times higher than the general population. Worse still, PBDEs react with other chemicals during a fire and yield even more toxic byproducts, like dioxins and furans. Firefighters can have levels of those toxins hundreds of times higher than the general population. One firefighter describes in a documentary film the toxicity unleashed by the average residential house fire as, "It's Love Canal, and it's on fire."[9] Foam treated with PBDEs gives off more carbon monoxide, soot, and smoke than untreated foam, and it's those three things, not burns, that are most likely to kill someone in a fire.

Of course the American Chemistry Council, the industry trade group, has come out defending flame retardants as necessary for public safety and dismissing studies linking them to adverse health outcomes. Only a few of these flame retardants have been taken off the market because of research suggesting serious health dangers. For example, chlorinated Tris, which replaced brominated Tris (mentioned before), after brominated Tris was voluntarily withdrawn, was itself voluntarily removed from children's pajamas in the 1970s because of studies linking it to cancer. But despite its danger, chlorinated Tris was not banned, and a recent study showed that 40% of couches manufactured between 1985 and 2010 still contained chlorinated Tris.[10]

The Great Brain Robbery – Brian Moench

A 2012 report, *Hidden Hazards in the Nursery*, from the Washington Toxics Coalition and Safer States and Maryland Public Interest Research Group, found toxic flame retardants in 17 out of 20 new babies' and children's products tested. Bassinet pads, nursing pillows, diaper-changing pads, and car seats were some of the items examined. The most prevalent flame retardant found was chlorinated Tris. California recently classified chlorinated Tris as a carcinogen, especially for kidney cancer, and evidence links the chemical to neurotoxicity as well as hormone disruption. The CDC estimates that 90% of Americans harbor flame retardants in their bodies. I wouldn't be surprised to see the chemical manufacturers try to spin this as a good thing and market them to treat "heart burn."

Because regulations in California played a pivotal role in launching the flame-retardant debacle, California became the focal point of the efforts to undo the damage. According to an investigative report by Environmental Health News, the chemical industry, specifically Albemarle, Chemtura, Tosoh, and Israeli Chemicals, spent at least $23.2 million to lobby California officials and donated to various political candidates from 2007 through 2011 so that fire safety regulations that launched their highly profitable, highly hazardous, and totally worthless flame-retardant business would be left untouched.

As the threat of regulation changes gained momentum, these companies hired the PR firm Burson-Marsteller, which has served such noble clients as foreign military juntas; tobacco and pharmaceutical companies; the guilty parties of the Bhopal, India, chemical disaster; and the Blackwater pseudo-terrorist private militias.

Burson-Marsteller are experts at creating "astroturf" groups, for the purpose of ginning up the false perception of public support for a point of view that would otherwise be unpopular, which is exactly what they did for flame-retardant manufacturers. They even paid a physician to fabricate emotional stories about tragically burned children to beat back any thought of regulatory change.

The *Playing with Fire* series revealed that the industry's front group bought the soul of a now infamous doctor and his false testimony for $240,000. In 2014, the physician, Dr. David Heimbach, who was facing disciplinary charges in Washington State, surrendered his license to practice medicine.

Kaiser Permanente, the country's largest health maintenance organization system, concluded that the evidence against flame retardants is sufficiently strong that it announced it will stop purchasing furniture treated with flame retardants. Kaiser released this statement: "Chemicals used as flame retardants have been linked to reproductive problems, developmental delays and cancer, among other problems. Concern over the health impacts to children, pregnant women and the general public has been growing in recent years, as scientific studies have documented the dangers of exposure."[11]

In response, pretending all the damning evidence didn't exist, the North American Flame Retardant Alliance of the American Chemistry Council asked Kaiser to reconsider its decision. "The use of flame retardants in upholstered furniture can help prevent fires from starting and/or slow the rate at which small fires become big fires, providing valuable time for persons to escape danger," Cal Dooley, the council's president and chief executive, wrote in a June 17, 2014 letter to Kaiser.

In Nov. 2013, California Governor Jerry Brown changed California's regulations so that furniture manufacturers were no longer required to use flame retardants but did not outlaw them. Because it will be decades before all furniture soaked with flame retardants is removed from homes and offices, this tragedy will continue to bring ill health, cancer, and death to thousands, if not millions, for many years into the future. Meanwhile, the retardant manufacturers enjoyed record profits as late as 2011 and global revenues of approximately $5 billion.

Despite California's progress on the issue of flame retardants, a recent investigation showed that virtually no furniture salespersons in California knew whether their furniture had flame retardants in them, and no manufacturers' labels indicated whether they were present. Predictably, a bill recently introduced in the California legislature to require disclosure by manufacturers is being fiercely opposed by the American Home Furnishings Alliance, the North American Home Furnishings Association, and the Polyurethane Foam Association. Beyond these and other industry groups, it is being fought by the National Federation of Independent Businesses and the California Chamber of Commerce.[12]

The differential effects of PBDEs based on sex was highlighted in a study that found higher levels had opposing effects on physical maturation. In girls, exposure delayed the onset of menarche, the hallmark of female puberty, but in boys it accelerated the onset of puberty.[13]

Numerous animal studies have found that prenatal exposures to PBDEs are associated with behavioral disorders.[14] Exposure to PBDEs during intrauterine development can impair mental and psychomotor development in children.[15] Exposure after birth is also neurotoxic, impairing spatial learning and memory.[16] Numerous studies in laboratory animals found similar results. A few studies showed a greater effect of PBDEs on males than females, but the differences were small and not consistent.

In case you are wondering about the plumes of red-colored flame retardants bombed by airplanes over forest fires, as was happening out my window as I wrote this, these are not the same chemicals as those that were used in furniture. Forest fire flame retardants are primarily water with about 10% commercial fertilizers, like ammonium polyphosphate, with thickeners and dyes (so that pilots can see where the product has landed). The fertilizer chemical reacts with the cellulose in trees and vegetation, which then releases water vapor as the temperature rises, creating a lower temperature burn, theoretically limiting spread of the fire. These chemicals are probably not toxic to humans but can be harmful to fish and other aquatic life, so standard policy on their use prohibits application within 300 feet of a known stream.

POLYCHLORINATED BIPHYENYLS (PCBs)

Polychlorinated biphenyls (PCBs) are a group of 209 synthetic organochlorine compounds that were introduced in the 1920s as industrial coolants and lubricants, and later used as ingredients in pesticides. Their hallmark characteristics were durability and resistance to fire, but those same desirable features make them environmental and public-health villains. PCBs generally do not mix with water, instead, settling on the bottom of lakes, riverbeds, and coastlines. From there, they enter the broader environment and ultimately, the food chain. Monsanto stopped making them in 1977; they have been banned in the U.S. since 1979 and were banned worldwide at the Stockholm Convention in 2001.

PCBs are known as persistent organic pollutants because they are superb at resisting degradation, and they bioaccumulate within the human body. So, despite the incomplete ban on these compounds, body burdens of PCBs in adolescents are still greater than in neonates. They are lipophilic, so they concentrate in fat. Despite far less production, the general environment continues to be contaminated with the compounds, and human exposure and the concomitant health consequences persist.

Current sources of PCB exposure include industrially farmed fish kept in high-density fish pens in the ocean, because they are fed fishmeal (from ground up small fish) that contains PCBs. In fact, farmed salmon is likely the most PCB-contaminated source of protein commonly available for U.S. consumers, with concentrations as much as 16 times higher than wild salmon, 4 times higher than beef, and 3.4 times more than other seafood.[17] Eating salmon is supposedly healthy for you, with one enormous caveat. If it's farmed salmon, and most of it is, as is all "Atlantic" salmon, then it is likely one of the most contaminated foods you can eat.

The EPA sets guidance limits on PCBs in wild salmon, but it's the FDA that sets limits on farmed salmon, and those limits are 500 times greater than those allowed in wild salmon.[17] This makes as much sense as regulating water pistols but not assault rifles, which I'm sure has been done by the Utah Legislature.

Significantly lower amounts of PCBs are found in industrially processed meat and dairy products. Cooking and preparation techniques can reduce the amount of PCBs consumed. Grilling or broiling is better than frying. Letting the fat drip away, and stripping away as much skin and fat as possible before cooking via any method is, at least, a safer way to eat farmed salmon.

PCBs act directly as neurotoxins and as endocrine disruptors, affecting brain development by both mechanisms. A common denominator in PCB neurotoxicity appears to be interference with the metabolism of thyroid hormone.[18]

PCBs are particularly toxic if exposure occurs during early brain development. In the Michigan Maternal Infant Cohort Study, children of pregnant mothers who ate Great Lakes fish, heavily contaminated with PCBs, had smaller head size, decreased birth weight, shorter gestational age, impaired visual recognition, and delayed muscle development compared with a group whose mothers did not eat the fish. Later on, examined at age 11, the same children were three times more likely to have decreased verbal IQ scores, worse reading comprehension, and greater attention deficits.[18] Older adults who consumed PCB-contaminated fish scored lower than average on memory and learning exams.[19] In lab animals, PCBs have been shown to impair learning, memory, and fine motor skills.[20,]

The microscopic effect that mediates the neurotoxicity from PCBs, seems to be a decrease in the plasticity of neuronal dendrites, the ability of a dendrite to change its shape in response to signals from other neurons, which is essential to processing information and developing memories. This is a microanatomic characteristic common to mental retardation, autism, and schizophrenia. More specifically, PCBs appear to lock up calcium channels in neurons in an "on" position, which in turn, locks the neurons in a state of over-excitation, overgrowth of dendrites, and an inability to prune neurons, a process essential to normal fetal brain development.[21]

Because of their effect on the neurotransporters dopamine and serotonin, it would seem plausible that PCBs might contribute to depression symptoms. Indeed, in a study of primarily adult males, greater PCB exposure correlated with the incidence of depression.[22]

PCBs have also been shown to alter the microbiome (bacterial population) of the GI tract. That is one way PCBs can contribute to poor neurologic outcomes, such as depression, anxiety, and impaired cognition.[23] The GI tract/brain connection is discussed in more detail in Chapter 8.

Numerous studies in lab animals have found that PCBs have a greater impact on males than on females, especially regarding behavioral disorders. Among the most surprising and disturbing conclusions from research on PCBs is that low exposure may be even more neurotoxic than higher exposure. The reasons for that are not yet clear. Unfortunately, we are not given much choice over the dose of our exposure. We get whatever our environment and corporate America have decided to throw at us.

FOREVER CHEMICALS: FOREVER BRAIN DAMAGE

In Janurary 2024, the Center for Desease Control and Prevention (CDC) made an unprecedented announcement. They advised physicians to start testing individual patients for blood levels of C8 chemicals, otherwise known as "forever chemicals," or the Teflon group. No federal or state health agency has ever made such a recommendation for any toxic chemical or group, and it is a manifestation of the increasing recognition that these chemicals are likely the most toxic chemical family in our environment today. The fact that there are about 12,000 different variants of these chemicals in production means that the worthy advice of the CDC is nearly impossible to be meaningfully implemented.

In 2005, chemical giant DuPont was given the largest corporate fine in the history of the EPA, $16.5 million, for a 40-year cover up of serious health hazards of C8 compounds which was one of their highly profitable, signature products. In the world of industrial chemistry, compounds that are composed of eight carbon atoms in a running chain are known as C8. (Little imagination went into naming that.) These are man-made chemicals not found in a natural environment. They are constructed for the specific purpose of repelling oil and water.

As part of the settlement with the EPA, DuPont voluntarily agreed to phase out manufacturing of C8 compounds over the next nine years. Given that Teflon sales that year had reached $1 billion, and given that many of those health consequences were fatal, that settlement reeked of about as much justice as offering your friendly neighborhood axe murderer a deal where he slows down his murdering of people over the next several years, ultimately agrees to start using a smaller axe, and pays a $50 fine.

The same year, DuPont entered into a $300 million class action settlement with 70,000 people who lived near its manufacturing plant in Parkersburg, West Virginia, where it made C8 and released its waste into the local air and water. DuPont refused to accept any responsibility or admit any guilt, and the fine and settlement barely scratched the surface of DuPont's perfidy. Neither has it done much to abate the global health hazard of this family of toxic compounds, given the broken system that utterly fails to protect public health from powerful corporations.

Teflon was supposed to be the poster child of the "miracle of modern chemistry"—a coating surface that does things that are almost too good to be true. It created a "wonderful, smooth, hard" surface that made cookware truly non-sticking, at least for a while. Close cousins of Teflon were the main ingredient in stain and water-repellent fabrics for clothes, carpets, and furniture. Similar chemicals were made for fire-fighting foam, dental floss, fast food wrapping, pizza boxes, microwave popcorn, ski wax, and over 3,000 products that consumers were exposed to routinely. These groundbreaking surfaces led to terrific profits for Fortune 500 companies like 3M and DuPont, but the way these compounds have behaved, they could have been manufactured by Lucifer in Dante's Inferno using a recipe from Edgar Allen Poe.

> This book was made in Utah, which is close to Amcrica, geographically

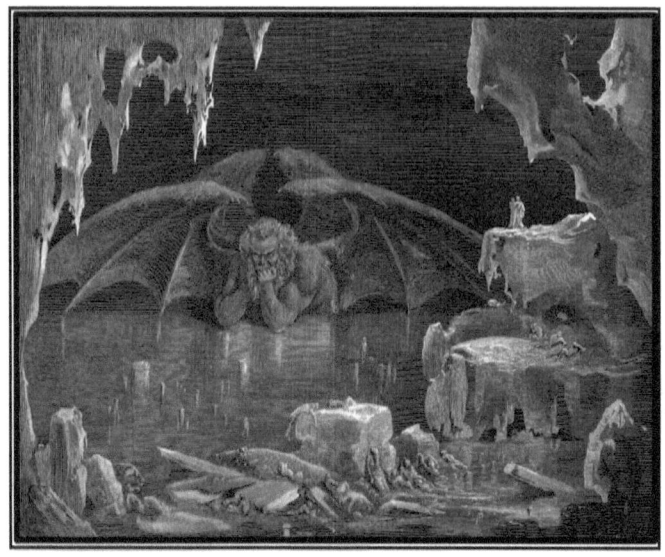

The plant in Ohio where C8 compounds were first produced.

Perfluoroalkyl substances such as PFOS (perfluorooctane sulfonate) and PFOA (perfluorooctanoic acid), are part of the C8 chemical family called per- and poly-fluoroalkyl substances (PFASs). They have found extensive modern-day utility because they are extremely resistant to breakdown anywhere—in the environment or in the plant and animal kingdoms, including humans—and they bioaccumulate in individual organisms and biomagnify within the food web (see page 157).

Like mercury, forever chemicals biomagnify and bioaccumulate. They are readily absorbed into the body when ingested, and in a third stage of a xenobiotic's journey, concentrate in certain organs, like the blood, liver, and kidneys. Longer-chained fluorinated alkyls also tend to degrade until they reach a derivative state of eight carbon atoms, and at that point, there is essentially no further breakdown. This means that even if all C8 compounds were banned, there would still be increasing levels in the environment. They are "Terminator" compounds—you can never get rid of them, and their toxicity persists as long as they do.

C8 compounds are now ubiquitous contaminants of virtually all ecosystems throughout the world. If in the last 20 years you have eaten anything cooked in non-stick cookware, eaten any fast food, worn any clothes, sat on any furniture, walked on any carpet, or flossed your teeth with anything other than barbed wire, then you have C8 chemicals in your body that will never leave. These compounds are found in newborn babies, in breast milk, umbilical cord blood, and every type of wild life ever tested. They contaminate the hair of Asian tigers and the brains of killer whales.

In America, 99.7 percent of people have C8 compounds in their blood.[24] Few of us are aware of our contamination, and none of us gave permission. One of the main companies that marketed and sold C8 compounds had put a safety threshold for PFOA in water for human consumption at 1 ppb. By 2003, tests showed that the blood of the average adult American had four to five times that amount. The average blood sample of people who lived in the Ohio Valley, where DuPont's main Teflon manufacturing plant was located, was 83 ppb. The median level for people living closest to the plant, whose drinking water was contaminated by the plant, was an astonishing 224 ppb.

In 2009, the EPA set a preliminary limit of 0.4 ppb for short-term exposure in drinking water. It was never finalized during the Obama or Trump Administrations, but it would later turn out to have been farcically inadequate anyway.

For the first several decades after its discovery of C8 chemicals, the 3M corporation, perhaps most famous for Scotch Tape, was the main manufacturer of C8 chemicals. When 3M was attempting to study exposure to Teflon in the late 1990s, they had intended to use as controls clean blood samples, found in blood banks taken from unexposed patients. Much to their own surprise, the only blood samples they were able to find that weren't contaminated with those Teflon chemicals were preserved blood from soldiers who died in the Korean War before the chemicals were ever manufactured and placed on the market. The company then realized that they had basically contaminated every person in the country, if not the world.[25] Shortly after, 3M issued a nondescript press release announcing that they would begin phasing out production of PFOS because of "new data" that showed low levels of the chemical had been widely found in the environment and in people.[26]

To the casual observer, this may have looked like a responsible thing to do—a corporation volunteering to sacrifice their business as a precautionary gesture to protect public health. But as we all know, looks can be deceiving. In 2010, the state of Minnesota filed a lawsuit against 3M because, it turns out, the company knew 40 years prior that their C8 chemicals were accumulating in humans and in fish. Within a few years after that discovery, their own research began showing toxicity to the immune system of humans. The suit claimed that 3M "acted with a deliberate disregard for the high risk of injury to the citizens and wildlife of Minnesota."[27]

After seeking $5 billion in damages, in Feb. 2018, Minnesota settled with 3M for $850 million. Documents revealed by the Minnesota Attorney General showed numerous examples, over the entire 40 years, of 3M altering or concealing their own research, and painting over the human disease potential of C8 and their other products with a deceptive veneer of safety. Moreover, according to an exhaustive report by *The Intercept*, it appears that 3M abandoned or failed to pursue other research that should have been precipitated by their own studies showing alarming results.[27]

If 3M managed their part in the C8 disaster with only a shred of conscience, Dupont managed theirs without burdening themselves with even a shred. Dupont's story of deception and culpability was told in the feature-length movie of 2020, *Dark Waters,* starring Mark Ruffalo. Documents unsealed during lawsuits involving 3,500 individual claims revealed that DuPont became aware of possible toxicity of C8 compounds as early as 1954. By 1961 DuPont's own researchers had confirmed that toxicity. Over the next several decades, DuPont's in-house scientists found that C8 compounds caused "enlargement of rats' testes, adrenal glands, livers, and kidneys."[28]

A 1965 DuPont study of rats found that just a single dose of the chemical could have a prolonged effect. Two months after such an exposure, the rats' livers were still about three times larger than normal. C8 compounds' resistance to degradation in the environment has parallels within the human body. They bind to proteins in plasma and are carried throughout the body, penetrating every human organ.

In the 1970s, DuPont's in-house studies showed that workers were accumulating C8 in their blood, they were showing increased rates of endocrine disorders, and their liver tests were more likely than not to be abnormal. Rhesus monkeys that were fed C8 compounds became chronically ill and died. DuPont's own studies showed there was no safe level of exposure to C8 compounds in animals. But the company did not alert any government regulators. By the 1980s, animal studies showed higher rates of birth defects, and a few of Dupont's pregnant employees gave birth to babies with facial birth defects, prompting the company to move its female workers out of the Teflon division.

Confronting the fact that C8 was toxic started presenting waste problems by the 1960s, so DuPont first buried 200 drums of it on the banks of the Ohio River not far from their plant. Then they came up with the brilliant idea of loading the drums onto barges and dumping them into the ocean; they continued to do that until 1965.[28]

DuPont then started disposing of its C8 waste in unlined landfills and ponds, sending it up company smoke stacks, and just dumping it into the Ohio River. Why not? That's how corporations with a long history of never facing accountability or consequences do things. By 1984, Dupont's own tests revealed C8/PFOA in the drinking water of communities downstream. Nonetheless, the corporation continued to increase production and told no one outside the company of the pollution of municipal water or the health risks revealed from their in-house studies.[29]

DuPont's in-house researchers had proven that PFOA could cross the placenta and expose fetuses to the chemical. They also knew that a 3M study in rats found the same facial birth defects as were found in the babies of some of their pregnant female employees. But DuPont didn't want to find any more damning evidence or deal with the implications of the evidence they already had. DuPont then terminated their studies and did not report their findings to the EPA, despite being required to do so by law.[30]

Instead of doing anything to reduce their toxic emissions or reconsider the basic safety of the chemicals, DuPont responded by doubling down on C8, ramping up their use of the product and keeping quiet about what they knew of its toxicity. In 1989, DuPont learned that the employees at their West Virginia plant had an abnormal number of leukemia deaths. Later that year, they found an abnormally high number of kidney cancers within their male employees. Still, they said nothing.

For over 50 years, DuPont studied and documented the health effects of C8 compounds in animals and humans—the testicular tumors, enlarged livers, kidney cancers, and the endocrine disorders. In 1991, DuPont knew that livestock were drinking from water downstream from one of their plants that they had contaminated with C8 compounds at a level 100 times greater than the internal "safety" limit the company had set for drinking water.[31]

In 1999, DuPont and 3M worked together on a study in monkeys in the hopes of establishing an exposure dose that could be classified as safe. Instead, they found that even the lowest possible doses of C8 compounds were making the monkeys sick; they concluded that there was not a safe level of exposure.[31] The results of the study prompted 3M to give up on manufacturing C8 compounds, but not DuPont. Studies showing the toxicity of C8 compounds were buried for at least 20 years by the companies that made and sold them.[32]

The most recent studies on C8 compounds have tied them to an extremely broad range of health effects, including cancers of the prostate and ovary, lymphomas, infertility, arthritis, ADHD, and immune disorders in children. An independent panel of epidemiologic experts that was formed as part of the settlement between DuPont and the 70,000 members of the nearby communities, studied the possible connection between C8 exposure and human diseases. After following 70,000 people over seven years and producing 35 peer-reviewed studies, the panel found probable links between exposure to these chemicals and 55 different diseases. In 2006, the EPA confirmed that PFOA is a likely human carcinogen.

In 2016, the EPA released an official, "voluntary" advisory for PFOA and PFOS exposure. In it, they warned against concentrations in drinking water exceeding 70 parts per trillion (ppt).[33] That concentration is equivalent to 70 grains of sand in an Olympic-size swimming pool. A study from The Department of Health and Human Services concluded that number is six times too high for infants and nursing mothers, but the study was suppressed by the Trump Administration.[30] Other reviews of the data indicated that those guidelines were "orders of magnitude" too high for lifetime human exposure.[34] In 2022 EPA reissued non-regulatory, non-enforceable advisories of 0.004 ppt for PFOA, and 0.02 ppt for PFOS.[70] Those concentrations are below the levels of detection and quantification, and the drinking water for most of the country exceeds those standards.

This means PFOA or PFOS are likely in your drinking water at levels that exceed these thresholds, even if testing indicates they are not there. So you will never know if your water supply is "safe," and if you find out your water supply is unsafe, that means it's really, really unsafe. The EPA was supposed to establish a national drinking water standard for the most common of these chemicals by the end of 2023, but timelines inevitably get pushed back by years, and sometimes decades…centuries actually. The bottom line is there is essentially no safe level of exposure to these chemicals, and yet we all have been exposed and still are, almost daily.

If there is any good news in this story, the levels of C8 compounds in the blood of the U.S. population is falling. But the bad news is that, once again, we are all victims of chemical whack-a-mole. As with so many other compounds, the law allows DuPont and other chemical companies to replace C8 compounds with similar chemicals with only minor changes, whose toxic potential has not been tested, and which may turn out to be just as dangerous to human health and may be even more. In 20 years, we'll likely repeat exactly the same cycle.

Rest assured, that cycle has already begun. DuPont is marketing a second-generation C8-type compound, a fluoropolymer they call GenX. DuPont filed 16 reports with the EPA showing evidence of numerous health effects from GenX in animals, "including changes in the size and weight of animals' livers and kidneys, alterations to their immune responses and cholesterol levels, weight gain, reproductive problems, and cancer."[35] In other words, the replacement chemicals have the same package of outcomes as the C8 compounds. In fact, regarding neurotoxicity of compounds with shorter chains than eight, presumed to break down faster, they may be even worse because they may penetrate the brain better, providing more opportunity to inflict biologic damage.[36]

A report sent by DuPont to the EPA shows that the biodegradation of GenX is essentially zero, the same as C8 compounds. Chemours, the chemical company spun off from DuPont in 2015, produces and sells GenX, releasing it into the environment in unknown quantities, because as with tens of thousands of other compounds, there is no current government regulation to stop it, minimize it, track it, or prevent human exposure to it. DuPont has handed off the toxic baton to Chemours and GenX so the cycle will continue. Inexplicably, the EPA's advisory level for GenX chemicals is 500 times higher than for PFOS, and 2,500 times higher than for PFOA.

Sewage sludge mentioned before has recently been shown to be contaminated with these C8 compounds. To no one's surprise, farmland where sewage sludge has been applied, yields crops forever contaminated with these "forever" compounds. That results in contamination not only of crops with these toxins[37] but also nearby water sources.[38]

The entire group of C8 chemicals are persistent toxins; they are broadly distributed throughout the environment and in virtually every human being. Their concentrations are somewhat higher in industrial areas. They disrupt multiple biologic processes, such as the normal metabolism of fats and amino acids. The disease consequences are far reaching and include endocrine and cardiovascular diseases, cancer, maternal and fetal developmental toxicity, and many others. But given the theme of the book, we'll stick with the evidence of neurotoxicity. These compounds decrease the levels of the neurotransmitter dopamine, and the number of dopamine neurons in invertebrates.[39] Higher levels of these compounds in the blood of pregnant mothers correlates with behavioral problems, and impaired executive functioning and problem-solving capability in their children when they became school age.[40]

The evidence for a gender difference in the neurotoxicity of forever chemicals is indirect. But females generally have lower concentrations of forever compounds than males do, at least until middle age.[71]

Because they impair thyroid function (and increase the risk of thyroid cancer), and normal thyroid function is critical to early-stage brain development and to later brain function, it seems likely that forever chemicals will be more definitively determined to be more toxic to the brains of males than females.

FLUORIDE: DENTAL CAVITIES VS. MENTAL CAVITIES

Indulge me in a detour from this depressing science into some depressing history. It has been called "America's Longest War." Not the Vietnam War. Not the War in Afghanistan that went on for almost 20 years. Not the War on Sanity still being waged by certain members of Congress, cable news pundits, and social media moguls. It started on Jan. 26, 1945, in Grand Rapids, Michigan. No one was shot, it didn't involve guns, tanks, bombs, protest marches, or a draft of civilians. And it's still going on. It's the War Over Fluoridation.

If one of your favorite hobbies is not starving to death and you have culinary preferences that extend beyond seaweed, you should consider Bone Valley in central Florida one of the most important places on earth you've never heard of and don't want to visit. This is not because it's littered with skeletons, at least not literal ones. It is home to one of the world's largest phosphate deposits, which is an essential ingredient in agricultural fertilizer. Highly toxic hydrogen fluoride and silicon tetrafluoride gases are waste by-products of Bone Valley's fertilizer production.

In the 1960s, the industry was forced to capture that pollution with scrubbers, which converted the noxious vapors into the liquid fluorosilicic acid (FSA). Fumes from FSA can cause severe lung damage or even death. Contact with bare skin can leave painful burns. Without the ability to rid themselves of FSA, the phosphate industry would have a serious and expensive waste-disposal problem. But the profitability of the phosphate industry, narrow priorities of public health officials, and the national security paranoia of the federal government during the Cold War Era converged to create a monumental public health mistake that continues to this day.

Ultimately, FSA, indisputably an untreated, toxic, industrial-waste product, is transported in large tanks throughout the country and dumped into the water supply of about 75% of American cities. Literally adding insult to injury, are trace amounts of arsenic and lead. I remind you that there is no safe level of lead for anyone to consume, and there is enough arsenic in FSA that a senior EPA scientist worried about its causing hundreds of cases of bladder cancer per year.[41]

Furthermore, even sodium fluoride, which provides a small amount of the fluoride for water fluoridation, has been used for a long time as rat poison, and it is also a waste product of the aluminum industry. Fluoride is among the most abundant natural elements on earth, but currently, water is almost the only dietary source of fluoride for most Americans. Nearly 99% of total body fluoride is deposited in our bones and teeth. The only risk of low fluoride intake is a risk of dental caries.

The ostensible reason the U.S. and only a handful of other countries in the world fluoridate their water is that it prevents tooth decay. But the fluoride in toothpaste has made that benefit obsolete, redundant, and counterproductive. How did it happen that we started dumping toxic industrial waste into America's water supply, and why are we still doing it? Like with so many other environmental transgressions, it was largely a crime of opportunity and complicity by government and corporate actors.

The Great Brain Robbery – Brian Moench

Poor dentition was a highly conspicuous embarrassment to people in the Americas, dating at least back to George Washington, who by the age of 57, when he was sworn in as our first President, had lost all but one of his teeth. To compensate, he used multiple dentures crafted from many different raw materials—his own pulled teeth, probably the teeth of some of his slaves, and even animal teeth from donkeys, horses, cows, and hippopotamus ivory (all true). Cadaver teeth were actually a hot commodity in America and England in the eighteenth century. After wars, soldiers not only lost their lives, but shortly after, their teeth—to scavengers for the morbid black market for dental implants.

In the early 20th century, widespread poor dentition was made even worse by the introduction of sugar to the American diet. Dentists commonly made full dentures for teenagers so they could look presentable at graduation. Army recruits in WWI and WWII were required to have at least six opposing teeth in order to be conscripted, and one-third of army recruits were turned away because they couldn't meet that standard. During WWII, improving America's smile became a nationwide priority.

Enter the Manhattan Project, the U.S. Government's top-secret endeavor to beat the Nazis in the race to develop a nuclear bomb, recently depicted in the movie, *Oppenheimer*. But showering the world with radioactivity was not the only public health menace to emerge from the Manhattan Project. Fluoride was the key element in atomic bomb production. Uranium hexafluoride was used to produce the fissionable material, and fluoride was a waste product of that process. Millions of tons of fluoride, known to be highly toxic, were used in the production of weapons-grade uranium and plutonium. From declassified documents, we learn that because of concern over probable adverse health consequences to workers and the environment from the fluoride, Manhattan Project scientists were pressured to obscure and deny what they knew or suspected about fluoride's toxicity.[42]

Fluoride accidents connected to the Manhattan Project resulted in the poisoning of crops, livestock, workers, and residents living near the manufacturing sites. In fact, the first lawsuits filed related to the Manhattan Project were not about radiation exposure; they came from New Jersey farmers who recognized the damage to their crops and livestock from environmental fluoride. Federal government officials worried the lawsuits would stymie production of the atomic bomb. Declassified documents show that officials from the U.S. War Department, the Manhattan Project, the Food and Drug Administration, the Agricultural and Justice Departments, the U.S. Army's Chemical Warfare Service and Edgewood Arsenal, the Bureau of Standards, and DuPont lawyers all met together to marshal all the necessary government resources to defeat the New Jersey farmers that had sued over fluoride damage. It became a matter of protecting the Manhattan Project that studies and information about the toxicity of fluoride be kept quiet. After the ending of the war, paranoia over communist Russia was used as justification for gross malfeasance by the government on many fronts, and the fluoride coverup continued.

Much of the "scientific data" used to demonstrate that low dose fluoride was safe for the public was created by Manhattan Project scientists who were literally ordered to come up with evidence defending contractors from any lawsuits from workers or the public about fluoride toxicity. Pardon anyone for concluding that the outcome of that research was predetermined. Those classified documents show that, in fact, the Atomic Energy Commission (AEC) censored the results of those studies for national security reasons. "Information was buried," concluded Dr. Phyllis Mullenix, former head of toxicology at Forsyth Dental Center in Boston, who eventually became a critic of fluoridation.[41]

Journalist Christopher Bryson writes in his book, *The Fluoride Deception*, that the post-war campaign to fluoridate drinking water was the end result of a PR ploy sponsored by industrial users of fluoride, including the government's nuclear weapons program, to divert attention from its toxicity to its ability to harden teeth. It was the lower-profile twin sister of the government's PR campaign to assuage the public's fear of another possible consequence of the Manhattan Project, ending the world in nuclear war. A narrative was manufactured to make us believe that "safe, abundant electricity, too cheap to meter," from nuclear power was a remarkable if not miraculous gift from atomic fission. In reality, that was "atomic fiction." Like nuclear power plants, fluoridating municipal water was born in a coverup. It has turned out to be a symbol of truth decay more than a cure for tooth decay.

Grand Rapids became the first American city to fluoridate its water supply. It was meant to be an experiment, but public health officials all over the country soon began calling for fluoridation almost as soon as the experiment began, under the assumption that it would be a public health boon, preventing community-wide tooth decay.[43] On the other side of the battlefield, at least initially, was a disparate, somewhat motley crew, including Christian Scientists, a few dentists, natural health food enthusiasts, and anti-Communist fanatics, especially the John Birch Society. But there were precious few voices with scientific expertise. Between 1950 and 1967, nationwide, there were 1,009 public votes on fluoridation. Forty-one percent of those fluoride proposals were adopted, and 59% were rejected.

Growing up in a politically liberal home, I overheard routine ridicule of the John Birch Society. The founder, Robert Welch, was a co-inhabitant of the ideological fox hole dug by paranoid anti-communist demagogue Joseph McCarthy. Welch was also obsessed with the "Red Scare," including the prospect of a communist hiding under every bed. I was in kindergarten during the height of the Red Scare, and I diligently kept an inventory of scary things hiding under my bed. Giant snakes were at the top of the list, following by Ronald Selby, who had tried to shoot my eye out with a BB gun. I tried communists for a while, but frankly, they just didn't do anywhere near the job that snakes did.

Decades before QAnon, Welch was instrumental in bringing conspiracy theories into mainstream public dialogue, and without the help of Facebook. As far as my family was concerned, "Birchers" were the original tin foil hat brigade. Of course, the reason the John Birch Society was opposed to fluoridation is that they were convinced it was a communist plot to destroy America—subtler and lower risk than nuclear war but every bit as effective and sinister.

The February 9, 1959, issue of *The Dan Smoot Report* channeled Aldous Huxley's dystopian novel *Brave New World*, in which a covert government plot subdues the population by giving them drugs en masse. "How could ruling authorities ever manage to give drugs to an entire population?" asked Smoot.[44] Obviously via water supplies, just like the proposals for fluoridation.

Fluoridation turned up as a key plot line in the satirical movie classic, *Dr. Strangelove*, as a Russian communist scheme to infiltrate America. General Jack D. Ripper justified nuclear war this way: "Have you ever heard of a thing called fluoridation? Fluoridation of water? Do you realize that fluoridation is the most monstrously conceived and dangerous communist plot we have ever had to face?" He railed that fluoridation was a poison to our "precious bodily fluids."

No doubt there is room for debate over which of our bodily fluids can be considered "precious," but it turns out, General Ripper was on to something, even though he didn't know what. By the 1990s, the movement for fluoridation hit full stride, winning 59% of public referendums. But the Birchers may have accidentally been on the right side of an issue, although not for the right reasons. If you were to tell me five years ago that I would side with the John Birch Society and against the CDC on any issue, I would say that was the first sign of the apocalypse. Of course, you can't throw a rock and not hit a sign of the apocalypse these days.

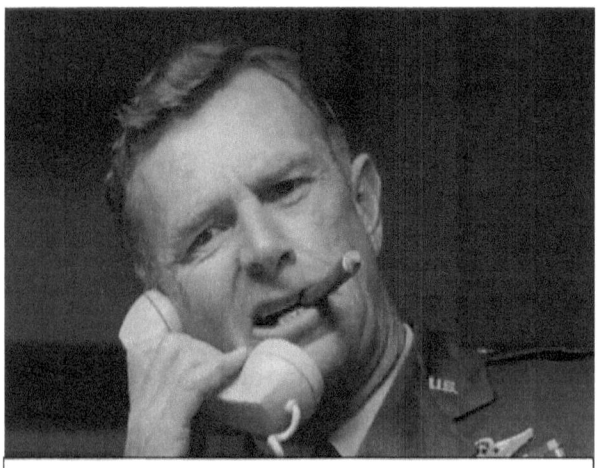

General Jack D. Ripper, promoter of fluoride conspiracy theory in *Dr. Strangelove*

Fluoride proponents love to brand their opposition as

"anti-science." They also like to round them up and put them in the same supposed anti-science corral with anti-vaxxers, anti-GMOers, climate deniers, conspiracy theorists, etc., in an attempt to establish guilt by association. In fact, dating back to the late 1940s, there was serious dispute within scientific, medical, and dental communities over whether fluoridation would be a net benefit to public health.[45]

But within about ten years, the opposition largely evaporated, and not because of any relevant or new science. The few scientists that maintained public opposition were shoved to the fringes of the debate and denigrated as quacks. A few of the remaining opponents published the *National Fluoridation News*, a *National Inquirer*-type yellow journalism rag sheet that embraced conspiratorial headlines, shocking revelations of pro-fluoridation tactics, harsh opinion pieces, and sarcastic cartoons. In today's social media dominated world it would fit right in. But any association with this tabloid tainted the credible scientific opponents of fluoridation merely by being on the same side of the fence. The fluoridation cheerleaders won, but the last battle in the war has not yet been fought.

The United States is one of only a few countries in the world that puts fluoride in municipal water supplies on a large scale. There are more people drinking fluoridated water in the United States than in the rest of the world combined.[46] Concerns about possible brain damage during fetal development led to the rejection of fluoridating water supplies in most European countries.[47] They also didn't have a phosphate industry to capitulate to and didn't warp their domestic public health policies to protect a nuclear weapons program.

Like lead, mercury, and aluminum, fluoride has no essential biologic function in the human body. There is no disease known to be the result of fluoride deficiency. Fluoridation of municipal water supplies, and to a lesser extent, the use of fluoride in medicine and industry, launched the era of living in an artificially fluoridated environment.

For most adults in the U.S., fluoridated water makes up about 80% of their fluoride ingestion, and over 74% of the U.S. population has been drinking water with fluoride added for the last

70 years, according to the CDC. In fact, the CDC named municipal water fluoridation one of the ten greatest public health achievements of the 20th century.[48] Their definition of "achievement," however, warrants, in medical parlance, a second opinion. Many researchers are ready to offer one.

Rates of tooth decay are no longer lower in fluoridated populations, undoubtedly due to the ubiquitous presence of fluoride in toothpaste, which provides as much as anyone needs. All the benefits of fluoride can be achieved by topical application, and there is no benefit whatsoever to fluoride exposure before a baby's teeth appear in their mouth.

Furthermore, communities that have stopped fluoridation have not seen a rise in rates of cavities. But fluoridation proponents are ideologically entrenched. The anti-intellectual, anti-science stigma successfully attached to opponents remains largely intact, and that has been extremely effective in preventing physicians from becoming engaged with or even studying the issue. It's long overdue that that dynamic be upended. Proponents ignore the disturbing history and the original impetus behind the practice, are refractory to being satisfied with the benefit of direct dental application of fluoride, and seem to cover their eyes and ears to avoid addressing the science that is rapidly building revealing fluoride's neurologic effects.

Children and infants retain higher proportions of absorbed fluoride compared to adults, i.e., about 80-90%, as compared to about 50-60% in adults.[49] Fluoride is toxic to the intrauterine developing brain. It crosses the placenta and enters the fetus, a concern magnified because of the immature BBB (mentioned in Chapter 2) at that stage of development.[50] Fluoride accumulates in those parts of the brain responsible for memory and learning.[51]

Scientific justification for the practice has essentially unraveled. The World Health Organization has broken ranks with the CDC, recently adding fluoride to the list of the ten chemicals of greatest public health concern. Fluoridation of water supplies is unique in this lineup of environmental neurotoxins, because it is the only one where exposure is intentional rather than an inadvertent side effect.

Since the 1930s, fluoride has been linked to systemic neurologic and psychiatric disorders, such as chronic fatigue, impaired cognition, poor muscular coordination, and depression.[52] Recently, researchers have found that fluoride reacts with trace amounts of aluminum (previously discussed) to form aluminofluoride complexes that can act as false neurotransmitters, with the "potential to modulate neurodevelopment, brain structure, structural plasticity, as well as higher neuronal functions."[53]

Fluoride at concentrations commonly found in the environment causes biochemical changes, including precipitating inflammation.[54] Research from the U.S. National Research Council (NRC) concluded that fluoride is an endocrine disrupter, and as such, it can impair thyroid function, which, at every stage of human life but especially at early stages of development, can harm brain function.[55]

Fluoride has been shown to inhibit or augment the activity of over 40 important enzymes. Fluoride neurotoxicity, like that from numerous other toxins, is not necessarily dose related. In fact, some studies found that, much like the toxic chemicals known as endocrine disruptors, lower doses can have an even greater effect than higher doses.[54] When the concentration of a chemical is not linearly related to its effect, i.e., the graph that describes the relationship is not a straight line, the relationship is called a "non-monotonic" dose response curve. These non-linear relationships occur in individual cells and tissues and in laboratory animals and humans. They have been observed with nutrients, vitamins, pharmacological compounds, hormones, and numerous toxins, including endocrine disrupting chemicals.[56]

Monotonic relationships are assumed in classic toxicology and are the foundation for virtually all government regulations of environmental toxins. Testing at high doses is extrapolated to lower and lower doses to deduce risk assessments and set safety standards.

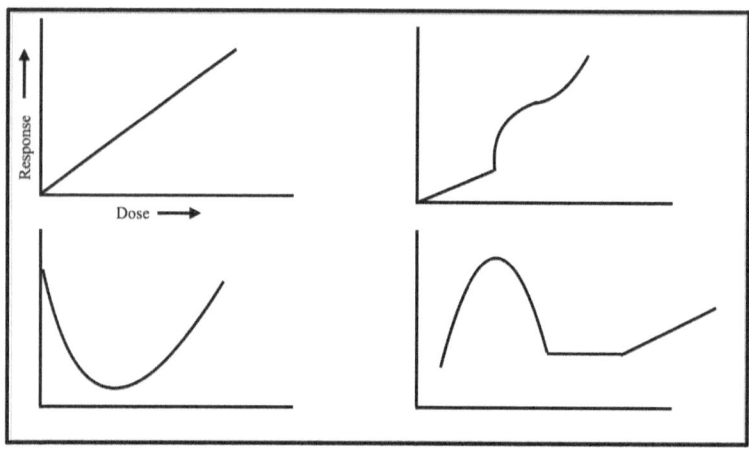

In the upper left-hand corner is a typical monotonic dose response curve. The other three are examples of non-monotonic curves.

But if, in fact, those relationships are not monotonic, then those safety standards are based on a false assumption. We don't know why these relationships occur; the possible explanations would depend on the compound, and for many endocrine disruptors, it is difficult to determine what constitutes a turning point where toxins have greater potency at lower doses. But what is clear is that toxicity is not always linearly related to the dose, and that may be the case with fluoride.

When I was a young, naive parent, part of the routine of good parenting was to give your children multi-vitamins with fluoride. I religiously abided by Newton's Second Law of Stuff I Made Up, which reads, "If a little of something is good, a lot must be better." I probably gave my kids enough fluoride that the tooth fairy could have made a nuclear bomb out of their baby teeth. Perhaps a non-monotonic dose response curve for fluoride is why my children have still been academically successful.

The NRC in 2006 reviewed fluoride standards of the EPA and concluded that fluoride can impair brain development both directly and indirectly, and as with lead, there was no safe threshold for exposure. Once within the brain, fluoride preferentially concentrates in the parts of the brain responsible for learning and memory.[51]

In a meta-analysis of 27 epidemiological studies before 2011, all but one of the studies showed that children exposed to high levels of fluoride suffered significant loss of intelligence, nearly 7 IQ points, compared to low- or non-exposed children.[57] In a second meta-analysis, adding 14 new studies published after 2012, every study showed dose-dependent cognitive deficits in children exposed to fluoride.[58]

Another prospective study of mothers and children in Mexico found that an increase of just 1 milligram per liter (mg/L) of fluoride in the pregnant mother's urine was associated with a loss of 5 IQ points.[59] The women studied had urine fluoride levels between 0.5 and 1.5 mg/L, almost identical to what is found in most women in the U.S.

Interestingly, after the findings regarding prenatal fluoride, this study did not find a relationship between fluoride exposure during childhood and IQ test performance. If this study is accurate, it speaks to the criticality of the timing of exposure, indicating that the fetal stage is the most vulnerable to the toxic impact of fluoride. A meta-analysis of studies in China revealed that children who grew up in an area of endemic fluorosis had a rate of decreased IQ five times higher than controls in an uncontaminated area.[60]

In an observational Canadian study, the children of over 500 pregnant mothers in communities with fluoridated water were tested. Compared to a control group, boys showed an average IQ loss of 4.49 points for every 1mg/Liter increase in the mother's urinary fluoride. No loss was found in girls.[61]

Having been published in one of the most prestigious medicals journals, the impact of the study was further enhanced by an accompanying editorial podcast from two distinguished journal editors, who described the results as "startling."[62] They compared the effect of fluoride to what would be found from lead exposure. One of the most disturbing studies looked for differences in the IQs of children who, for the first six months of life, were fed formula reconstituted with water in communities with added municipal fluoride. Compared to formula-fed newborns in non-fluoridated communities, the investigators found a difference in IQ of 8.8 points. No difference was found in infants who were breastfed.[63]

The recommended fluoride level in U.S. water supplies is 0.7-1.2 mg/L, orders of magnitude higher than what is found in breastmilk. Incidentally, tea plants concentrate both fluoride and aluminum and likely contribute to high levels in humans.[64] Regular tea consumption in countries like the UK and the U.S. may be one reason why Boris Johnson and Donald Trump were once elected to lead the world's sentinel democracies.

Other studies show that elevated prenatal fluoride exposure was associated with increased risk of ADHD.[65] Studies of aborted fetuses in parts of China where natural fluoride levels are high, show brain abnormalities, including abnormally smaller brains and a decreased concentration of neurons.[66] Endemic fluorosis is a public health problem in many countries, especially China, where fluoride exposure comes from drinking water, even more from tea consumption, and from the emissions of coal-fired power plants. Fluorosis causes both dental and skeletal disorders. Skeletal fluorosis is a serious bone disease caused by excessive intake of fluoride. Adults with the disorder also show a wide array of cognitive deficits.[67]

Autism is more prevalent in cities where the water supply is fluoridated. A very credible argument is made that fluoride exposure from artificial addition to municipal water supplies may be acting synergistically with aluminum adjuvants in vaccines to increase the poor neurologic outcomes, including an increased risk of autism.[68]

As of May 2020, 73 studies have looked at the connection between fluoride and brain function in humans. Sixty-five of those studies found that fluoride is associated with reduced IQ. More than 60 studies found a similar impact on learning and memory in animals. What should be accepted as the definitive word on fluoridation came in October 2020 from the U.S. National Toxicology Program (NTP). They released an extensive review of all the available human and animal studies on the possible neurotoxicity of fluoride and its effect on brain development and cognition. They concluded, "fluoride is presumed to be a cognitive developmental hazard to humans."[69]

Most of the research that could be used to exonerate fluoride from neurotoxicity is either anachronistic or born from clear pre-existing agendas. It is long overdue that public health officials allow the recent science its due and willingly acknowledge this enormous mistake that has been going on for more than half a century. The best that can be said for mass fluoridation of public culinary water is the one-time rationalization for it that has disappeared, just like the rationalization for the electoral college. But a more honest evaluation is that it is as much of a scandal as flame retardant chemicals and with similar dark elements. We don't have to choose between tooth decay and brain decay. Even if we did, you can drill and repair or even replace a tooth. You cannot drill, enhance, repair, or replace a brain, Dr. Frankenstein's efforts notwithstanding. And as with so many of these toxins, boys are likely more victimized than girls.

Old habits and ways of thinking are hard to break, even among those who want to think of themselves as committed to science and empirical evidence. The American Dental Association is still firm in advocating for fluoridated municipal water. The American Academy of Pediatrics remains supportive. Frankly, their responses to all this damning research demonstrates that their preconceptions overshadow their objectivity. Dr. Philippe Grandjean explained it like this: "These new prospective studies are of very high quality and, given the wealth of supporting human studies and biological plausibility, leave little doubt that developmental neurotoxicity is a serious risk associated with elevated fluoride exposure, especially when this occurs during early brain development."[58]

Fluoridation opponents among health care professionals are rapidly growing in number. I never expected to be among them or on the same side with the John Birch Society on any issue, advertently or inadvertently. But the evidence that I must join them is too compelling, even though it will cause both of my parents to roll over in their grave.

Environmental Attacks on the Brain

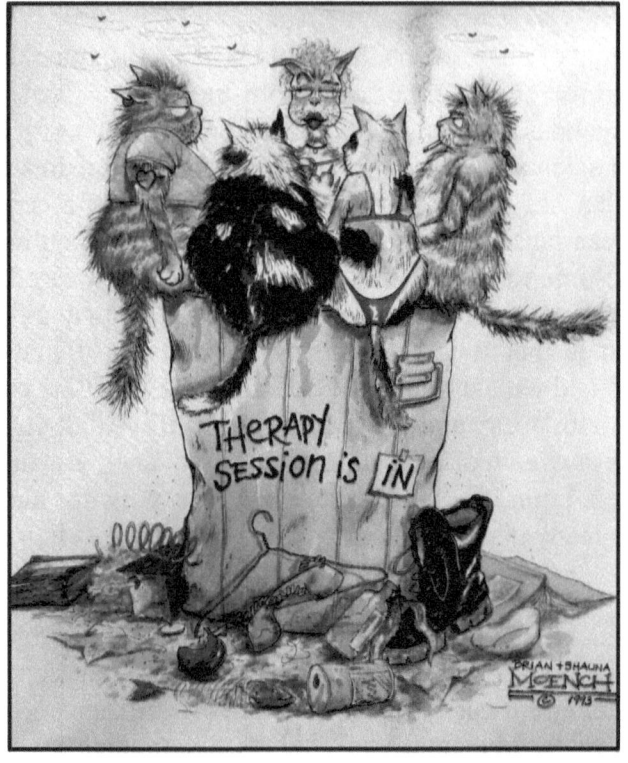

"You wanna hear something really disgusting? They're putting fluoride in our drinking water."

AGAINST ANIMAL TESTING

However, if they do have to be tested, we believe essay exams are the only fair way

Chapter 5

MORE ENVIRONMENTAL ATTACKS ON THE BRAIN

"I never understood wind. You know, I know windmills very much. I've studied it better than anybody. Gases are spewing into the atmosphere. You know we have a world, right? So the world is tiny compared to the universe. So tremendous, tremendous amount of fumes and everything."

—Donald J. Trump

"I guess that makes our biggest weakness lack of strength."

— Gene Stallings, Texas A&M football coach after hearing TCU head coach Abe Martin claim his team's biggest strength is its lack of weakness

"It depends upon what the meaning of the word 'is' is. If the—if he—if 'is' means is and never has been, that is not—that is one thing."

—President Bill Clinton in his testimony to the grand jury on the Monica Lewinsky affair

As a board-certified male, and likely the owner of some XY chromosomes, there is little in this book that makes me very happy. My wife believes my philosophy in life is best summed up by Roger McGough's poem, ***Survivor***

Every day…..I think about dying… About disease, starvation…

violence, terrorism, war… the end of the world….

It helps keep my mind off things.

More Environmental Attacks on the Brain

Thank you, Roger, for being a kindred spirit. This chapter is guaranteed to help you keep your mind off things as well.

The Flynn effect, named after James Flynn, the psychologist whose work described it, refers to the observation that during the 20th century, average IQ test scores steadily increased in the developed world. Numerous possible reasons account for or at least contribute to the trend that saw IQ test scores increase about 3 points per decade. Those likely IQ boosters included improved nutrition and education and reduced infections or "pathogen stress." But in recent years, the Flynn effect has stalled, and in many countries has actually reversed.[1] Results of recent elections, irrationality, violence, and the wide spread of conspiracy theories in the U.S. and Europe certainly would be prima facie evidence to call into question the higher intelligence of humans in what should be the most advanced countries on earth.

The stalling and reversal of the rise in IQ scores began with those born in the mid 1970s, and it's not been an insignificant drop. The IQ scores of young people have been dropping by 7 points per generation. Some observers discount the drop, believing that traditional IQ tests are no longer very relevant as measures of intelligence because of cultural and lifestyle changes among the young people who are taking these tests. But even if that were true, the average IQ of a country's population is still linked to economic strength and innovation. Flynn himself has published research showing that the Flynn effect has stalled or reversed, and that much of the loss has been occurring among those at the top of the IQ curve.

Two of the prominent hypotheses set forth to explain this fall of IQ scores have been 1) A dilution effect of the tested population in richer, developed countries by poorer, less well-educated immigrants, 2) Something researchers call the "dysgenic fertility" effect, which means there is a negative correlation between intelligence and the number of children. A harsher way of putting it is—the less intelligent people are having the most children. I refer you to the satirical comedy *Idiocracy*, from the creators of South Park, for what a continuation of that trend would look like 500 years from now. Hint—the President of the United States is a TV wrestling star, Dwayne Elizondo Mountain Dew Herbert Camacho, and America is irrigating their crops with an energy drink called Brawndo. In other words, it's almost a documentary.

Idiocracy notwithstanding, recent research does not support either of those politically incorrect explanations. Mounting environmental neurotoxins, like the ones in this and the previous chapter, are likely contributors.

ORGANOCHLORIDE PESTICIDES (DIELDRIN, ENDOSULFAN, HEPTACHLOR, DDT, DDE)

When I was a teenager, my father gave me a copy of Rachael Carson's sentinel book, *Silent Spring*. I remember the book better than almost any other book of my adolescence. It probably deserves credit as the impetus for the modern environmental movement. The message that lingered with me for decades was that DDT was dramatically reducing the populations of our iconic birds, like our national symbol, bald eagles, because it made their shells too thin, and baby chicks were being born prematurely. DDT had been a mainstay of mosquito-control strategies, but in response to Carson's clarion call about its dangers, the EPA under Richard Nixon banned DDT in 1972, followed by bans in most other developed countries in the ensuing decade. Nearly 50 years later, we are still suffering the consequences of the once widespread use of DDT.

The Stockholm Convention on Persistent Organic Pollutants (POP) is an onging global treaty between 186 countries to minimize exposure to toxic chemicals. The chemicals addressed in this treaty have been singled out because they resist break down, persist in the environment, and bioaccumulate in the fatty tissue of humans and wildlife, reaching ever higher concentrations in the upper reaches of the food chain, causing a long list of poor health outcomes. Think of them as the most toxic of the 140,000 industrial chemicals humans are exposed to. Of the 41 chemicals officially recognized as POPs by the Stockholm convention, 18 are pesticides.

Pesticides are detected on every continent, in every lake and ocean, and in rainfall from the sky.[29,30,31] For just about every human on earth pesticides now contaminate our air, drinking water, food and soil. The toxicity of pesticides has become more recognizable and broad-based in the last two decades because many of them are now known to be endocrine disruptors.

We are all exposed to a battery of endocrine disrupting chemicals (EDCs) on an almost daily basis, because they have become omnipresent in plastics, personal care products, food packaging, pesticides, and many other products. EDCs are chemicals that mimic or inhibit key human hormones at very small doses. Another defining characteristic of EDCs is that the adverse human health effects may not be apparent for many years after exposure and therefore cannot be assessed using traditional dose response models that are the key to toxicology risk assessments used for determining safe thresholds. Their toxicity may reach future generations even if they are unexposed, because of the harm they do to epigenetic integrity and male and female reproductive systems.[26,27]

A recent review by 12 of the most knowledgeable researchers on EDCs, concluded that, "Whether low doses of EDCs influence certain human disorders is no longer conjecture, because epidemiological studies show that environmental exposures to EDCs are associated with human diseases and disabilities," and that, "For every chemical that we looked at that we could find a low-dose cutoff, if it had been studied at low doses it had an effect at low doses."[32]

Toxicologist Linda Birnbaum, the director of the U.S. National Institute of Environmental Health Sciences (NIEHS), stated that "existing US regulations have not kept pace with scientific advances showing that widely used chemicals cause serious health problems at levels previously assumed to safe."[33] At the top of the list of chemicals of concern are pesticides (insecticides and herbicides) because they function as biological poisons to all living cells, from pest insects to humans, and everything in between.

The same technology that fueled the devastating world wars of humans against each other in the first half of the 20th century, also fueled the rise of a much longer, and still ongoing, devastating war of humans against nature. Historian Edmund P. Russell III argues, "…the science and technology of pest control sometimes became the science and technology of war [WWI and WWII] and vice versa.[28]

Pesticides (insecticides and herbicides) share the same chemical heredity as pre-WWII organophosphorus nerve agents. Many insecticides are merely derivations of those warfare chemicals. In perhaps a supreme irony, chemicals judged to be too hideous for war were diluted and altered slightly and declared just fine for peacetime.

DDT was first used to against mosquitoes and lice in in WWII to fight off malaria and typhus among troops. Needing a transition to peacetime relevance and profitability, after WWII the chemical industry campaigned for a war against pests and the use of DDT in all walks of life. In 1944, Popular Mechanics ran an article, "Our Next World War –Against Insects": "This one will be a long and bitter battle to crush the creeping, wriggling, flying, burrowing billions whose numbers and depredations baffle human comprehension." Profitability, not science, has been the driving force on this war against insects and nature that has continued ever since.

Most insecticides work by causing disruption of the brain and nervous system of insects. Human beings share the same basic biologic blueprint and biochemical metabolic processes with other living organisms. In fact, a 2006 EPA review declared that animal studies of pesticides are relevant to human health because most insecticides act on functions of the nervous system common to the animal world. More specifically, insecticides as a group disrupt the passage of chemical neurotransmitters, prohibiting transmission of electrical signaling between nerve cells. Moreover, pesticides can reach the fetus by passing through the placenta.[2]

It should not be a bridge too far then, that human nerve cells could also be affected, especially when considering that at the critical embryonic stage, the human fetal brain is no larger than many insects. Research confirms that mothers more exposed to commonly used, "safe" pesticides bear children with lower intelligence,[3] structural brain abnormalities,[4] behavioral disorders, compromised motor skills,[5] higher rates of brain cancer,[6] and even smaller head size.[7] Adult neurologic diseases like Parkinson's and an acceleration of cognitive decline are more common in adults with even modest exposure to "legal" pesticides.[8] Pesticides almost certainly are contributing to a decline in America's collective intellectual prowess that I would go so far as to characterize as spiraling toward catastrophe.

Unfortunately, the banning of DDT continues to generate controversy, primarily among anti-environmental and anti-science crusaders who try to blame the ban for hundreds of millions of malaria-related deaths, mostly among poor children in the third world. For many years, articles have appeared with titles like, "The Murderous Church of Rachael Carson," and "Rachael Carson's Deadly Legacy." These assessments are myopic in the extreme, ignoring the broad reach of DDT's toxicity, and the cascade of consequences throughout the biologic world. Critics of the ban on DDT ignore a simple and obvious reality; that humans are part of that biologic world, and depend on it for their own health and surivival. And that myoptic view can be found even among sophisticated, well-educated elites.

The Daily Beast, not exactly a conservative megaphone, ran an article in 2017 titled, "How Rachael Carson Cost Millions of People Their Lives," written by Paul A. Offit, MD, a professor of pediatrics and director of the Vaccine Education Center at The Children's Hospital of Philadelphia.[9] Dr. Offit is an expert on vaccines, no argument there. In fact, he was in the news in that role during the COVID pandemic. But he is not an expert on DDT or environmental contamination, and that's an important distinction. Dr. Offit included a critique of the EPA's banning of DDT in his book, *Pandora's Lab*, a supposed exposé of seven examples where "science" got things wrong. In doing so, he joined forces with right wing, anti-science groups funded by free market, libertarian think tanks like the Cato Institute, famous for carrying water for their corporate sponsors, like the chemical and tobacco industries. Offit and the Cato Institute claim millions have died of malaria because of the banning of DDT.

The Great Brain Robbery –Brian Moench

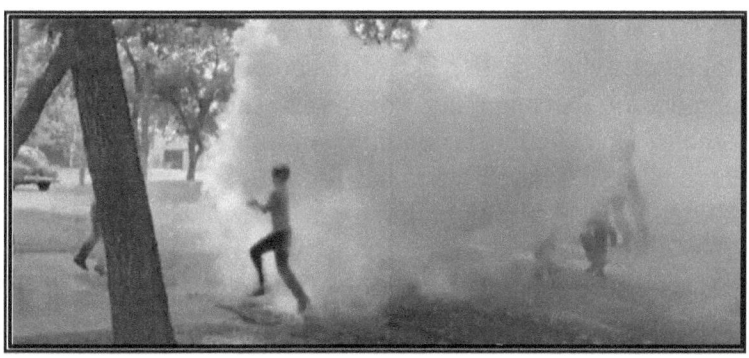

Children playing behind a DDT truck in the 1940s

While it is not my intent to engage in a side battle over all the reasons why the defense of DDT is myopic and disingenuous, it is appropriate in the context of this book to point out that the argument that "DDT saves lives" is pushed by people and organizations that meander in a fog of willful ignorance of the dark side effects of DDT that go well beyond thinner egg shells. In joining that club, Offit ironically commits the very sin he accuses others of committing as the theme of his book, i.e., becoming blinded by his own scientific capability such that he renders himself oblivious to his own limitations. This goes to show that the Dunning Krueger Effect can even plague very intelligent and accomplished people.

Mosquitoes quickly develop resistance to insecticides, as they have done with DDT, and the use of it grew increasingly counterproductive. The more DDT sprayed, the more the mosquitoes developed a resistance to it, and the greater the spread of malaria.

But DDT was never a binary choice between saving the lives of birds or the lives of poor African children. Because of the long half-life of DDT and similar organochloride compounds and their continued use in parts of Africa and developing nations plagued by malaria, virtually the entire globe and every human being on earth is contaminated with DDT and its metabolites. Chemically, insecticides are poorly selective biologic poisons, toxic to numerous "non-target" species including humans.

Given the exquisitely sensitive process of fetal brain development, which is dependent on precise coordination of and communication between nerve cells, it should be intuitive that exposure to such chemicals could impair human brain development. Research since Rachael Carson has linked DDT to an extensive list of human diseases including cancer, diabetes,[16] obesity,[16] hypertension,[17] and fetal and reproductive toxicity. Women exposed to DDT before puberty, especially in infancy, have much higher rates of breast cancer.[18]

Beginning in 2006, studies emerged showing a connection between DDT and neurologic diseases like Alzheimer's[19] and Parkinson's and harm to the brain development of children. Mothers with the highest levels of DDT in their blood give birth to children that, at 12 and 24 months, scored 7 to 10 points lower on Bayley mental tests compared to children of mothers with the lowest levels of DDT.[20] Pregnant mothers with high blood levels of the metabolites of DDT have a significantly increased risk that their children will be diagnosed with autism.[21]

Prenatal DDT exposure is associated with a much higher rate of behavioral disorders in children.[22] DDT triples in breast milk after one household spraying.[23] Adults with high levels of DDT metabolites are four times more likely to have Alzheimer's.[24] DDT is the only well-studied neurotoxin in this group that found greater impact on females than males. There is a substantial body of research in animals and humans that most of these organochlorine pesticides--endosulfan, dieldrin, and heptachlor, for example, affect males more than females.[25]

ORGANOPHOSPHATE PESTICIDES (CHLORPYRIFOS, DIAZINON, MALATHION, PARATHION, AND NALED)

Organophosphates (OPs) are acetylcholinesterase inhibitors, progeny of nerve gas agents originally used in WWI. Acetycholinesterase (AChE) is an essential enzyme in all mammals, including humans, because it rapidly breaks down the nerve transmitter acetylcholine. Inhibition of AChE provokes a marked acceleration of nerve impulses and an excessive build up of acetycholine. Sarin gas caused paralysis in humans via this mechanism. While AChE is essential, there certainly can be too much of a good thing, just like with plastic surgery.

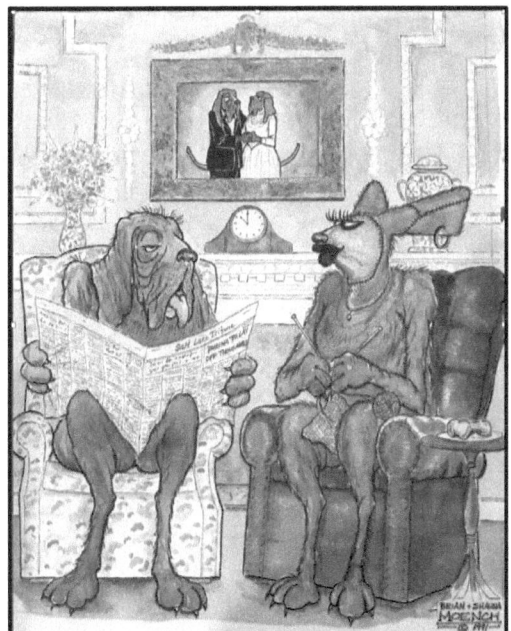

OPs were adapted from these chemical weapons to be lethal to insects at low doses via the same mechanism. It was a default assumption that low doses meant they would be harmless enough to humans and wildlife, and everyone should be happy. The chemical companies certainly were.

Over 30 years ago, the Office of Technology Assessment (OTA) of the US Congress (not exactly a household name) released an extensive report entitled "Neurotoxicity: Identifying and Controlling Poisons of the Nervous System." One of the two primary targets of the report was chemical pesticides. They stated, "Of particular concern are the delayed effects of some of the organophosphate pesticides."[1]

In 2018, a meta-review of data and literature on OPs analyzed and cross-referenced numerous reviews and epidemiological studies with a UN database that includes 71 countries, and other research material.[2] The lead of author of the panel of experts involved in the study, Irva Hertz-Picciotto, Director of the UC Davis Environmental Health Sciences Centre, said, "We have compelling evidence from dozens of human studies that exposures of pregnant women to very low levels of organophosphate pesticides put children and foetuses [British spelling for fetuses] at risk for developmental problems that may last a lifetime. By law, the EPA cannot ignore such clear findings: It's time for a ban [on] all organophosphate pesticides."[3]

Bruce Lanphear, one of the paper's co-authors and a scientist at Vancouver's Simon Fraser University, said: "We found no evidence of a safe level of organophosphate pesticide exposure for children. Well before birth, organophosphate pesticides are disrupting the brain in its earliest stages, putting them on track for difficulties in learning, memory and attention, effects which may not appear until they reach school-age. Government officials around the world need to listen to science, not chemical lobbyists."[3]

In 2021 researchers at NYU concluded that 81% of the cognitive loss in children from environmental neurotoxins came from exposures to polybrominated diphenyl ethers (PDBEs) and organophosphate pesticides, far eclipsing that caused by heavy metals like lead and mercury.[4]

I have met with the Chemical Divison of the EPA to discuss with them the human health hazard represented by mosquito abatement pesticides, including organophosphates, in my home town, Salt Lake City. We had sent them a 73-page report with over 300 scientific references from mainstream medical journals challenging their approval of these insecticides for mosquito control. The outcome was, predictably, a disappointment in that they took no action on their approval. But it was infuriating that they made no attempt to even hide their complete disinterest in reviewing the science we presented. I have no doubt had we been lobbyists from the chemical industry that their interest level in our presentation would have been starkly different.

I have served as an expert witness in several lawsuits over poor health outcomes and environmental contamination. One of the most heartbreaking involved a family that sent me a letter, some excerpts of which follow.

The Great Brain Robbery – Brian Moench

My husband and I began building what we thought was to be our dream house. We did much of the work ourselves and spent hundreds of extra hours and tens of thousands of extra dollars in customizations we thought would be perfect for our family. We'd only lived in the home for just over a year when our autistic son starting getting sick...episodes of dizziness and [he] began falling...Headaches, lethargy, seizures-like shifting of his eyes, and muscle tremors. He was sleeping 17-18 hours a day and was becoming almost unresponsive at school and at home. Within several months, other members of our family began developing symptoms. Headaches, slurred speech, stinging eyes, sweats, diarrhea, respiratory problems and general malaise. Our pets developed strange infections and tumors.

An entire family developing neurologic problems strongly suggested an infectious or environmental etiology. It turned out there wasn't a lot of mystery about what was the cause. Their next-door neighbor was a pesticide contractor who would often bring trucks to his home, store pesticides, dispose of some, and rinse out his truck on his property. Neighbors would often comment on the odor. The letter went on:

"The local health department found VOCs [volatile organic compounds] *coming from a sump hole* [in the family's basement].... *The house that we spent almost two years and all of our savings building now sits empty, unsafe to live in.... The system is broken.... While there are measures and laws in place to protect the sprayers and businesses, there seems to be no concern for the families being affected."*

Many of the neighbors had similar but less severe symptoms. After fleeing their "dream house," which turned into their nightmare house, some of the family members started to improve. Unfortunately, the husband developed progressive, debilitating symptoms of a neurodegenerative disease and peripheral neuropathy, much like multiple sclerosis. All of the males in the family were more affected than the females.

The letter I wrote to the attorneys on behalf of the family included these passages:

> *"One of the most well-established consequences of pesticide exposure are symptoms and diseases of the nervous system. Insecticides are biologic poisons, most of which target the nervous system of insects. Because human nerve cells share the same basic metabolic processes as insect nerve cells, it is not surprising that insecticides could cause various types of nerve damage in humans. Indeed, numerous studies show a wide range of poor neurologic outcomes among humans exposed to insecticides—decreased cognition and memory, depression, impaired anatomic and functional brain development in children, higher rates of autism, worse motor skills, and higher rates of neurodegenerative diseases like Parkinson's and Alzheimer's.*
>
> *"That the family's autistic son had the most severe neurologic symptoms is consistent with the medical research, because children are affected more than adults, and males are usually affected more severely than females.*
>
> *"Chronic, repeated exposure is not required for a person to be permanently harmed. A recent study showed that just one significant pesticide 'event' was associated with decline in cognition equal to almost four years of aging.*
>
> *"Studies dating back to 1957 show that combined exposure to several different types of pesticides, as was the case with this family, can have a cumulative and synergistic effect (greater than the*

sum of the individual effects). For example, exposure to one pesticide at a dose thought to be safe, combined with exposure to a second, or third pesticide at doses thought to be safe, does not mean that the combined exposure is indeed safe. In fact, the combined exposure can be much more toxic than the additive impact of each individual chemical (synergism)."

They never found out what specific pesticides the contractor had kept on his property. It probably included multiple chemicals, and it probably doesn't really matter; they all have similar toxicity, quantitatively and qualitatively. The family eventually settled out of court but almost certainly for insufficient compensation, given what they went through and what they may yet face, given that their cancer risks will increase over the next several decades.

Made by Dow Chemical beginning in 1965, chlorpyrifos used to be the most commonly used insecticide in American homes. It was commonplace for poor families to routinely spray chlorpyrifos to control roaches. Thirty years later, the EPA fined Dow a whopping $732,000 (that's less than the loose change they have in the cushions of their couch, another example of industry capture of regulatory agencies) for not revealing over 200 reports of poisoning with the chemical.

It was found that after a single broadcast use of the pesticide by professional pest control teams in apartment rooms, chlorpyrifos continued to accumulate on children's toys and hard surfaces for 2 weeks afterwards. Following such a spraying, the levels of the pesticide could reach up to 119 times what was thought to be a reasonably safe level of exposure. Evidence became overwhelming that the insecticide was toxic to the brain, and it was banned for widespread residential use in 2001. However, it was still allowed to be used in large volumes for agricultural use.

Toward the end of the Obama Administration, the EPA was poised to finally prohibit its use everywhere. But the Trump Administration reversed course and withdrew the ban, ensuring that farm workers, their children, and everyone that eats fruits and vegetables (which excludes Trump himself) will continue to be exposed.

The Biden Administration's EPA finally banned the use of chlorpyrifos on food crops in 2022, representing 90% of its commercial use. But the chemical industry and Big Ag fought back because, of course, profits were at risk, and convinced the US Court of Appeals to capitulate to their hysterical demands to vacate the EPA's rule which would have revoked all food tolerances for the chemical. The battle to protect the public has now gone on for over 20 years and counting, and your children's Cheerios are still plastered with these neurologic poisons, and many others.

Naled is an organophosphate routinely used for mosquito abatement via aerial delivery systems because it's considered too toxic to be used by applicators on the ground, i.e. trucks, ATVs, humans with backpacks. Naled has been banned in the European Union because of its neurotoxicity, but it is applied throughout the US using ultra-low volume (ULV) sprayers mounted on drones, planes or helicopters, dispensing very fine aerosol droplets containing small quantities of insecticide that drift through the air and kill mosquitoes on contact. Because the insecticide is highly diluted (1-2 tablespoons per acre sprayed) it is assumed to be safe at the population scale.

That assumption ignores numerous lines of research. Naled leaves a breakdown product, dichlorvos, which is also an insecticide with similar acute and chronic effects and a much longer half-life. In various types of water, dichlorvos can last up to 6 months. Dichlorvos, is classified by EPA as a group C (possible) human carcinogen, while, inexplicably, naled itself is not. Dichlorvos exposure during pregnancy or childhood has been linked to an elevated incidence of brain tumors and leukemia.[5] Naled is far more toxic by inhalation exposure than by ingestion, maybe as much as 20 times more toxic.[6] Nonetheless, EPA states there are no risks to inadvertent bystanders, a bewildering, critical omission, made even worse because EPA has not bothered to calculate the potential for "bystander" exposure. The EPA's position is, literally, people may prefer to stay inside and close windows and doors when spraying takes place from the skies over their neighborhoods, but it is not necessary. That's like saying people may prefer to run and hide when a mass shooting is taking place, but it is not necessary.

Within a population of 25.5 million children 0 to 5 years of age, researchers calculate a total loss of 16.9 million IQ points due to common background exposure to organophosphates alone. This estimation does not take into account all the other known environmental neurotoxins like heavy metals, PCB, flame retardants, many other neurotoxic chemicals, including other pesticides, which only add to that total.[7]

In Japan, between 1957 and 1971, school children saw a huge increase in impaired vision eventually tied to the use of an OP in agriculture. One town near an agricultural area now has an eye disease named after them, "Saku disease." In that town 98% of the children had visual acuity problems linked to the regular application of an OP on near-by agricultural fields.[8] In California a boy became blind after being outside while a helicopter was spraying an OP.[9] I'm guessing the boy and his family would have something to say about EPA's lack of concern over direct exposure to aerial spraying.

Recall that OPs kill insects by the same biochemical process that sarin gas kills humans, provoking a marked acceleration of nerve impulses. They also cause brain damage at exposure levels commonly found in the broad environment, even at levels below the threshold for secondary toxicity. That indicates an additional mechanism of toxicity beyond its known chemical effects on insects.[10]

Multiple studies of children with in-utero or post-natal exposure to this group of insecticides have shown reduced IQ, impaired memory, and behavioral disorders.[11] Proximity to an agricultural area where organophosphates were used was found to significantly increase the risk of autism and developmental delay, even more for third-trimester exposure.[12]

Let's get back to the theme of males being harmed more than females. In vitro nerve cells from male animals show greater chemical toxicity from exposure to these pesticides compared to nerve cells from females.[13] But the researchers also found that chlorpyrifos was more potent in reducing the IQs of male children than females.

Use of fumigants and organochlorine insecticides is associated with significantly increased rates of depression and suicide among pesticide applicators.[14] Just one significant pesticide exposure event is enough to precipitate significant cognitive decline among pesticide applicators.[15] Several studies show that as a group, organophosphate chemicals (nerve agents and pesticides) cause greater neurotoxicity in male animals than females.[16]

I can't help but wonder if the pesticide contractor in the lawsuit mentioned above—using the poor judgement and impaired cognition to mix, rinse, and dispose of all his chemicals at home—wasn't also victimizing himself with the same chemical toxins that had ruined the lives of his neighbors.

For more detail on the neurologic damage from organophosphates see the Appendix at the back of the book.

PYRETHROIDS: COGNITIVE ABATEMENT

Not long ago, a young man in his late teens came to my door trying to sell me "pest control." When I asked how what he was selling would accomplish that, he said his company used an all-natural chemical that was completely safe—that it was made from flowers. The only people who don't like flowers are the holy trinity of evil, Dracula, Darth Vader, and Marjorie Taylor Greene. Great, sign me up! With a picture of a photoshopped pot of chrysanthemums, it was a slick sales pitch. There was only one problem—everything. He didn't know the names of the chemicals he was selling or anything about what they did, how they worked, or anything about those safety claims. It wasn't his fault, of course. He was a high school kid doing a summer job. In a gentle way, I tried to persuade the boy that he needed to get another job, and that he should have greater aspirations, like becoming an Elvis impersonator.

I took his brochure and later called the company and gave them a piece of my mind, perhaps overly generous on my part given how many pieces I have left. The miracle pest control made of photoshopped chrysanthemums was in the chemical family, pyrethroids. It just so happened that I knew something about how wonderful pyrethroids weren't, which gave me ample reason to crank up my righteous indignation and terrify some poor secretary at company headquarters.

Pyrethroids are the most often used insecticides in mosquito abatement, a euphemism for spreading poison over a large area in hopes that more things die that you don't like, such as mosquitoes, than things that you do like, such as your children or their brain cells. But pyrethroids are hardly specifically selective for mosquitoes. They work by disrupting a mosquito's nervous system just like numerous other insecticides. It doesn't require every neuron in your frontal lobes to consider that anything that attacks the nervous system of an insect could also attack other nervous systems, like those of beneficial insects, wildlife, and human beings, especially at the stage where human beings are as small as mosquitoes, i.e., at the embryonic stage.

Community fogging with pyrethroids is promoted under the premise that mosquito-borne diseases like West Nile Virus (WNV) are significant public health hazards. While WNV and the other mosquito-borne diseases are not trivial, they are also not the only public hazard in this equation. Unfortunately, mosquito abatement agencies are usually staffed by people who have very little understanding or even curiosity about the health consequences of the pesticides they use. It is the rule, not the exception, that those who order their widespread application assume they are safe for public use merely because they are available. Under both Republican and Democratic administrations, the EPA's permitting the use of a chemical is not even close to a scientific exoneration of its toxic potential.

Pyrethroids seep indoors within any residences near where spraying is conducted, and they accumulate in dust and on household surfaces because they don't break down indoors like they do in sunlight outdoors. Children end up with higher blood concentrations of these chemicals than adults do because they spend more time near the floor and engage in much more hand to mouth activity. Human exposure also occurs because these chemicals linger on vegetables and fruit. Pyrethroid fogging is now considered by many health experts to be a seriously flawed public policy because the danger to human health caused by the indiscriminate spraying of pesticides is far greater than the danger of acquiring a serious disease from the WNV carried by mosquitoes.

Those subgroups of the population most susceptible to serious consequences from WNV are the very young, old, and otherwise immunocompromised. Yet these are exactly the people whose immune systems are compromised further by the insecticide spraying intended to protect them. In other words, exposure to chemical pesticides may actually be counterproductive by increasing the risk of developing a serious case of WNV encephalitis.

Community fogging often is further counterproductive, because mosquitoes can quickly become resistant to it and can even become more aggressive after being exposed to it. Moreover, not only does repeated spraying fail to eradicate the mosquitoes, but repeated spraying leads to the survival of more aggressive mosquitoes that are resistant to pesticides and have increased prevalence of the WNV within their bodies. This resistance is passed on to new generations, leading to endless cycles of increased pesticide spraying each year. It creates a pesticide arms race.

Pyrethroids' mechanism of action is similar to organophosphates and DDT, causing damage to insect neurons by increasing impulse conduction, overloading the nerve pathways and blocking the passage of sodium ions across nerve cell membranes, resulting in paralysis and death of insects. Pyrethroids also act as endocrine disrupters because they mimic the action of estrogen in both males and females.

In humans, long-term exposure of children to pyrethroids is documented by an increase in their metabolites in the urine. Higher levels of those urinary metabolites is associated with behavioral changes, like increased aggressive behavior.[1] Some research has found that consuming food containing permethrin (a type of pyrethroid) causes loss of short-term memory and inability to concentrate.[2]

Safety claims regarding pyrethroids do not adequately take into account cumulative exposures from a repeated, often seasonal spraying program. If a woman conceived a child at the beginning of mosquito spraying season, her baby in utero is likely to be exposed to multiple and perhaps constant doses of the insecticide for several months during the most critical stages of embryonic development. Furthermore, because no one is exposed to just one toxic chemical or even just one pesticide, the toxicologic studies on chemical exposures never adequately assess the clinical consequences of our cumulative exposures, especially in fetuses and infants.

Implicating the risk of pyrethroids to fetuses are studies showing toxicity to small invertebrates at concentrations of as little as two parts per trillion (2ppt). In addition to contributing to neurologic diseases, impaired intellect, and endocrine disruption, constant spraying of neighborhoods in mosquito abatement programs creates problems for chemically sensitive individuals.

A few years after I co-founded the physician group, Utah Physicians for a Healthy Environment (UPHE), a family that lived about 100 miles away asked if they could meet with me in person to see if I could help them. I agreed, and when they arrived it became clear who needed help; their adult daughter who appeared to be in her late 20s and who used a wheelchair. She had pale skin, a very pretty face, and a thin frame.

I learned that the cause of her debilitation was primarily profound fatigue. The family felt like she was reacting adversely to chemical exposures, primarily pesticides. In their town, the owner of a pesticide company had a far too cozy relationship with a key county commissioner, and the end result was that their neighborhood was targeted by a "mosquito abatement" program that ended up sending a truck around several times each summer, bombarding a mist of pyrethroid insecticide all over homes and yards throughout the town. Every time the truck came by, the family would hurry to close the windows, and she would retreat to the most protected part of the house. But it was never enough. She would feel profoundly distressed, fatigued, and have difficulty breathing for days if not weeks afterwards. And then the truck would come by again. It was a nightmare for her and the entire family. Pesticides weren't the only trigger, but they were the most consistent and most severe.

The family told me in detail how they had attempted to get the local officials to apply more restraint to the mosquito abatement program and consider how it was affecting her daughter and others in the town. But the local officials weren't interested in offering deference to their complaints.

At first, I, too, was a bit skeptical. I probably did what so many other doctors have done to other similar patients, primarily women. I was tempted to dismiss her complaints as "supra-tentorial," all in her mind, driven by emotion for whatever motivation, perhaps to get attention. Then I felt like I owed it to her to be more objective. I didn't have an answer, a cure, or even good advice. But regardless, I did know that those pesticides weren't doing anyone any favors in that town. Almost all of Utah is a desert and hardly a haven for mosquitoes. For the county commissioners and others to ignore their complaints was essentially bullying of their constituency.

On behalf of the family, I wrote blistering letters to multiple layers of government, the county commissioners, the Utah Department of Agriculture, and EPA. I wrote, "In my opinion, it is a callous and ignorant disregard for the rights and safety of county residents to continue systemized fogging of residential areas with pyrethroid pesticides simply because the government has not prohibited such conduct yet." This pesticide program was probably doing more harm than good to public health, and it certainly was to this family.

I also started investigating more about what might be the cause of this young woman's distress. Pesticide-provoked allergic reactions are not uncommon. I believe this unfortunate young woman also has "multiple chemical sensitivity syndrome," which can afflict as much as 10-15% of the adult population. The diagnosis is one of exclusion, because there is no real objective test to establish it. For these patients, chemical exposures can be a debilitating nightmare that includes profound fatigue, nausea, coughing, bronchospasm, rashes, severe headaches, and impaired mentation. Insecticides are the most common triggers for the syndrome, which can be precipitated by as little as one exposure event. It is a travesty that these individuals must endure physical suffering from these exposures, most of them unnecessary. Adding insult to injury, they also often have to deal with psychological pain inflicted on them by others who dismiss their complaints or look upon them with condescension or contempt.

The research showing the toxicity of pyrethroids to human health is extensive. Most pyrethroid compounds are endocrine disruptors, and as such, can interfere with human reproduction and act as carcinogens. Adults exposed to higher levels of pyrethroids over 14 years were found to have significantly higher rates of mortality, including cardiovascular mortality, compared to groups with less exposure.[3]

Due to their fat solubility, pyrethroids pass through the BBB.[4] After birth, the next round of pyrethroid exposure is probably from its presence in breast milk.[5] Low level, prenatal, and perinatal pyrethroid exposure affects learning, motor activity, and sexual behavior in lab animals that persists into adulthood.[6] Studies on neurotoxicity in children show that prenatal permethrin exposure is linked to delayed neurodevelopment at 36 months and loss of intelligence of about 4 IQ points.[7] In total, the research on pyrethroid exposure and intelligence tests, memory, visual acuity, behavioral problems, and motor function in children show deficits with a severity comparable to what is seen with lead exposure.[8] Animal studies suggest males are more affected than females.[9]

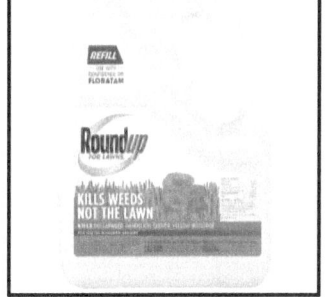

ROUNDUP (GLYPHOSATE)

More Environmental Attacks on the Brain

In Benton, Yakima, and Franklin Counties in Washington State, beginning in 2010, a mysterious mini-epidemic of a fatal brain birth defect, anencephaly and severe spinal cord birth defects emerged at rates 4 to 8 times the normal rate. Toxic environmental exposures almost certainly had to have been the cause, and pesticides have to be at the top of the list of suspected environmental exposures. Coincidently, also beginning in 2010 and continuing for four years, Benton County started a noxious weed eradication program, spraying glyphosate along the Yakima River, which all three counties used for irrigation water. No one bothered monitoring glyphosate concentrations in the water. There is the distinct possibility of a direct causal link between the ability of glyphosate to inhibit folic acid production, and a deficiency of folic acid in pregnant women which is a known contributor to the risk of anencephaly.

Birth defects of the brain and spinal cord (neural tube defects) occur in one in about 1,000 births, which make this category the second most common birth defect. Both industry-sponsored and independent research have shown that glyphosate interferes with development of the brain and skull, collectively known as the cranium.[10]

The Washington State Health Department investigated the epidemic and has come up with no answers. But Sarah Barron, the nurse who first made the observation and alerted authorities, wonders if perhaps they didn't find anything because they were halfhearted in their search for the culprit. The state hasn't spoken to any of the families who had the babies with birth defects. Not a single one. They never asked key questions like what they ate or if they'd been exposed to pesticides sprayed in this agricultural area.

Andrea Jackman, whose daughter, Olivia, was born with spina bifida, another type of serious neural tube defect, is outraged. "Nobody's asked me anything," said Jackman. "It's almost like the state doesn't want to know."[11] It's hard to imagine that the health department was not aware of research that showed that maternal residential proximity within 1,000 meters of glyphosate applications occurring around the month of conception was found to be associated with an increased risk of exactly this type of devastating birth defect.[12]

Every night during the spring, if you are watching TV you will likely see an ad for Roundup, the best-known glyphosate-based herbicide (GBH). The 2020 edition of the ad had cartoon graphics on a white screen symbolizing simplicity and purity. It had a backdrop of peppy, upbeat music intended to make you feel good, comfortable, "homey," and safe. And it told you that Roundup is what you need to get those "low-down, dirty little scoundrels—weeds," and has been "trusted for over 40 years." I agree there is something low-down and dirty in those ads, but it's not the weeds.

Ironically, those ads encouraging us all to use more Roundup ran in the spring of 2020 at the very same time that Bayer, the manufacturer, had lost several individual lawsuits, most of them judgements that indeed, Roundup caused people's cancers. Numerous multi-million-dollar verdicts have already been handed down, with likely many more to come. Bayer just recently agreed to pay nearly $11 billion dollars in a class action lawsuit that charged Roundup with causing cancer. I guess they're trying to sell a lot more Roundup to pay for the judgments for the cancer they've caused with the Roundup they've already sold. As cynical and callous as that sounds, the rest of the story is just as jarring.

Glyphosate was originally patented as a chelating agent, a pipe cleaner—think of Drano. It was discovered to act as an herbicide secondarily in 1974. Its ability to bind metals is relevant to its prevention of plants' absorbing nutrients from the soil, and it also inhibits the absorption of nutrients in pregnant mothers.

Use of GBHs increased 100-fold in the 40 years after 1974.[13] It is used on 150 different crops. Even greater use in the future is expected, however, because of the rapid evolution of increasingly resistant weeds, more Roundup Ready genetically modified crops (crops planted from seeds genetically modified by the maker of Roundup to be resistant to Roundup), and the growing adoption of an industrial agriculture technique we should call "Death Star Harvesting."

More Environmental Attacks on the Brain

Roundup is being sprayed directly on crops shortly before harvest to facilitate what is referred to in the industry as a "clean harvest" (love the irony) by uniformly killing off all plants (including the crops, mind you) on the field. If maturation of the crops has been compromised by excessive moisture, as is sometimes the case, herbicides are used to bring the crops to maturity by means of a "death-spray"—Big Ag's "Death Star." The technique accelerates the drying out of the crops and kills the weeds at the same time.

For example, as late as seven days before wheat is harvested, milled into flour, and sold to bakeries, Big Ag soaks the wheat in Roundup to dress the kernels up in the appearance of uniform maturity. In today's world, "looking good" is priority number one. As for you, the consumer, it is exactly the same as adding glyphosate—again, think "poison"—as a flavoring ingredient right into the bread dough, as if it were maple syrup. If you're in the habit of having a bowl of oatmeal for breakfast and like to sprinkle it with brown sugar, maybe some raisins or sliced almonds so that it's tastier and more nutritious, know that the good folks of Quaker have already added their special ingredient. They had their corporate farm sprinkle it with a little Roundup just before the oats were harvested. GBH cannot be removed from food by washing and is not broken down by the heat from cooking or baking. Glyphosate residues in food can remain stable for at least a year, even if the foods are frozen or processed.

The Death Star strategy is now common for staples like potatoes, grains, canola, and legumes, and even for crops that are not genetically modified organisms (GMOs). To facilitate the Death Star technique, the European Union raised the legal limit of glyphosate in wheat and bakery items to 100 times the legal limit for vegetables with no scientific justification. For livestock feed grains, it was raised even more. Never mind that enforcement of even these loose limits is essentially nonexistent.

Desiccating crops with Roundup just before harvest is undoubtedly a primary reason Americans are showing more Roundup in their bodies than ever before. In the last twenty years, the number of people that test positive for the ingredients in Roundup shot up 500%, and the amount in their bodies increased more than ten times, 100 times more than what was found in lab rats, by comparison. Even more worrisome is that children are generally showing higher levels than adults. Roundup isn't just in the food you eat; it's undoubtedly in the water you drink. Tests done by the U.S. Geological Survey found glyphosate in more than 75% of rain and rainwater samples across the Midwest.[14]

The EPA under the Trump Administration showed absolutely no concern about Americans' consuming more Roundup. To be fair, the EPA under Barak Obama didn't show much either. Given the longstanding bipartisan capitulation to corporate agriculture, it remains to be seen if under a Biden Administration, EPA will be more concerned about the toxic chemicals we are subjected to from what we eat and drink.

The efficacy of glyphosate as an herbicide is the result of inhibition of a key plant enzyme, 5-enolpyruvylshikimate-3-phosphate synthase, which is involved in the synthesis of aromatic amino acids. Since this enzyme is not present in vertebrates, the sales pitch from glyphosate manufacturers has been that it would not harm humans, most of whom are vertebrates, except of course, the lizard people that have been discovered by researchers at the University of QAnon. However, QAnon zombies aren't the only ones getting this wrong. Lack of that enzyme in humans does not mean that humans can't still be harmed by glyphosate through a different mechanism than the one that kills plants, much like organophosphates are toxic to humans through an auxillary, undefined mechanism.

Furthermore, when trying to make a stew of poison, everyone knows you don't use just one ingredient. Research has shown that the non-glyphosate ingredients (adjuvants and surfactants) in formulations like Roundup may be even more toxic than the active ingredient. Concerning as well is a recent investigation that found Roundup formulations contain neurotoxic heavy metals, like arsenic, chromium, cobalt, lead and nickel.[15] It is no surprise that those commercial formulas have been shown to be more toxic than glyphosate alone,[16] undermining the contention that Roundup is not a threat to vertebrates.

In January 2020, EPA released this statement: *"EPA has concluded its regulatory review of glyphosate—the most widely used herbicide in the United States. After a thorough review of the best available science, as required under the Federal Insecticide, Fungicide, and Rodenticide Act, EPA has concluded that there are no risks of concern to human health when glyphosate is used according to the label and that it is not a carcinogen."*

The world's most expert and independent scientific body on cancer and environmental toxins, the International Agency for Research on Cancer (IARC, a branch of the World Health Organization), ruled in 2015 that GBH was a probable human carcinogen. The chemical industry went apoplectic. What the dirty, low-down scoundrels at Monsanto (bought in 2018 by Bayer) did to fight back against the IARC has been exposed in numerous articles, most comprehensively in the French magazine, *Le Monde*, and their multi-part series and documentary, *The Monsanto Papers*.[17]

The EPA has a long history, across multiple administrations of both political parties, of acting as a handmaiden of the chemical industry rather than as a guardian of public health. The extensive documentation of that dysfunctional and likely corrupt relationship has been addressed in other books. For now, suffice it to say that many independent scientists would vigorously disagree about their glyphosate conclusions and about whether EPA used the best available science.

Monsanto, now Bayer, thinks that glyphosate shouldn't be restricted at all. Monsanto has long put pressure on EPA to stop investigating the health hazards of Roundup, their flagship product. Under pressure from the chemical companies and Big Ag, EPA dramatically increased the allowable glyphosate contamination of food in 2013. The new regulation raised permitted levels anywhere from 2 to 25 times higher than previous safety thresholds depending on the type of crop. There was no scientific "Paul on the road to Damascus" moment that justified the changes, just industry pressure.

The Great Brain Robbery – Brian Moench

On a wide array of issues, California has a long history of being more proactive in protecting public health from environmental toxins. California's proposed No Risk Level for glyphosate consumption is 1.1 mg daily for an adult weighing 70 kg (~150 lbs). The EPA Reference Dose (supposedly safe level) is 2 mg per kg. For a 70 kg person, that is 140 mg a day, or 127 times higher than California's safe level. The Environmental Working Group believes that even California's limit is 100 times too high, especially to protect children and developing fetuses. Any rule inadequate to protect a fetus is inadequate to protect society at large and is a moral and scientific failure.

The research EPA has used for establishing supposedly safe amounts of GBH for human consumption, such as through traditional toxicology risk assessments, is largely 30 years old.[18] The overwhelming majority of the studies used to establish glyphosate's safety were company funded, unpublished, and non-peer-reviewed. In those 30 years since, scientific methods have actually advanced; perhaps that's news to EPA. More than 1,500 studies on glyphosate have been published in just the last ten years, but these have been largely ignored in safety evaluations. An essay in one of the most respected medical journals in the world says, "It is incongruous that safety assessments of the most widely used herbicide on the planet rely largely on fewer than 300 unpublished, non-peer-reviewed studies while excluding the vast, modern literature on glyphosate effects."[19]

Thanks to the extremely loose federal regulatory standards, the acceptable level of glyphosate in U.S. drinking water is an absurd 700 ppb, 7,000 times more than the permitted level in Europe of 0.1 ppb. Even at Europe's "acceptable level," genotoxicity and organ damage in animals has been found.

Roundup causes liver and kidney damage in rats via changes in the functions of 4,000 genes at exposure levels of only 0.05 ppb. Cheerios breakfast cereal has been found to have glyphosate residues as high as 1,125.3 ppb.[20] At that concentration, you might just as well sprinkle Cheerios over your yard to kill the weeds rather than spraying Roundup. GMO soybeans, a ubiquitous ingredient in processed foods on nearly every shelf of every grocery store in the country, have been found to be contaminated with an average of 11,900 ppb.[21] Even Monsanto considers residue levels of 5,600 ppb to be extreme.[22]

Virtually every human tested has shown Roundup in their urine at concentrations between 5 and 20 times the level considered safe for drinking water.[23] Roundup has been classified by EPA as "low toxicity," and they have resolutely refused to join the IARC in ruling glyphosate a probable human carcinogen. But as I noted, that is more a result of the chemical industry's capturing the levers of the government's regulatory infrastructure than an expression of independent and objective science. Much like the targeted weeds, numerous, persistent, and troublesome health consequences have emerged between the cracks in industry's narrative.

The likely health consequences of GBH compounds are widespread and involve most major organ systems. But you might have noticed that this book is about the brain, so I'll focus just on the neurologic outcomes. Numerous animal and tissue studies have found diminished neuronal cell count, decreased cellular glutathione content, excitotoxicity, degeneration of neurons, and numerous developmental brain abnormalities related to GBH exposure.[24] Clinical outcomes for humans include increased risk of ADHD, Alzheimer's, anencephaly, autism, brain cancer, depression, ALS, multiple sclerosis, and Parkinson's. Many of these disorders are related to glyphosate's endocrine disruption action.

The National Socialist German Workers' Party sounds like it might be a solid advocate for worker's rights. But known by its other name its true identity is easily revealed; the Nazi Party. Likewise, The *Genetic Literacy Project (GLP): Science not Ideology,* sounds like an altruistic, credible organization, just trying to help make the peasantry scientifically literate. The GLP is, in fact, the opposite; a chemical industry front group. You can pick any name you want, but that doesn't change who you are. It repeats the standard industry line that glyphosate "undergoes little metabolism in the human body. If accidentally consumed, glyphosate is excreted mostly unchanged in feces and urine, so it doesn't stay in the body and accumulate." If that were true, then you wouldn't see effects like this: several studies found that "glyphosate residues in the kidney, liver and lung were comparable to those found in the urine."[25] Animals exposed to low doses of glyphosate in adolescence showed altered activity levels, malabsorption of nutrients, weight loss, and failure of the critical organs, including the brain, to grow to a normal size and weight.[26] Indeed, it is safe to say the chemical is certainly affecting these animals, contrary to the claims of the GLP. Similar experiments with other pesticides—deltamethrin, fenvalerate, and diazinon—showed similar results.[27]

Male lab animals prenatally exposed to glyphosate showed immediate decreased overall activity in the womb.[28] Studies in animals show that glyphosate increases glutamate levels, which provokes excitotoxicity and oxidative stress in parts of the brain.[29] Parents who frequently use pesticides at home or are occupationally exposed, have nearly double the risk of their child having a brain tumor.[30] Rats exposed to glyphosate showed decreased levels of the neurotransmitters 5-HT and dopamine in several areas of the brain and depressive behavior.[31]

> The Fake News Media is spreading the lie that this book, the most tremendous book in the history of books, did not win the Pulitzer Prize. Everyone knows that this book won by a lot, but the vote was rigged by very corrupt people that allowed millions of literary scholars to pour across our border to vote against it. So we have to ban all the other books but this one, or we won't have a country any more.

Laboratory studies of the microscopic effects of Roundup formulations showed a significant demyelination effect on nerve cells.[32] There is strong evidence that glyphosate shifts the balance between beneficial and pathogenic microorganisms in the GI tract to favor the pathogenic organisms. The medical dictionary word for it is dysbiosis. The overgrowth of pathogenic intestinal bacteria can generate toxic metabolites that have neurologic consequences.[33]

As yet, there is not enough research to determine whether GBHs cause more neurotoxicity in males compared to females.

NEONICOTINOIDS

In the last 15 years, neonicotinoids (neonics) have become the most widely used insecticides in the world. They are nicotine analogues, so they act like super-charged nicotine (think of insects flying around smoking 100 packs of cigarettes in an hour), and bind permanently to nicotinic acetylcholine receptors in the central nervous system of insects. They quickly trigger overstimulation of nerve cells, paralysis, and death. As pointed out with organophosphates, mammals have those same acetylcholine receptors, so again, it is easy to see that they might be toxic to humans as well.

Crop seeds are treated with neonics prior to planting. As a result of that process, the pesticides become systemic, meaning they permeate the entire plant from the roots to the stems, flowers, and leaves. They are highly mobile and have relatively long environmental half-lives in water and soil. Neonicotinoid residues are present in most edible parts of fruits and vegetables unless they are organic. Washing them off does nothing to remove the chemicals before you eat the produce. Neonics have contaminated almost all the consumable corn in the U.S. and a large percentage of soybeans.

As with most of the other pesticides, the greatest concern about human toxicity pertains to the intrauterine stage of brain development. Studies in mammals found that exposure to neonics can harm brain development by inhibiting the growth of neurons and the action of microglia.[34] In 2013, The European Food Safety Authority ruled that neonicotinamides may adversely affect the development of neurons and brain structures in unborn babies.

PETS AND PESTICIDES

The EPA banned many of the pesticides used in flea and tick treatments from other household uses years ago but overlooked them in pet products. Neonics, pyrethroids, and organophosphates are just some of the pesticides used by manufacturers of flea and tick collars that pet owners drape around their cats' and dogs' necks. Most pet owners have no idea that these collars are impregnated with pesticides that eventually spread throughout the household. That is a particular risk for children, who are invariably in close contact with the pets and who often put their hands in their mouths after petting an animal. High levels of pesticides can remain on a pet's fur for weeks after a collar is applied. Young children are particularly susceptible to conventional pesticides' effects because their nervous systems and brains are still developing, and their ability to metabolize these chemicals is weaker than in adults.

The nervous system of pest insects is the intended target of these insecticides, but beneficial insects, such as pollinators, are just as vulnerable. They disrupt the bees' homing behavior and their ability to return to the hive. "Bee Autism" is a perfect description of what these pesticides do to bees (see Chapter 8). Chemicals that interrupt electrical impulses in insect nerves will do the same to humans. Just like nicotine can disrupt brain development in humans, these nicotine analogues can as well.

But you may think to yourself, humans are much bigger than insects, and the doses to humans are miniscule, right? It is worth repeating that during critical first trimester development, a human is no larger than many insects. There is every reason to conclude that pesticides could wreak havoc with the developing brain of a human embryo.

Because of the mounting evidence of toxicity to beneficial insects and humans, the European Union banned these insecticides. In the U.S., the EPA under the last two administrations made no such move; it remains to be seen what the Biden Administration will do.

THIS IS YOUR BRAIN ON RADIATION

Ionizing radiation (IR) includes a group of subatomic particles and electromagnetic waves, or photons, which are capable of creating electrically charged particles such as alpha and beta particles, gamma rays, and X-rays, causing ionization of atoms, altering molecules, affecting cells, impairing tissue function, and harming organ function. Radiation increases DNA damage and mutations, changes gene expression, alters levels of cellular proliferation, and causes apoptosis. Unless you are Bruce Banner (and the Incredible Hulk for 20 hours per week, with no benefits), radiation at any level is a threat to your health, including your brain.

Radiation damage is cumulative, and each successive dose builds upon the cellular mutation caused by all the previous exposures. It can take years for radiation damage to manifest pathology. The genetic mutations cause endocrine and immune disease, heart and lung disease, birth defects, and cancer.

A new study suggests nuclear radiation causes slightly more boys than girls to be born. While effects were seen to be regional for incidents on the ground, like Chernobyl, atmospheric blasts were found to affect birth rates on a global scale.[1] The likely cause is that eggs insulate their chromosomes better than sperm. Because the sex of the baby is determined by the father, that means both the X and Y chromosomes from the male are more at risk for radiation damage. Furthermore, the X chromosome is a much larger target for radiation. That means a damaged X from the father is more likely to be fatal to a female embryo. This is strong evidence of damage to humankind's genetic pool by ionizing radiation.

Radiation-induced genetic mutations tend to be recessive, and in those cases, the large majority of genetic damage does not become manifest until several generations after exposure. Many of the diseases caused by radiation were found in the children and grandchildren of those exposed, i.e., soldiers, uranium miners, workers at uranium mills, radium factories, the Manhattan Project, Nevada Testing Range, and nuclear submarines. According to many scientists, like Dr. Arthur Upton, director of the National Cancer Institute, and the scientists that wrote the seventh report of the National Academy of Sciences (BEIR [biologic effects of ionizing radiation] VII), as is the case with many other environmental toxins, there is no safe level of exposure to radiation.

The BEIR VII report is widely considered the gold standard analysis of the health threat of radiation. The fundamental precept established by the report is the linear no-threshold (LNT) assumption, meaning there is no level of radiation below which it can be written off as safe. Most of the attention given to radiation's risks focuses on cancer. But because radiation has broad impacts on the integrity and expression of genes, the health effects extend far beyond cancer.

Hermann Muller, winner of the 1943 Nobel Prize for discovering the genetic mutations caused by x-rays, wrote a paper in 1964 titled, *Radiation and Heredity,* predicting the gradual reduction of the survivability of the human species as the exposure to ionizing radiation from numerous sources increased. Throughout the Western world, sperm counts are dropping,[2] likely due to many environmental factors that Muller didn't anticipate, but one of which is radiation exposure that he warned about. Fertility rates are dropping precipitously, below replacement levels,[3] likely due to both environmental and socio-economic factors. The trend indicates that by the end of the 21st century, every country in the world will see a declining population. In 1950, women were giving birth to an average 4.7 children in their lifetime (not sure what a .7 child looks like, other than a couple of my buddies in high school). If that number falls below 2.1, the population will decline. Fertility rates are on pace to fall to 1.7 by 2100. If all that were simply a matter of choice, some may interpret that as good news, in that the world's population would peak at around 9.7 billion by 2064. But the reasons for that decline are likely not good news.

About one in eight couples in the U.S. are having difficulty conceiving or sustaining a pregnancy,[4] and environmental toxins are likely culprits. Toxins not only decrease natural fertility but also make in vitro fertilization (IVF) much less likely to succeed. Toxins, like chemicals and radiation, can affect fertility in four different ways: endocrine disruption, damage to the female reproductive system, damage to the male reproductive system, and impaired fetal viability.[5]

One of the most sinister and egregious examples of government authorities' willingness to knowingly harm public health for a feeble rationalization was the way the federal government's AEC conducted the Nevada nuclear testing program. The only military force that ever dropped nuclear bombs on American citizens was their own government.

More Environmental Attacks on the Brain

The Korean War prompted the federal government to move their nuclear weapons testing program from the Pacific Ocean in favor of a less expensive, continental location. A site 65 miles north of Las Vegas, Nevada, was chosen for multiple reasons: the sparse population, prevailing easterly winds that would normally blow towards another sparsely populated state, Utah, and hundreds of miles of flat, government-controlled land.

On January 27, 1951, a one-kiloton bomb was dropped from an airplane and exploded over Frenchman Flat, launching America's post–Manhattan Project domestic nuclear testing program, which continued until 1992. In those four decades, 1,021 nuclear bombs were donated, including 100 atmospheric tests during the first 12 years. Even the underground tests released radioactivity into the atmosphere. One of the largest underground detonations left a crater 320 ft deep and 1,280 ft wide, displacing 12 million tons of earth. The AEC assured the public that the tests would be conducted "with adequate assurances of safety." Declassified documents revealed that the federal government knew even before the bombs were dropped on Japan that radioactive products of nuclear fission were deadly carcinogens, and they could spread over thousands of miles. Yet not only were they undeterred, not only did they make no effort to protect or warn the public, they waged a deliberate campaign of deceit and denial about the danger.

In the early part of the program American troops were often deliberately placed within a few miles of "ground zero" of the tests, acting as guinea pigs so the armed forces could assess how the soldiers would react psychologically. Within hours of the explosions, many of them were ordered to conduct war games at the actual ground zero sites, including parachuting directly into the sites. In all, hundreds of thousands of U.S. soldiers were exposed. Many others were similarly exposed decades later during cleanup operations of the explosion sites at the Marshall Islands in the Pacific. Years later, America's "atomic vets" suffered a wide array of medical problems, especially cancer. Some eventually received government compensation. Many of their children and grandchildren have suffered similar maladies as well as birth defects, but the government essentially washed their hands of any responsibility to the progeny of our atomic vets.

For years, radioactivity drifted over the entire United States. Most of the entire population of the United States, 160 million people, were exposed to some degree. The youngest children were the most at risk. Residents of my home state of Utah undoubtedly received the highest doses. Those conducting the tests routinely waited to make sure that the prevailing winds would carry the radioactive isotopes towards Utah rather than further south toward Las Vegas, or west toward Southern California. The unwritten implication was that Utahns were more expendable in the name of national security.

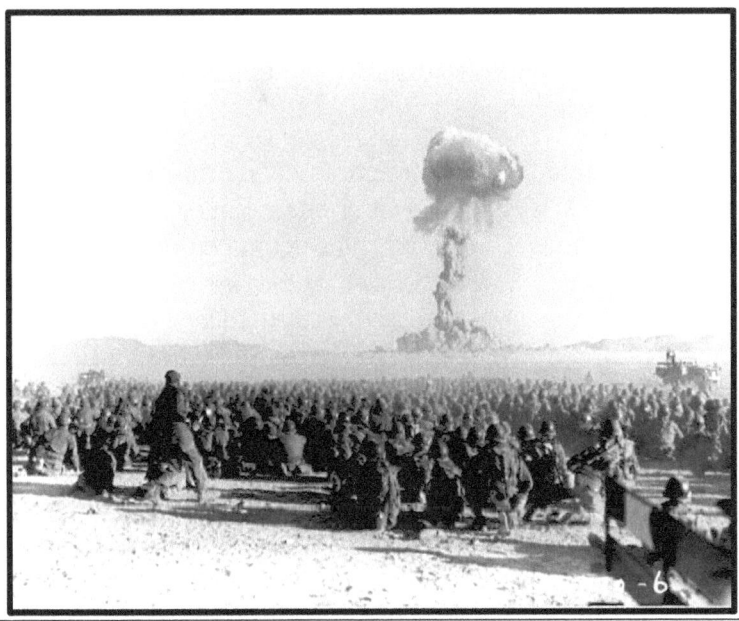

Operation Buster-Jangle Dog test, at the Nevada Test Site, November 1, 1951, with troops participating in exercise Desert Rock afterward. It was the first U.S. nuclear field exercise conducted on land. Troops shown are only 6 miles from the blast. After detonation, troops were ordered to move toward the blast site. The advance was halted when troops were 900 meters from ground zero.

One of the small Utah cities in the most direct path of much of the fallout was St. George, 144 miles from the Nevada test site.

More Environmental Attacks on the Brain

St. George residents could feel the percussion of some of the blasts, and they could see the intense glow on the western horizon. Hours later radioactive debris would fall down upon the residents. The government announced over the radio to St. George residents that the radiation was safe. Nearly half a century later, a study of 102 samples of soil in the area found Cesium^{137} (one of the more toxic of radionuclides) in every sample but one, giving strong evidence that the damage to public health continues.

Cancer receives the most attention for radiation-induced disease, but it is long overdue that we look at the evidence of radiation's effects on the central nervous system. Those effects include cell death, altered migration of neurons, impaired capacity to establish correct connections among cells, and/or alterations in dendritic development. These structural changes are associated with behavioral and cognitive disorders manifesting themselves in adolescence or adulthood.

In 1957, the largest amount of nuclear radiation measured in the United States was spread over the country from the highest kilotonnage of nuclear weapons ever detonated at the Nevada test site. Radioactive iodine, I^{131}, was taken up by the thyroids of pregnant mothers where it would retard their growth and brain development of their babies in utero even if only slightly. Eighteen years later, in 1975, when these children took the SAT tests, the percentage drop in scores nationwide, from the year before, was the largest ever seen in one year. The New York Times article that reported the drop in test scores dealt with the information by raising just about every other possible explanation—deterioration of American schools, too much TV watching, not enough discipline and studying by the students, more disadvantaged students taking the test, and civil unrest over the Vietnam War.[6] The decline raised public alarm such that a commission was appointed by then Secretary of Labor, Willard Wirtz, to study the possible causes. Two years later, the commission came up empty handed. But they failed to consider what is, in retrospect, the most likely explanation. A pretty clear pattern emerged on closer examination and in the following years.

The Great Brain Robbery –Brian Moench

In 1963, 18 years after the first Nevada nuclear test was detonated in 1945, national SAT scores given to high school seniors started to decline slightly, 2-3 points on average. It also happened that after decades of steady decline, in the early 1950s, during the heaviest nuclear testing fallout, national infant mortality rates stopped declining. Rates of birth defects and infant mortality spiked in 1957. The plot further thickened. Between 1959 and 1961, a truce on nuclear testing was reached, and 17-18 years later, in 1976 and 1977, verbal SATs only dropped three and then two points.

Nuclear fallout was not evenly distributed throughout the country, nor was the drop in SAT scores. Comparing 1976 SAT scores with 1975 scores, Western states, i.e., those closest to Nevada, saw a drop of 19 points in the verbal test, compared to 9 points in the Midwest, 13 points in the MidAtlantic states, and 13 points in the South. Again, this followed the pattern of nuclear fallout not just from Nevada, but also from the Pacific and from Siberia.

The results from individual states, however, were truly alarming. The most immediate downwind state from the Nevada test site was Utah, my home state, where the drop in verbal SAT scores was a shocking 26 points. The fallout pattern then went north but largely spared Ohio, where the drop was only two points. As Dr. Ernest Sternglass said, "There was just no way that such an enormous difference in the sudden drop could be explained solely by socio-economic factors, differences in the quality of teachers, school curricula, television viewing, amount of cigarette smoking, drug use, alcohol consumption, or other gradually changing physical factors in the environment such as air pollution or pesticides."

In fact, Utah, with its heavily Mormon population, had an advantage over other states in almost every one of those other potential confounding sociologic variables, as Mormons typically avoided tobacco, alcohol, and recreational drugs. Furthermore, in SAT tests taken in 1963, Utah had by far the highest verbal SAT score average of any state, 532, perhaps because of those advantages. Eighteen years before was the last year before the nuclear testing era began.

More Environmental Attacks on the Brain

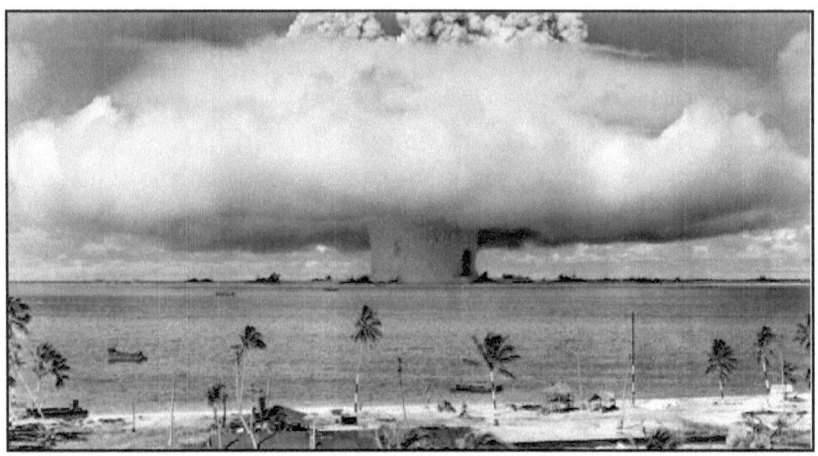

The Castle Bravo hydrogen bomb sent waves of radioactive fallout over much of the continental United States.

This followed a pattern seen elsewhere and in other years with radiation exposure. In 1954, on the Bikini Atoll near the Marshall Islands, the U.S. blew up the Castle Bravo hydrogen bomb, 1,000 times more powerful than the bomb dropped on Hiroshima. The island has been uninhabitable since. On the island of Rongelap, 150 miles away, virtually all the children developed thyroid disease, showed significant growth retardation in their bodies overall, and had much smaller brains.

But the damage was felt far beyond the Pacific Ocean. For American students born in 1952-53, 189,300 students scored above 600 in the verbal test. For those born in 1957-58 there were only 110,300, a drop of 42%. The number of students scoring over 700 saw an even steeper decline: 33,200 fell to only 14,800 for those born in 1957-58, the years of the heaviest fallout from our weapons testing.

Prior to the signing of the atmospheric nuclear test ban treaty, a second wave of nuclear testing occurred in 1962. Seventeen years later, in 1979, the same pattern emerged. Utah showed the largest drop in SAT scores of any state, 11 points, and the drop declined the further away from Utah that the students were. For example, New York dropped 5 points, Connecticut, 3 points, and Rhode Island just 1 point. For those children born well after 1963, when atmospheric testing in Nevada ended, the decline in mental acuity had ceased. Fewer children were born with birth defects, and there were fewer cases of childhood leukemia and brain tumors.

A 2007 study of Swedish children exposed to fallout from Chernobyl as fetuses between 8 weeks and 25 weeks gestation found that the reduction in IQ at very low doses was greater than expected, given a simple LNT (linear, no threshold) model for radiation damage. This indicated that the LNT model may be too conservative when it comes to neurological damage.[7] Studying patients in Norway after the Chernobyl accident, researchers found that low-level radiation exposure before 16 weeks gestation showed a loss of verbal IQ measured at adolescence.[8] Forty-five percent of children born to mothers surviving Hiroshima and Nagasaki showed intellectual impairment. There is little research that has been able to differentiate the neurologic consequences between males and females.

A study of Gulf War veterans who have depleted uranium shrapnel in their bodies showed that they test more poorly on general brain cognitive exams of "performance efficiency and accuracy."[9] Females and children are considered more sensitive to radiation's overall health consequences, cancer vulnerability in particular. Nonetheless, female mice are better at reducing neuronal damage from radiation. Microglia from female animals are more adept at reducing ischemic damage, as shown by transplanting female microglia into male brains depleted of microglia.[10]

Studying low-dose scatter irradiation from x-rays, researchers found anatomic changes occurred in the morphology of neurons in the prefrontal cortex of females but not males. On the other hand, in a different area of the brain, the hippocampus, the males were affected but not females,[11] suggesting that male mice have a more pro-inflammatory immune response. A few other studies have shown the brains of female animals are more affected than those of males.

Sex differences aside for the moment, all this research should have implications for physicians and their eagerness to order high-radiation exams like CAT scans. Those exams have become the go-to investigative tool for just about every symptom a person in the emergency room might have. For example, they are the preferred tool now used to diagnose appendicitis. Because of trends like this, the average person's lifetime dose of diagnostic radiation has increased seven-fold since 1980. The number of scans has increased about 30 times over that time period. Diagnostic imaging has become an industry worth more than a $100 billion. The FDA believes 30-50% of CAT scans are unneeded.[12] This is a particularly acute issue for children because they are at greater risk for radiation-related disease, especially cancer. Radiation from CAT scans can vary widely depending on technique, equipment, and the skill of the technician. On average, a CAT scan uses the radiation equivalent of about 200 chest x-rays. CAT scans cause as much as 2% of all cancers, nearly 30,000 cases, and 15,000 deaths annually.[13]

Healthcare workers are often not as careful as they should be in covering up the parts of the body that don't need to be x-rayed with lead shields, unnecessarily increasing exposure. During the nearly 40,000 surgeries I have been a part of during my career, I have observed that the physicians and operating room personnel have often been too cavalier about the radiation exposure of patients, staff, colleagues, and even themselves.

A few years ago, my eight-year-old granddaughter fell in a playground, broke her elbow, and needed a surgical repair. I had to go over with the charge nurse, the surgeon, and the anesthesiologist how I wanted her entire body covered with lead except where the break was because I had seen far too many examples where those precautions were not taken. Avoiding exposing children to radiation is even more important than exposing adults because they have longer post-exposure lifespans, and therefore, more cellular divisions at risk for carcinogenic mutations. Furthermore, radiation exposure to the gonads of males or females prior to conception may cause infertility, miscarriages, birth defects, or other genetic mutations in future generations.

In my experience, total radiation exposure is seldom a part of the conversation or consideration by healthcare providers when deciding among diagnostic options. It is long overdue that our healthcare system pays as much attention to patients' history of cumulative radiation exposure as they do their vaccine, medication, and family histories.

Radiation toxicity has implications for nuclear power, because every single stage of the nuclear fuel cycle—from the mining of uranium to the milling, concentration, and production of nuclear fuel rods, the routine operation of the nuclear plant, and the unsolvable problem of long-term storing of nuclear waste— releases radioactivity into the general environment, exposing all of us.

In the climax of the popular 2023 movie, *Oppenheimer*, J. Robert Oppenheimer asks Albert Einstein if he remembers a conversation they had in the past—one depicted earlier in the movie—where some of the Manhattan scientists calculated that there was at least a small possibility that detonating an atomic bomb could wind up igniting the earth's atmosphere, destroying every living thing on earth. "I remember it well," Einstein says. "What of it?" Oppenheimer replys, "I believe we did." While nuclear war is obviously the implied apocalypse in that conversation, the spin off of the nuclear weapons industry, the nuclear power industry, may end up coming just as close to accomplishing the apocalypse of "destroying every living thing on earth" as nuclear weapons.

CELL PHONE RADIATION

Cell phones send signals back and forth from nearby cell towers (base stations) using radio frequency waves. Cell phones emit pulsed microwave radiation, a form of energy in the electromagnetic spectrum that falls between FM radio waves and microwaves. Older 2G, 3G, and 4G technology emits RFR (radio frequency radiation) in the range of 700 to 2,700 MHz (microwaves), which can penetrate 3-4 inches into the human body. The fifth generation of cell phone technology, 5G, is the presumed future of cell phone technology, and that will include the lower frequency radiation of older technology, but will also expose users to frequencies as high as 60,000 MHz. This allows the transmission of much more and faster data, like 1-10 gigabytes per second. That's an ability to download an entire plotless, poorly acted Hollywood movie within a minute.

Five G will use new "beam-forming" antenna that create multiple signal streams from each fixture. Each installation site may have over a thousand antennas that are transmitting simultaneously, creating radiation that will be difficult to even measure. You cannot turn a cell tower off. FiveG and 4G cell towers near homes and apartments means constant exposure, 24/7, 365 days a year.

Nonetheless, despite industry claims that 5G will be faster, 5G is turning out to be no faster or even slower than 4G. So far 5G is bringing no communication benefit, but is bringing increased health hazard. Numerous cites and local governments throughout the world are trying to halt the deployment of 5G due to health and safety concerns. For example, in Italy over 600 cities have passed such resoutions.

Given the reduced reach of much higher frequency radiation, 5G technology will require orders of magnitude more cell antennas, approximately one every 100 to 200 meters, which is around 800,000 new antenna sites, literally in many backyards. Proximity to a radiation source is proportional to risk. Other new technological features of 5G will include such things as active antennas and massive inputs and outputs, all of which will expose many more people to millimeter wave radiation.

These higher frequencies (also called millimeter waves) travel shorter distances and do not penetrate the body as much as lower-frequency wavelengths; they go only few millimeters into the skin and the cornea. But that means more concentrated energy, and therefore risk, in shallower areas. Generally speaking, the higher the frequency, the more damage the radiation can do.

Unfortunately, scientific research on cell phones is often dominated by large telecom companies who have a vested interest in the outcome and control the research agenda, the funding, and the release of the results. Almost all the studies sponsored by industry show no health risk from cell phones. Almost all the independent studies in animals and humans have much different results. Any cancer or other health effects demonstrated to be caused in animals, especially mammals, should be assumed to be caused in humans until proven otherwise.

Neither 4G or 5G have been studied much for their possible effects on human health. Researchers found a ten times higher rate of broken DNA with the new 3G phones compared to 2G.[15] If there are synergistic effects from simultaneous exposures to multiple types of RFR, our overall risk of harm from RFR may increase substantially with the widespread deployment of 5G.

New phones are smaller, and they come with three or four antennas (for GPS, e-mail, phone, texting) built directly into their backs. In other words, the more bells and whistles and the more power to your phone, the more exposure to RFR inside the brain, and the greater the danger. Another reason for concern is that the cell phone radiation test used by the FCC is based on the devices' possible effect on large adults, not children. Children's skulls are thinner and can absorb about twice as much radiation as an adult. The bone marrow in a young child's skull can absorb up to ten times more radiation than adults can. This is obviously of concern with the cultural trend of more and more children having access to cell phones, almost before the umbilical cord is clamped.

Radio frequencies can unleash free radicals, disrupting the cellular bonds that hold molecules together. That means they can alter living cells, creating the types of damage known to cause cancer and neurologic disease.

RFR from a phone held to the head is absorbed by the brain and can induce local changes in cell membranes. This facilitates the passage of electrically charged particles in and out of nerve cells, and in electrical brain activity measured by electroencephalogram (EEG).[16] It is well established that holding a cell phone to the head heats up brain tissue.[17] Cell phone radiation increases the permeability of the BBB, which allows more toxins in the blood to reach brain tissue,[18] and breaks DNA bonds proportional to the amount of exposure.[19] Eighty percent of the radiation absorbed comes from holding the phone to the head, and the right side of the head, for unknown reasons, seems to be more vulnerable. One study showed that holding the phone pressed against the ear increases the metabolism and energy demands of the brain next to it. In the region of the brain closest to a cell phone's antenna, a significant increase in glucose metabolism occurred when the phone was turned on and held next to the head for 50 minutes.[20]

Recall that autophagy is the medical dictionary term for physiological garbage collecting. Damaged or aged cells or cell components need to be cleaned up to maintain organ function and good health. Circumstantial evidence of the biologic stress and damage done by cell phone radiation is revealed by an increase in autophagy in various areas of the brain in animals exposed to cell phone radiation.[21]

Recall as well that like electrical wires, nerve cells need insulation. Specialized Schwann cells form the myelin sheath to provide that insulation, which is very important in both the development and function of a healthy brain and nervous system. Exposure to cell phone radiation damages the myelin sheaths in the brains of animals.[22]

How do these changes at the microscopic level translate into clinical outcomes? Studies in animals and humans paint a disturbing picture. A study in mice showed that prenatal exposure to cell phone radiation resulted in hyperactivity and impaired memory.[23] Other studies in rats showed prenatal and postnatal exposure to wireless radiation caused damage to the brain and a decrease in the number of brain cells.[24]

Researchers found decreased figural memory among teenagers with higher cell phone exposures to the brain after one year of repeated exposure. Figural memory is primarily located in the right hemisphere, and the memory loss was more pronounced in those adolescents that used the phone on the right side of the head. Notably, non-call cell phone usage, i.e., texts, playing games, and internet browsing, did not impair memory.[25] Extensive use of cell phones in medical students impairs their ability to concentrate and their ability to suppress competing stimuli.[26] Clinical studies have found a correlation between cell phone usage and a wide range of neuropsychiatric disorders.[27] Several studies have shown that cell phone use can magnify the neurotoxic effects of other known brain toxins, such as lead.[28] Short-term cell phone radiation exposure can have adverse physiological effects in the peripheral nervous system, the immune system, and the cardiovascular system.[29]

Numerous independent studies have shown increased rates of cancer with long-term cell phone radiation, especially brain cancer and other cancers of the head and neck. That fact is made even more remarkable given that solid tumors typically take decades to develop. For example, the increase in brain tumors that were caused in survivors of the atomic bombs dropped on Nagasaki and Hiroshima did not show up in significant numbers until 40 years later.

In 2018, the NTP concluded that their research showed there is clear evidence that high levels of the type of radiation used in 2G and 3G technology precipitated malignant tumors (Schwannomas) of the heart in rats but only in males.[30] They described some evidence for causing brain tumors (malignant gliomas), and benign and malignant tumors of the adrenal glands in male rats. They also found that three regions of the brain, the liver, and blood cells all showed DNA damage from cell-phone radiation. More specifically, the study found DNA damage in the frontal cortex and hippocampus of only male rats and in the blood cells of female rats. The highly respected Ramazzini Institute in Italy confirmed the principal finding of the NTP using a different carrier frequency and even much weaker cell phone radiation over the life of the rats.

In 2011, the WHO classified cell phone radiation as a Class 2 B Carcinogen "possibly carcinogenic to humans"—in the same category as lead, engine exhaust, DDT, and jet fuel. Almost certainly it deserves a higher classification.

If a person starts as a teenager, after more than 10 years of cell phone use, the risk increases for multiple cancers, especially brain cancer.[31] Cell phone use for ten years increases the rate of acoustic neuroma 250%, and cancer of the pituitary gland 200% after only five years of use.[32] Several other studies have shown increased rates of malignant and non-malignant brain tumors among people who began using cell phones before adulthood.[33]

More Environmental Attacks on the Brain

Cell phone radiation causes significant decreases in sperm counts and quality of sperm, decreases in testosterone and male fertility, and changes in testicular architecture.[34] Use by pregnant women may result in learning disabilities and attention deficit/hyperactivity disorder in the children to whom they give birth.[35] This is another manifestation of fetal brains being especially vulnerable to neurotoxins. Because female eggs are especially sensitive to radiation, even third generations are at risk.

Most cell phones come with this warning: "Do not hold closer than one inch from your body," the same warning that comes with a hot dog from your local 7-11. It is notable that insurance companies refuse to provide insurance coverage to cell phone companies. All radio frequency can pass unnoticed through anything not encased in metal and deposit energy into anything that contains water, i.e. all human tissue. The current worldwide recommended maximum exposure for man-made RFR is over one trillion times the natural level that we were exposed to 100 years ago.

The FCC has failed to update the RFR exposure limits they adopted in the 1990s, which was based on research from the 1980s. The research used to set those limits assumed the length of a call to be 6 minutes, virtually irrelevant to how cell phones are used now, and were based on the radiation impact on a large, adult male, which hardly represents the vulnerability of the entire population, especially children. Since then, the majority of more than 500 studies have found harmful biologic or health effects from exposure to RFR at intensities below those known to cause significant heating, which had been the presumed mechanism of physical harm from RFR.[36]

More than 246 scientists who are likely the world's experts on the biologic and health effects of non-ionizing electromagnetic fields (EMF), and have published over 2,000 peer-reviewed research papers on the issue, signed the International EMF Scientist Appeal that calls for stronger exposure limits on cell phone radiation[36] and a halt to the deployment of more 5G infrastructure until more research is done.[37] They are concerned about characteristics of the cell phone signal not yet considered for their health impact, like pulsing and polarization. They said:

> *Numerous recent scientific publications have shown that EMF affects living organisms at levels well below most international and national guidelines. Effects include increased cancer risk, cellular stress, increase in harmful free radicals, genetic damages, structural and functional changes of the reproductive system, learning and memory deficits, neurological disorders, and negative impacts on general well-being in humans. Damage goes well beyond the human race, as there is growing evidence of harmful effects to both plant and animal life.*[38]

Many of these scientists believe that cell phone radiation deserves a higher risk classification for causing cancer. Of course, you haven't heard any of that on the jazzy TV ads extolling the unmitigated virtues of 5G. Just "Trust us: it will all be fine."

The American Academy of Pediatrics has warned about the danger of cellular radiation, linked to headaches, memory deficits, dizziness, sleep disorders, and depression.

In 2024, Dr. Devra Davis, of the Environmental Health Trust, slammed the National Toxicology Program of the National Institute of Environmental Health Sciences after they very quietly disclosed that they will stop studying the biological and environmental impacts of cell phone radiation. "This decision comes despite results from the program's carefully engineered and reviewed decade-long $30 million animal studies that found cancer, heart damage and DNA damage associated with exposure to cell phone radiofrequency radiation at levels comparable to those experienced by Americans today."[39]

The behavioral advice of non-industry funded experts to protect yourself from cellular radiation includes:

- Do not hold a cell phone up to your head.

- Use the speaker option, ear pieces, or Bluetooth.
- Do not keep it on your body, i.e., in your pocket or if you are a woman, in your bra.
- If you have to carry it on your body, have the keypad facing toward you because the antennas are on the back side.
- Pregnant women should not use it or carry it on their abdomen.
- Try hard to not use it inside a car or other areas with weak signals.
- Don't leave it near your bed while you sleep, and never put it under your pillow.

Volkswagen of Europe has warned that cell phone usage inside a car can be "injurious to health due to the extremely high electromagnetic fields generated." Parents should significantly limit cell phone use by children. Most of the research on the neurotoxicity of cell phone radiation does not differentiate between the sexes, but the majority of the ones that do show a greater effect on males, consistent with most of the other toxins addressed in this book.

BPA AND OTHER ENDOCRINE DISRUPTORS

In the previous chapter, I mentioned that wholesale contamination of the global environment with toxic chemicals justifies renaming Earth, the Chemosphere. We could just as well rename it the Plasticsphere.

Microplastics have so thoroughly penetrated all ecosystems that our food, water, and air is contaminated with nano-sized plastic particles. Some of the first places that microplastics were found in wild animals were in birds, insects, and fish, where one study found it caused neurotoxicity.[1] It would be naive to think that somehow this contamination bypasses humans. Rest assured, it does not. The average person inhales and ingests, at a minimum, 50,000 particles of microplastics per year.[2] Like glyphosate, it is even contaminating rain water. As microplastics are found in human stool,[3] it is obvious they arrive there by ingestion, but also by inhalation.

In a 2024 published study, researched found microplastics and nanoplastics embedded in the carotid artery [main artery to the brain] plaques removed for stroke prevention in the majority of the patients. Electron microscopy revealed "visible, jagged edged particles" embedded in the plaques. Those patients had a significantly higher risk of subsequent heart attack, stroke, or death.[19]

Human organs are now ubiquitously contaminated with nano-sized plastic particles. Researchers looked at 47 samples of human organs and tissue in a tissue bank and found microplastics in every single sample from every single organ. Just as alarming, they found the plasticizer, endocrine disrupting chemical, bisphenol A (BPA), in every tissue sample as well.[4] Hundreds of chemicals fall into the category of endocrine disruptors, meaning they mimic or block endogenous human hormones like estrogen, testosterone, and thyroid hormones. Your home is full of them, your bathroom and kitchen especially. Unfortunately, your body is as well. It is impossible to address all the research on each chemical, so I'll focus on one of the most well-known, most controversial, and most thoroughly studied.

Bisphenol A (BPA) was first synthesized in 1891 with the intention of making a drug that mimicked estrogen. It is little wonder, then, that when it was ultimately found to be useful in making hard plastic, epoxies, and resins, that it behaved as its original research suggested, like estrogen. As a primary substrate for numerous synthetic, polycarbonate plastics, it was commercially produced in the early 1950s. It is a clear solid, making objects almost shatterproof, and it has become one of the highest-volume chemicals in production. It became a ubiquitous part of a wide variety of consumer products—water bottles, food and beverage can linings, flooring, electronics, dental sealants, tableware, and receipt paper. It easily leeches into food and water from containers.

More Environmental Attacks on the Brain

When studies began to appear that challenged the presumed benignity of BPA in the early 2000s, images of toxic baby bottles in the mouths of America's infants began to haunt millions of mothers. Americans soon realized that with virtually every can of food and every bottle of water, they were swallowing something toxic. The emerging BPA controversy stirred a pot filled with politics, health sciences, toxicology, and economics. In response to the research and public outcry at the time, the U.S. Food and Drug Administration banned the use of the chemical in baby bottles and cups in July 2012. However, recent research has found that BPA is still detectable in the atmosphere attached to air pollution particles, and in municipal water supplies, making our exposure to it impossible to avoid unless you are willing to not drink or breathe.[5] Ninety percent of the population has detectable levels of BPA in their urine.[6] This is all the more remarkable because BPA is broken down quickly in the body, which means that virtually all of us are continuously exposed.

The research on very low dose exposure to BPA shows estrogen-mimicking effects with a wide range of poor health outcomes—increased rates of cancer, DNA damage, cognitive and behavioral disorders, and metabolic diseases such as glucose intolerance, all related to endocrine disruption. BPA's adverse health effects are the result of its ability to play both offense and defense on the body's hormonal system. While it mimics estrogen, it also blocks receptors for testosterone.

Over an eight-year period, from 1997 to 2005, 115 BPA studies examining low-dose exposure, conducted by many different laboratories in several different countries, showed extensive human impacts. It affected prostate and mammary gland development; caused chromosomal damage, behavioral disorders, immunosuppression, and endocrine disorders; and altered brain function. In fact, 90% of the studies that were funded by the government found some of these disturbing effects at or below doses previously presumed safe. Some studies found adverse effects at doses orders of magnitude smaller than doses previously considered safe.

Concerns over BPA include chromosomal damage that interferes with the production of sperm and egg cells. Making matters worse, this genetic damage continued to appear in as many as two generations of unexposed lab animals who were progeny of the exposed group.[7]

BPA also suppresses the functioning of a certain gene, *Kcc2*, critical to nerve cell function and the proper development of the brain and nervous system.[8] By interfering with that gene, BPA causes neurons to accumulate abnormal amounts of chloride inside the cells.

BPA can cross the placenta and the BBB and contaminate the entire process and duration of intrauterine brain development. Fetal levels can be even higher than maternal levels.[9]

Locus Coeruleus (LC) is not the name of the most demented Roman emperor. It is the area of the brain that might have gone missing in the most demented Roman emperor. Specifically, it is the primary production site for norepinephrine, a critical neurotransmitter. And because the LC has more connections than a Mafia don, it distributes norepinephrine throughout the brain. In case you're wondering why you should care about norepinephrine and your LC, they are like the brain's in-house Starbucks, providing a critical jumpstart in arousal, vigilance, and focused attention. The number of neurons in the LC diminish as a person ages, and particularly in age-related neurologic diseases. Alzheimer's, Parkinson's, and chronic traumatic encephalopathy (CTE, the football players' disease) all feature an abnormal loss of LC neurons.

Prenatal BPA exposure changes brain architecture of male animals, specifically abnormally enlarging the LC, probably related to its estrogenic properties, which are typically larger in females.[10] Moreover, prenatal BPA exposure causes changes in the expression of certain brain-related genes, which changes animal behavior, primarily in males.[11] BPA has been shown to have a wide range of clinical health effects in humans beyond the scope of this book (meaning I was too lazy to write about it). But those effects include overall increased risk of death from all causes.[12]

More Environmental Attacks on the Brain

Limiting the discussion to its effects on the brain and nervous system, exposure to BPA, especially prenatally, is associated with a greater risk of attention deficit disorder, anxiety, depression, aggressive behavior, and memory deficits. Although evidence is mixed, the preponderance of studies found a greater affect in boys.[13]

Mice exposed to BPA during pregnancy gave birth to pups that showed atypical brain development and abnormal behavior later in life. The dose the mice were exposed to was 10-20 times lower than the recommended daily exposure limit for humans.[14] Even at that low dose, BPA abnormally accelerated the growth of neurons and impaired the ability of those neurons to engage in self-renewal.

Recently, researchers found a significant correlation between levels of BPA in pregnant mothers and alterations in the microstructure of white matter, assessed by MRI scans, when the children they gave birth to were 2 to 5 years old.[15]

Thyroid hormone is essential for normal prenatal and postnatal brain growth and development. Small decreases in thyroid hormone, even if it remains in a normal range, can still have an effect on the end result. Boys born to pregnant mothers exposed to more BPA had lower thyroid levels than girls.[16] For every doubling of BPA in the pregnant mother, researchers found almost 10% less thyroid stimulating hormone in the boys to whom they gave birth but not the girls. This study was even more worrisome because the mothers that were studied were mostly low-income, Mexican-American farm workers who had 42% less BPA exposure than the average American female of child-bearing age.[17]

Pressure on manufacturers and the chemical industry to abandon the use of BPA led to replacement chemicals with very little difference from BPA, such as bisphenolS (BPS). Not surprisingly, the health consequences, including the neurologic consequences of BPS appear to be similar to and just as significant as those from BPA. Researchers found that exposure during fetal development of as little as pico molar concentrations (less than one part per trillion) of BPS can change how a cell functions in ways that can lead to "diabetes and obesity, asthma, birth defects or even cancer" later on in life.[16] Eighty-one percent of Americans now test positive for BPS in their urine.[18] From the chemical industry's standpoint, the problem has been successfully swept under the rug for another ten years at least, because they can claim their products are BPA free.

PERCHLORATE

Someone walking away from an explosion without looking back has become such a movie cliché I can't remember the last time I saw a movie that didn't have at least two of these scenes. Maybe *The Notebook*. After learning about perchlorate, perhaps you'll want to skip explosions altogether.

Whenever you light a sparkler, watch a fireworks display up close, or enjoy any kind of explosion other than on your TV screen, you are inhaling or absorbing through your skin a basket full of chemicals and heavy metals that should numb your enthusiasm for the celebration just a bit. Probably the worst of that basket of deplorables (apologizes to Hillary Clinton) is perchlorate. A similar basket of deplorables is also contaminating the air and groundwater of most of American military installations around the world, foreign and domestic, and many of the nearby neighborhoods.

Perchlorate is a negatively charged molecule made of one chlorine atom and four oxygen atoms. Nearly all the food you eat comes with a little frosting of perchlorate. There is enough of it in most foods that it could serve as an entrée. It arrives there via hypochlorite bleach (an antimicrobial that degrades into perchlorate), perchlorate added to plastic food packaging, and in perchlorate-contaminated drinking water. That contamination comes from military and aerospace industrial activities involving the use of rocket fuel, munitions, ignition devices, fireworks, and from agriculture's use of fertilizers. It also occurs naturally in the drinking water in some states in the Southwest.

Perchlorate is one of 10,000 chemicals approved for use in food processing and packaging according to the Environmental Defense Fund. The amount of perchlorate in your food has been increasing since at least 2003.[1] In 2005, the FDA approved it to prevent the build-up of static charges in plastic food packaging, then expanded its approval to include dry-food handling equipment. Perchlorate is also a degradation chemical from hypochlorite used to disinfect food-processing equipment, meaning it is also found in organic food. Perchlorate levels in children's food increased about one third after 2005. The Trump FDA rejected a 2017 petition from numerous health and environmental organizations to ban the use of perchlorate as a food additive.

Perchlorate inhibits the uptake of iodine into the thyroid, reducing the production of thyroid hormone, or T4. Even brief exposure during intrauterine life or infancy can have lifelong consequences.[2] For the first 18-20 weeks after conception, fetal organ development, including the brain, is almost completely dependent on thyroid from the mother.[3] A pregnant mother's exposure to perchlorate will reduce the amount of free thyroxine available to the fetus.[4] This risk is magnified in one in five pregnant women who are deficient in dietary iodine, enhancing the ability of perchlorate to reduce thyroid production, irreversibly affecting her baby's brain development, lowering IQ, impairing motor skills, and inhibiting cognitive and language development.[5]

For the last 24 years, EPA has declined to add any new chemicals to the group they regulate in our drinking water, despite the increasing awareness of the myriad of neurotoxins that now permeate our environment. Under President Obama, EPA was finally developing enforceable limits for perchlorate in drinking water, and then President Trump pulled the quintessential putting "the fox in charge of the chickens" maneuver and installed a former coal lobbyist, Andrew Wheeler, as EPA's administrator. In a gift to the American Chemistry Council and defense contractors, the Trump EPA announced in May 2020 that they intended to brush off both the science and a court order, and wouldn't regulate the amount of perchlorate your kids will be drinking. In 2022 under Biden, EPA has once again refused to regulate this potent toxin in drinking water. The American Academy of Pediatrics lambasted EPA for even considering not regulating perchlorate. In a letter, they wrote:

Perchlorate causes goiters and damages the nervous system of fetuses and children. Research has identified a well-established causative association between perchlorate ingestion and thyroid hormone disruption...When fetuses are exposed during pregnancy, perchlorate endangers a child's development. Children born with even mild, subclinical deficiencies in thyroid function may have lower IQs, higher chances of being diagnosed with attention- deficit/hyperactivity disorder (ADHD), and visuospatial difficulties.[6]

This is just the latest of EPA's abdication of their mandate to protect public health. Wheeler says that up to 90 ppb of perchlorate in drinking water would be acceptable, even though EPA has admitted that children in those critical developmental windows exposed to 56 ppb would experience an average IQ loss of 2 points, with even greater effect on those who already would be on the lower end of the IQ bell curve. Illustrating just how detached Wheeler chose to be from the science, experts in California have recommended their state standard should be reduced to 1 ppb. Massachusetts's standard is 2 ppb.[7] Perchlorate is another toxin for which there is not enough research to distinguish a disparity between its effects on male versus female children.

Andrew Wheeler is just one of countless powerful people in government (mostly men), who seem to be unable to marshal the intelligence necessary to stop harming their own intelligence. Thus, the degenerative downward spiral accelerates.

PHTHALATES

By now, you may be getting a little discouraged, thinking, "Hell, everything's bad for my brain. I might as well go drink a mercury martini, gargle with Roundup, and get some of that *Old Spice Fresh Radioactive Scent* for deodorant." Isn't there anything I can enjoy that won't burrow its way into my frontal lobes? The short answer is no. We have a few more toxins to get through. Actually, we have a lot more scary toxins to get through.

More Environmental Attacks on the Brain

Phthalates (pronounced "ffffffffffftttttttttthhhhhhhhlllllllll—ates") are another class of endocrine disruptors found in common fragrances like perfumes, personal care products, pharmaceuticals, scented candles, toys, vinyl products, and air fresheners. Basically, anything that smells good is bad for you, just like anything that tastes good or feels good is bad for you, just like they told you at church.

Air fresheners have become an easy, almost mandatory substitute to cleaning up an apartment or a home. And who doesn't want their abode to smell fresh, clean, sweet, just like your mother or Mother Nature intended? Well, phthalates have little in common with your mother or nature. An investigation by the National Resource Defense Council found that of 14 top-selling air fresheners, despite none of them listing phthalates as an ingredient, these chemicals were found in 12 of the 14, including those they labeled as "all natural," or "unscented."[8] Because these chemicals are not covalently bound to these products, they evaporate into the atmosphere and can migrate just about anywhere. Contact with phthalate-embedded products can result in absorption through the skin, ingestion, and inhalation. Ingestion is likely the main route for contamination because of their use in the creation and packaging of processed foods.[9]

These chemicals can cross the placenta, and after birth, they will be found in breast milk. Research from Columbia University found that children whose mothers were in the highest phthalate-exposed group during their pregnancy had IQ test scores a shocking 6 to 8 points lower than the children of mothers in the lowest exposed group.[10] The kinds of phthalates tracked in this study were typically found in average household products such as cosmetics and personal care products, shampoo, nail polish, lipstick, hair styling products, soap, shower curtains, and dryer sheets. The levels of exposure in the study were consistent with what the CDC has found in its National Health and Nutrition Examination Survey:[11] in other words, at levels common in American households.

Other researchers measured phthalate metabolite concentrations in the urine of 153 pregnant mothers in a study from several different centers. Examining the children those mothers gave birth to several years later, the researchers found that higher concentrations of those metabolites correlated with higher rates of attention deficit, aggression, and rule-breaking behavior.[12] A similar study found a significant correlation between IQ loss and phthalate levels in the children themselves, but not with the levels found in their mothers during the pregnancy.[13]

A recent experiment in rats might make you feel like you should opt for smelling like a rat rather than use cologne or perfume to disguise it. Researchers divided rats into three groups: a control group, a group given a low-dose phthalate exposure, and a group given a high-dose exposure. Exposure in both high- and low-dose groups was comparable to the range found in humans, and in fact, below the daily tolerable intake limits of some countries' government agencies. The phthalate exposure was delivered in the form of a daily cookie. (Rat Oreos are available at all major grocery stores in case you were wondering). Actually, and this is true, the cookies were *Newman's Own* organic alphabet cookies, vanilla flavored, that the researchers laced with phthalates. These rats were given these cookies during pregnancy and for ten days after birth, during lactation.

Both low- and high-dose prenatally exposed rats had significant deficits in cognitive flexibility when they were tested as adults. When rat psychiatrists interviewed the test subjects, they asked them how long they had been feeling that way...sorry that didn't happen—they died before they could get an appointment. When microscopic examinations of their brains were performed, they showed that neurons, synapses, and overall tissue volume were significantly decreased in the medial prefrontal cortex (mPFC), an area important for cognitive and proper executive functioning, and where pathologic changes are associated with many psychiatric disorders and autism. This was a clear signal of permanent brain damage.[14] The authors wrote: "These results may have serious implications for humans given the mPFC is involved in executive functions and is implicated in the pathology of many neuropsychiatric disorders."

A Canadian study of 2,000 pregnant mothers found an association between exposure to higher levels of phthalates and an increased chance of autism-like traits in the boys the mothers give birth to, but not in the girls. The good news, however, if there was some, was that folic acid supplements during the pregnancy attenuated that risk.[15]

More recent research shows that prenatal exposure to phthalates is associated with impaired motor scores in female children in infancy, in toddlers, and persisting into older childhood. Exposure after birth is associated with impaired motor development in boys.[16]

AIR POLLUTION

My hometown of Salt Lake City, Utah, is positioned in a geographic bowl in a valley between two mountain ranges. In the winter, when the storm track bypasses Utah and there is snow on the ground, a meteorologic inversion sets up, trapping pollution. Within a few days, the buildup of pollution in the major urban areas of the state can be intense. Salt Lake City frequently ranks in the American Lung Association's top ten worst polluted cities in the country for acute, 24-hour spikes in particulate pollution.

A few years ago, my physician's group UPHE organized what turned out to be the largest anti-air pollution rally in the modern history of this country. About 5,000 people turned up on a Saturday in January demanding that the governor and legislature take more serious action to reduce air pollution in Salt Lake City. The turnout could be attributed to many years of an extensive media campaign we mounted to educate the public about the full extent of the health consequences of air pollution and the frustration of the public on the ineffectual response of the state government.

Air pollution is often presumed by the public and the media to be primarily, if not exclusively, a problem for the lungs. But the microscopic particles that constitute air pollution common to the global atmosphere, urban areas in particular, can find their way into virtually any cell in the body, and when they do, an immune response is generated and all critical organs are affected. The inflammation affects the brain, causing neuronal damage, neuronal loss, loss of brain mass, cortical stress measured by EEG, enhancement of Alzheimer-type abnormal filamentous proteins, and cerebrovascular damage. Many of these changes can be found in children and young adults.[1] The inflammation can cause the BBB (see Chapter 2) to lose its normal function of acting as a barrier preventing foreign particles, chemicals, and the body's own molecules of inflammation from entering the brain.[2]

The immune response to the inflammation can also include the release of antibodies to nerves themselves. Reduced blood flow can be the result of this inflammatory process, and anatomic evidence of blood- and oxygen-deprived areas of the brain appear on MRI scans as spots of white matter hyperintensities (WMH), found throughout the brain, but primarily in the pre-frontal cortex. The WMH interfere with nerve-to-nerve signaling and impair brain function, creating essentially dead zones in the brain. The presence of WMH doubles the risk of dementia and triples the risk of a stroke. WMH impair physical coordination, increase the risk of depression, and are inversely associated with intelligence. WMH used to be considered an expected hallmark of advanced aging. Now we know these pathologic findings are present long before that.[3] These foreboding WMH are found even in children and young adults exposed to high levels of air pollution and are seldom found in children breathing clean air.[4]

Air pollution nanoparticles and their attached heavy metals and toxic chemicals can actually end up inside the brain from two routes. One is through inhalation by the lungs, translocation to the capillaries in the lungs, then distributed by the blood stream with greater access afforded by this disruption of the brain's normally protective blood vessel barrier, the BBB. But another is through the nose. Pollution particles can attach themselves to the lining of the nose, then to the olfactory nerve fibers in the nose, and then, as if on a conveyer belt, can migrate directly back to the brain stem itself.[5] If you've heard the phrase "cutting off your nose to spite your face," with air pollution you could modify that to "cutting off your nose to save your brain." That may not catch on, however.

More Environmental Attacks on the Brain

Toxic, nano-sized particles called "magnetites," resulting from high-temperature fossil fuel combustion, have been found at autopsies in the brains of people as young as three years old.[6] People with higher concentrations of these metallic nanoparticles are known to be at higher risk for Alzheimer's, and the kind of brain damage these magnetites can cause is consistent with the disease. These particles, including iron oxide, platinum, nickel, and cobalt can originate from industrial smoke stacks, vehicle tail pipes, or other sources of pollution from high temperature combustion. British researchers studying numerous brain tissue samples found "millions of these particles per gram of brain tissue" in every brain, including those of children. The lead author of the study said these results are "dreadfully shocking."[7] These pollution-generated magnetites were responsible for $1/100^{th}$ of the weight of the brain in some patients. Think of magnetites as an energy-zapping, havoc-wreaking "kryptonite," contaminating the brains of all us, starting from the moment of birth or even much earlier.

Remarkable research in both humans and animals has shown that prenatal exposure to pollution harms the architecture of the brain. In mice, prenatal exposure to diesel exhaust results in impaired behavior later on when they are adults.[8]

There is a linear relationship between the amount of exposure of a pregnant mother to a common group of toxins in air pollution, PAHs (polycyclic aromatic hydrocarbons, i.e., multiple benzene-ringed compounds), and the loss of brain white matter, primarily on the left hemisphere. As yet, we don't know the reason the left hemisphere suffers the most loss. The researchers found no safe level of PAH exposure.[9] The loss of white matter, brain volume, and PAH exposure, in turn, all correlated directly with cognitive loss and behavioral disorders measured later on in childhood.[10] Loss of gray matter and reduced cortical thickness were documented in 12-year-olds if they had been exposed to more traffic-related air pollution during their first year after birth.[11]

Numerous other studies show a link between pregnant mothers' exposure to the full range of air pollution components—PAHs, traffic pollution, coal combustion emissions, carbon monoxide, benzene, and nitrogen oxides—and decreased intelligence measured in their children later on in childhood.[12] Animal studies examining the effect of pollution inhalation during what would correspond to the first month of human life, show loss of brain mass around the ventricles (pockets of cerebrospinal fluid in the center of the brain), causing abnormal enlargement of the ventricles, primarily in the male animals.[13] In humans, this anatomic anomaly, in turn, is associated with schizophrenia, autism, attention deficit disorder, developmental delays, and cognition handicaps.[14] White matter loss in the elderly also corresponds to air pollution exposure.[15]

Zebra fish are a minnow-sized fish found in Asian fresh water streams. They have zebra-like black and white stripes: thus, the name. Aquarium owners love them, but so do researchers. According to carbon dating (which is only for adult singles over 10,000 years old), around 300 million years ago zebra fish and humans shared a common ancestor. This was even before the first prehistoric Twinkies were discovered. Having a common ancestor means that humans and zebra fish are genetic "bros," making them much more important than just aquarium celebrities. They are absolute rock stars for human genetics researchers. Zebra fish reach adulthood extremely quickly, i.e., in about three months. A single female fish can produce hundreds of eggs at a time, like an aquatic version of the Duggars on steroids. But the best part is that when they are young, they are almost completely transparent. This unique feature allows researchers a window into embryonic development almost like no other, because researchers can study what is happening to the fish without touching them, and even better, without killing them, as is often required with other laboratory animals.

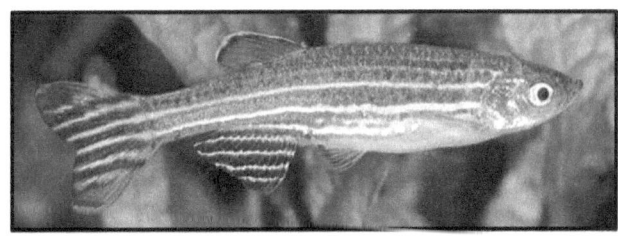

The genetic overlap between zebra fish and humans is about 70%. I guess that means the love scene in *The Shape of Water* wasn't as creepy as it seemed. For genes that play a role in human disease, the overlap is even greater, about 84%.[16] Researchers can use the zebra fish to study the proteins genes produce. (Producing proteins is the primary function of genes.) Using these fish proteins, researchers can determine which chemicals cause genetic mutations or could be used as therapeutics. Researchers expect to discover the function of 80-90% of all human genes by studying zebra fish. Next time you see a zebra fish, compliment him/her for those awesome-looking genes.

Neurons in a zebra fish brain interact in similar ways to those in the human brain. To study if pollution in diesel exhaust can precipitate Parkinson's disease, researchers added low doses of chemicals in diesel exhaust to the water environment of zebra fish. The chemicals not only changed the behavior of the fish, the transparency of the fish allowed researchers to document that neurons were dying off in the brains of the fish.[17] Then they set out to detect how that damage occurred.

I have mentioned before the importance of the brain's garbage collection or "autophagy" service. Obviously, some brains produce more garbage than others, some put out nothing but. Parkinson's disease is at least partly the result of toxic accumulation of brain garbage called alpha-synuclein proteins.

Clumps of alpha-synuclein build up around neurons, eventually strangling them. Clinically, this becomes evident as tremors and muscle rigidity, hallmarks of Parkinson's. The researchers could then see, literally, that in the presence of diesel exhaust chemicals, the garbage of the brain was not being picked up. To confirm the relevance to humans, the researchers then conducted a similar experiment on cultured human neurons, and diesel exhaust chemicals had a similar effect in that setting. A recent headline of *Science* magazine reads, "The Polluted Brain—Evidence builds that dirty air causes Alzheimer's, dementia." Alzheimer's and Parkinson's disease are characterized anatomically by abnormal brain architecture, loss of brain volume, aberrant biochemical and neurotransmitter function, and the deposition of abnormal protein tangles and plaques in the brain, such as tau and beta amyloid. Air pollution is associated with all of these kinds of brain abnormalities, even in children,[18] and is likely a contributor to the growing worldwide epidemic of Alzheimer's, responsible for about 20% of the disease, according to one study.[19]

The latest research examined the brains of 203 people, ranging in age from 11 months to 40 years old. At autopsy (causes of death were usually trauma), every single brain but one showed those abnormal Alzheimer proteins, even in the 11-month-old, and the amount of these abnormal proteins was proportional to the amount of air pollution where the subjects lived. The principal author, probably the world's expert on this type of research, said, "Alzheimer's disease hallmarks start in childhood in polluted environments, and we must implement effective preventative measures early. It is useless to take reactive actions decades later."[20]

Well over 150 clinical studies confirm that pollution exposure is associated with almost the full range of neurologic disorders throughout the age spectrum, including lower intelligence, diminished motor function, attention deficit and behavioral problems, accelerated dementia, memory and cognitive loss in elderly adults, higher rates of strokes, relapses in multiple sclerosis, impaired olfactory sense, Parkinson's and other neurodegenerative diseases, anxiety, and depression.[21] Air pollution is associated with higher risk for developing and seeking treatment for virtually all mental disorders and a much higher mortality risk for those with mental health and behavioral disorders, including suicide.[22]

| Rated **PG-13** | Sale of this book to anyone who has been pregnant thirteen times is ~~strictly prohibited,~~ highly recommended. |

Recently, a criminal defense attorney reached out to me because she was wondering if her defendant might have developed homicidal urges because of the air pollution where he grew up. Almost as a reflex I told her I was slow to sign on to a theory that "the air pollution made me do it." Experts in science always want to be publicly cautious about a radical discovery or an outlier opinion, even if supported by the evidence. However, the attorney may have been on to something. We do know that CTE, the brain disease found in 99% of NFL players studied at autopsy,[23] is characterized by many of the same kind of pathologic findings as are present in Alzheimer's. CTE-like changes are linked to air pollution, and are associated with loss of impulse control, antisocial aggression, and violent behavior. Furthermore, the WMH are predominantly found in the prefrontal cortex, an area of the brain impaired in people who manifest poor decision-making ability, aggression, and antisocial behavior.[24] I intend to engage in my own research to prove that WMH and CTE are also caused by listening to country western music and sitting through the entire play of *Waiting for Godot*.

Another fascinating study showed that in addition to increasing depression and suicidal tendencies, air pollution is associated with an increased tendency to criminal activity and unethical behavior.[25] The childhood lead exposure of the attorney's client would likely be even more relevant than the air pollution he had breathed, but it would be impossible to determine what that may have been decades later without pulling teeth (literally) or taking a piece of his bone marrow.

The same vascular changes that are responsible for heart attacks are also responsible for pollution-related strokes. Numerous studies show significantly higher rates of strokes with chronic and acute exposure, even within only hours after the onset of a spike in pollution.[26]

"Air pollution is stunting our children's brains, affecting their health in more ways than we suspected," says Dr. Maira Neira of the WHO.[27] More than 90% of the world's children breathe air known to be toxic to their health and development every day. Because they have higher metabolic rates, children breathe more frequently and inhale more air pollution than what would be expected of an adult of the same size. They also have a higher heart rate, and those two features combine to disseminate more pollution particles throughout their bodies.

Children's smaller size means they also live closer to the ground where air pollution levels are typically higher. While this may seem trivial, it's actually not at all. Researchers in the UK's Surrey's Global Centre for Clean Air Research measured air pollution at the height of infants riding in baby strollers pushed by parents and compared it to the exposure of the parents, whose upper airways would be presumably only a few feet higher. They found that the infants breathed 44% more air pollution than the adults pushing the strollers.[28] However, when the strollers added covers, that reduced the infant's exposure significantly.

Children are more vulnerable to air pollution than adults. The protective barriers from specialized cells lining the lungs, the BBB, the nose, and the GI tract are less developed than those of an adult. These factors increase a child's exposure, subjecting them to a chronic state of environmental stress, provoking dysregulation of genes that control inflammation, immune response, cell viability, and communication between brain cells. At the same time, because of the "in progress" developmental status of the fetal, infant, and childhood brain and nervous system, the damage can be much greater.

Childhood brain disorders associated with pollution have been well documented by a robust body of experimental, clinical, epidemiological, and pathology research. Furthermore, the impact on brain function can be almost immediate. One study showed that attention span in school children was impaired by the air pollution they breathed that day on the way to school.[29]

PON2 (paraoxonase/arylesterase 2) is a common intracellular enzyme. It functions as an important anti-oxidant. Mutations in the gene that codes for the enzyme have been shown to cause a wide variety of diseases, like atherosclerotic vascular disease and diabetes. PON2 interacts with estrogen to provide a protective effect on the brain. Because of that enhancement, across multiple species—mice, rats, non-human primates, conspiracy species knuckle draggers, and humans—females have more PON2 activity than males.[30]

Higher gene expression that creates PON2 and the presence of estrogen combine to give females an advantage in protection from neurotoxicity and neurodegenerative diseases.[30] More active PON2 may explain why, among multiple brain cell types—neurons, astrocytes, and microglia—females demonstrate less vulnerability to the toxic inflammatory effects of one of the most potent types of air pollution—diesel exhaust.[31]

Numerous studies show that air pollution has a more potent toxic effect on the male brain than the female. Representative of these studies was one published in the prestigious Proceedings of the National Academy of Sciences that tracked both chronic and transient air pollution exposure of a population in China. The researchers found that intelligence test scores decreased in all age groups with more pollution exposure, but the population that demonstrated the strongest correlation was less well-educated elderly males. They also found the greatest drop was in verbal tests, and less so, math tests. Verbal capability is more dependent on the white matter part of the brain, math calculations are more dependent on gray matter. Air pollution has a stronger impact on white matter. The researchers commented, "Since men have a much smaller amount of white matter activated during intelligence tests, their cognitive performance, especially in the verbal domain, tends to be more affected by exposure to air pollution."[32]

I have been contacted by numerous people over the last several years seeking an expert opinion to evaluate and hopefully validate their concerns, and sometimes their cases in court, that an acute episode of air pollution or chemical exposure has precipitated chronic neurologic symptoms. Their stories are often tragic and devastating. An all-too-common event invovles someone already with struggling with a disability, such as autism, who, after a toxic exposure, has their symptoms worsen, sometimes dramatically.

Not long ago a truck driver contacted me seeking someone who could offer a supportivie opinion that a several-day exposure to high levels of diesel exhaust from a leak in his truck could be the cause of debilitating, chronic and persistent headaches, visual distrubances, attention deficit, and cognitive and memory loss, all of which started right after the leak. When I told him I thought that was indeed plausible, if not likely, he broke out in tears. Despite receving what appeared to be excellent care (including hyperbaric oxygen therapy, see Chapter 9), and extensive rehabilitation sessions, none of his other physicians seemed to be willing to make the case that his exposure had caused his symptoms. His story speaks to an ongoing, serious gap in the education and expertise of the medical community on the connection between disease and environmental contaminants. And this patient's toxin related brain damage is likely worse because he is a male.

NEWBORN ICU ENVIRONMENT

Among 184 of the world's major countries, the rate of preterm birth (before 37 weeks' gestation) ranges from 5% to 18%. In the U.S., as of 2018, it is 11-12% of all births, or about 450,000 premature infants per year, about two thirds of whom end up in newborn intensive care. In Chapter 3, I addressed the increased vulnerability of male infants to premature birth and its complications, many of which are related to delayed, incomplete, or impaired brain development. It is also worth addressing in more detail in this chapter, the adverse environmental circumstances and toxins that a premature infant is exposed to, because here again, male infants are likely to suffer greater consequences.

Advances in perinatal medicine and newborn intensive care over the last 20 years have improved survival of severely premature infants. But they remain victimized by, among other health problems, persistent neurologic deficits. Very low birthweight infants (<1500 gram) experience loss of brain function and/or behavioral disorders at alarming rates, 50-70%.[1] Even moderately preterm infants, born anywhere from 28-36 weeks gestation, have significantly higher rates of behavioral disorders and intellectual deficits compared with term infants.

Prematurity affects the brains of males and females differently. Both sexes suffer loss of overall brain volume, but male brains suffer more overall loss, and more particularly, loss of gray matter.[2] Females suffer more loss of white matter. Recall from chapter 2 that gray matter is responsible for muscle control, the senses, memory, speech, and emotion, while white matter connects different regions of gray matter to each other.

More Environmental Attacks on the Brain

In general, studies with brain imaging of children born prematurely show more abnormal brain structure in males compared to females, examined either as neonates or later on in childhood.[3] Overall, boys suffer greater clinical neurologic deficits related to prematurity.[4] Nonetheless, gestational age is not necessarily linearly correlated with deficits, to the point where researchers believe other factors are at play. Iron deficiency is detrimental to brain development in infancy, and boys have lower iron stores than girls.[5]

When a premature newborn has to trade its mother's womb for a newborn intensive care unit (NICU), it is thrown into a world much different, much more stressful, and much more riddled with toxins than the one it just left. A NICU exposes a baby directly to an array of chemicals, medications, light, noise, sleep disruption, radiation, heavy metals, stress, isolation, and other environmental factors proven to be detrimental to brain development. In other words, the prematurity itself impairs brain development, but the new environment necessary for survival only adds to it.

Babies in a NICU are subjected to multiple procedures that involve the use of medical equipment and devices that come into direct contact with their bodies, including their lungs, blood, and other bodily fluids. Researchers analyzed 50 items in that setting, including plastic medical devices, oxygen masks, endotracheal tubes, syringes, IV tubing, medicines, fabrics, personal care products (including topical creams), and nutritional supplements. They found 60% of the items contained BPA, and 80% contained parabens; both are potent endocrine disruptors. Metabolites of these compounds in the urine of these babies were up to 30 times greater than in healthy babies out of the hospital.[6]

Through leaching, migration, and evaporation, plastics used for IV bags and tubing can release even more neurotoxic chemicals, such as phthalates (mentioned earlier in this chapter) into the IV fluid and blood transfusions being dripped into a baby.[7] Because of immature liver and kidney function, premature infants are unable to adequately rid themselves of phthalates and phenols, so they're more susceptible to the potential toxicity. Studies have documented higher levels of exposure for these infants compared to infants requiring less care or no hospitalization.[8] Metals such as silver are often added to IV components for anti-microbial purposes. Aluminum, mentioned in the previous chapter, used to be added to intravenous nutrition for these infants, but a study showed worse neurologic outcomes compared to infants for whom the aluminum was eliminated. The practice of adding it, we hope, has ended.

Every one of the 40 trillion cells in the body operates with an electric potential. Furthermore, internal electromagnetic fields and currents are assumed to facilitate and direct cell migration during development. This electric potential can be altered by the charged elements in the outer membrane. External sources of electricity and electrical fields can have an impact on cells, adversely affecting human health, especially those vulnerable humans, premature babies. Some animal studies, but not all, have validated that concern.[9] For neonates, the largest source of electromagnetic fields is the incubator.

Babies in the NICU are exposed to radiation from the x-rays performed on them and the scatter radiation from x-rays done on other babies near them. While the radiation exposure from a single x-ray is small, many babies require multiple x-rays, and the exposure couldn't happen at a worse stage in life. As alluded to earlier in this chapter, physicians should be very cautious about ordering x-rays and especially CT scans in these babies because of the large amount of radiation involved.

We do not yet have the ability to determine how much neurologic damage is the result of prematurity and how much is due to the neurotoxicity of the known toxins in the NICU environment. But the end result, unfortunately, is that premature brain deficits are significant and are worse in boys than in girls.[10]

More Environmental Attacks on the Brain

Men just don't have the right temperament to be librarians

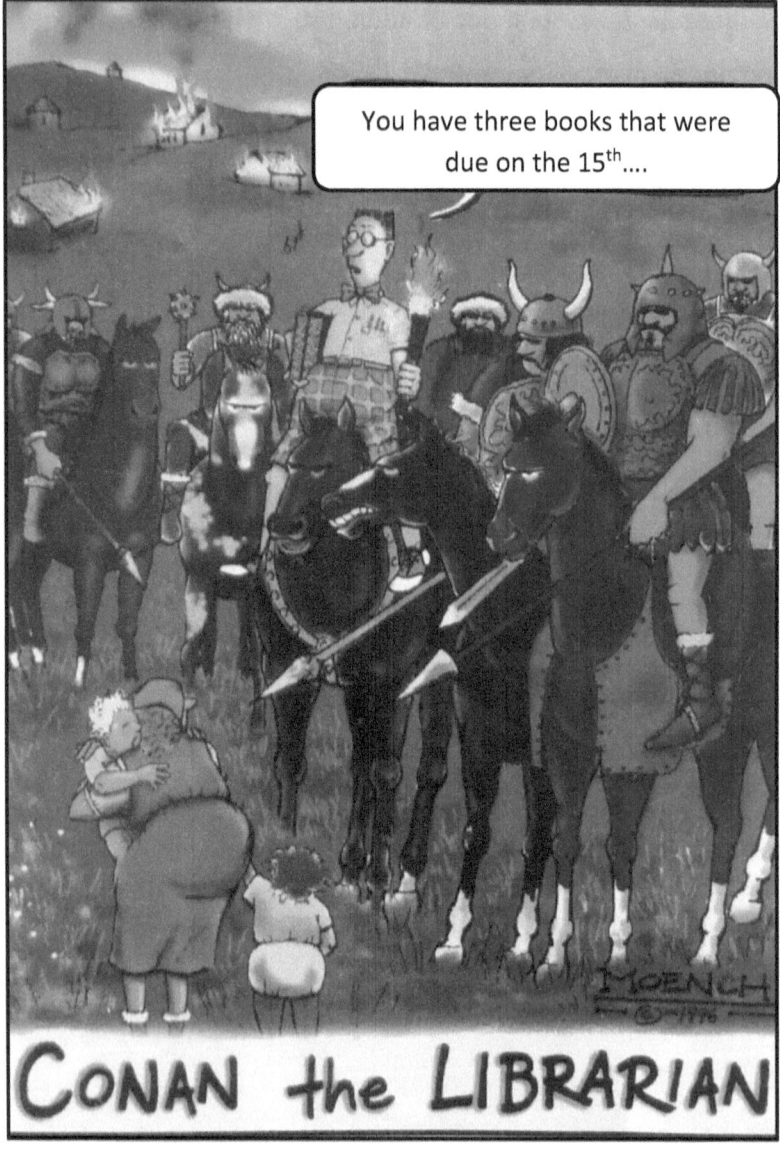

Chapter 6

FEMALE HORMONES—THE GREAT BRAIN PROTECTORS

"What's another word for Thesaurus?"

—Comedian Steven Wright

"...it's kind of like marriage when you say it's not a man and a woman any more, then why not have three men and one woman, or four women and one man, or why not somebody has a love for an animal?"

—Texas Representative(R) Louie Gohmert, explaining how in his mind, gun control leads to sex with animals

"There are many other states that embrace those conservative values, the approach that we've taken over the years. I'm in one today, in Florida."

—Texas Gov. Rick Perry, delivering a speech in Louisiana

The first draft of this chapter got me sent to a re-education camp for the politically incorrect. The second draft got me sued by Donald Trump for gloater fraud. This is the third draft, the hard work of a committee consisting of all my multiple personalities, edited by the My Pillow Guy.

Undercutting everything I've said about women being smarter than men, is the life and times of Rep. Marjorie Taylor Greene. In fairness, Hillary Clinton revealed a rather surprising lack of understanding of third grade–level physiology. In her book, *What Happened*, Secretary Clinton writes:

> *I did yoga with my instructor, Marianne Letizia, especially breath work. If you've never done alternate*

Female Hormones—The Great Brain Protectors

> *nostril breathing, it's worth a try. Sit cross-legged with your left hand on your thigh and your right hand on your nose. Breathe deeply from your diaphragm, place your right thumb on your right nostril and your ring and little fingers on your left. Shut your eyes, and close off your right nostril, breathing slowly and deeply through your left. Now close both sides and hold your breath. Exhale through the right nostril. Then reverse it: inhale through the right, close it, and exhale through the left. The way it's explained to me, this practice allows oxygen to activate both the right side of the brain, which is the source of your creativity and imagination, and the left side, which controls the reason and logic.... It may sound silly, but it works for me.*

Ms. Clinton is obviously a very smart woman, but, yes, this sounds not only silly, but it is medically absurd. You can sit with your left elbow in your right ear, your right foot wrapped around your left kidney, your right knee jammed up your left nostril, and you may look awesome doing that, but it will not change how your brain get its oxygen. The oxygen to both sides of your brain comes from what you inhale through your lungs and it is then delivered to your brain via your heart and arterial system. You do not, and cannot, oxygenate one side of your brain at a time, whether you breathe through one nostril, alternating nostrils or through someone else's nostrils (which can be awkward on a first date). New research also indicates she is wrong about one side of your brain being more creative and the other side being more analytical.

There are several likely microbiologic, hormonal, and chemical contributors to why women are smarter than men. The real answer probably includes elements of all these considerations. First, males and females differ notably in their ability to produce glutathione (GSH). You may have never heard of glutathione before opening this book, but you can't live without it. Some of you may be thinking this sounds like the name of your wife's Italian personal trainer. But it's actually much more important than that. Anyone can ditch their personal trainer, and the worst that could happen is you'd probably save money. But you'd be hard pressed to ditch your glutathione, and if you did, when you looked in the mirror you probably wouldn't like the results. Without glutathione, you would have the jowls of a blood hound, the intellectual prowess of Forest Gump, and the muscle tone of Jabba the Hut.

Glutathione is a tripeptide, γ-L-glutamyl-L-cysteinyl-glycine, and is "the most abundant intracellular low molecular weight thiol in cells and tissues, and plays an essential role in numerous cellular processes, including antioxidant defenses, the regulation of protein function, protein localization and stability, DNA synthesis, gene expression, cell proliferation, and cell signaling."[1] The emoji for glutathione was created back in the 15th century by the famous surreal painter, Hieronymus Bosch, whose tortured mind must have been exposed either to toxic levels of lead, fluoride, or the editorial pages of the Wall Street Journal. Here it is:

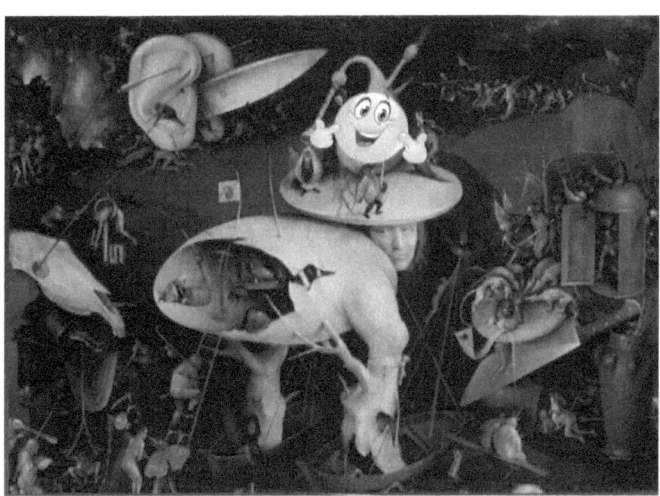

In simplified English, glutathione is a critical antioxidant composed of three amino acids (cysteine, glycine, and glutamic acid) that neutralizes free radicals. More about that shortly. There are dietary sources of glutathione (the things you're supposed to eat but don't, like fresh vegetables), but your liver is its primary manufacturer and exporter. Many of the biologic processes for which glutathione is a critical ingredient show gender differences. (The academic word for that is sexual dimorphism).

Men and women appear to have an equal amount of glutathione when they are first born. Unfortunately, production of

Female Hormones—The Great Brain Protectors

GSH declines quickly with age, but it is well documented that it declines more in males in than females.[3] Why that is the case is not clear: perhaps payback for men not giving women the vote until 1920. Nonetheless, young males have lower levels of GSH than females in the parietal cortical region.[4] In fact, reduced levels of glutathione can be used as biomarkers of autism.[5] Reduced production or accelerated depletion of GSH is the major contributor to neurodegenerative diseases.[6] Male versus female differences in GSH metabolism have been found in neurodegenerative diseases like Alzheimer's and Parkinson's. For example, GSH concentrations in red blood cells are diminished in men with Alzheimer's compared to a control group, but that decrease was not found in women.

A second chemical difference between the sexes is the availability of sulfate chemical groups.[7] You might think of sulfur only as the smell of rotten eggs, what bubbles from the 10,000 hydrothermal features in Yellowstone National Park, or the official perfume of *Dante's Inferno*. But you wouldn't do well without this rotten-egg element. Sulfur is a critical element in important biologic molecules like amino acids (specifically methionine and cysteine), proteins, enzymes, and vitamins, essential for all organisms. It is the third most abundant mineral in the human body after calcium and phosphorus. Sulfate is required for many biologic activities, and sulfate depletion can reduce detoxification capability and increase the toxicity of xenobiotics (chemicals that are found in an organism but not produced by that organism). Sulfate is an essential component of glutathione.

Studies in lab animals, like centaurs...rats, actually, found that males are about twice as dependent on sulfate for detoxification of phenolic compounds (such as acetaminophen) as females. Any deficiency in sulfate would, therefore, affect males more than females. Important dietary sources of sulfur include nuts, legumes, seafood, dried fruit, eggs, dairy, asparagus, broccoli, Brussels sprouts, oats, and wheat. In other words, the opposite of the typical American male diet of deep-fried Oreos with cheese, Doritos with cheese, and Mountain Dew with cheese.

If God played a role in the creation of humans, He/She also gave females a much more difficult role to play in that creation. Nothing that a male experiences is comparable to a female being pregnant or giving birth. Anyone should be able to see the disconnect of women's reproductive rights being legislated by primarily men. But at the same time there are some distinct advantages to being female. When it comes to brain protection, He/She gave most of those advantages to females.

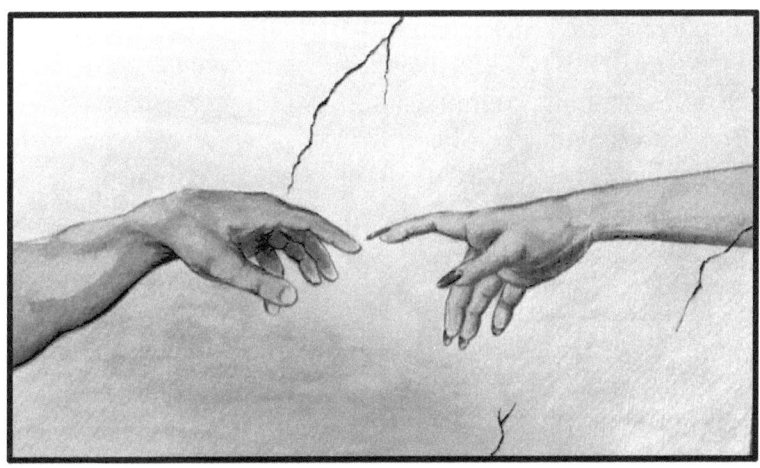

ESTROGEN $C_{18}H_{24}O_2$

β–Estradiol

There is abundant evidence that the hormones estrogen and progesterone may provide neuroprotection, whereas testosterone may enhance neurotoxicity. In short, estrogen regulates the menstrual cycle and progesterone supports pregnancy. Females have longer life expectancies than males in most developed countries, and that is not explained by men's having more dangerous occupations, faring worse psychologically after a divorce, or women's poisoning their unfaithful husbands. It is also true in mammals in general, which also leads to the conclusion that it is not a manifestation of socioeconomic factors.[8] Estrogen is central to the chemical profiles of males and females.

There are three different natural estrogens in females; estrone (E1), 17β-estradiol (E2) and estriol (E3). Estradiol is the most potent and most abundant estrogen and is produced by the ovaries during childbearing years. Estriol is produced only during pregnancy. Estrone can be produced after menopause, albeit in much lower doses. After menopause, small amounts of estrogen are produced locally in fat cells like the breast, in bone, and in the brain, which helps maintain cognitive abilities.[9] Recent research has found that the hypothalamus in the brain can produce estradiol in larger quantities than previously thought, enough to raise the levels throughout the body.[10]

Approximately 1.7 million people suffer a traumatic brain injury (TBI) every year. About 275,000 are hospitalized, about 33% of those have long-term disabilities, and about 18% of those requiring hospitalization die from the head injury. Lower estrogen leaves males more vulnerable to head injuries. Moreover, women recover from comparable brain injury about three times faster than men, according to some studies. Women also have a lower incidence of residual morbidity and mortality after TBI compared with age-matched men. Controlled experiments eliciting head trauma in animals have shown improved survival and cognitive function among females. Many animal, laboratory, and clinical studies show that from the eighth week after conception and throughout the remainder of life, estrogens are neuroprotective.[11] Estrogen promotes nerve repair and replacement after neural injury.

Even in male rats subjected to brain trauma, pre-treatment with estrogen improved neurologic outcome. In contrast, the same pre-treatment with estrogen had the opposite effect in female rats,[12] an example of too much of a good thing. Apparently, it is possible to have too much estrogen for brain repair. Estrogen administration after injury in male lab rats also improved neurologic outcomes.[13] Other studies also showed less neuronal cell death in similar experiments, reduced brain swelling, and less disruption of the blood-brain barrier.[14]

Researchers analyzing 72,000 patients over 5 years found that women older than 45 years and postmenopausal women (older than 55 years) had better neurologic outcomes and lower rates of mortality after moderate-to-severe TBI compared with men of comparable age.[15] One of the most troubling aspects of treating brain trauma is that after neuronal injury, microglia secrete pro-inflammatory chemicals, cytokines, that increase and spread tissue damage. Some studies found that estrogen decreases the release of these inflammatory mediators.[16] There is also evidence in animals that estrogen improves outcome with spinal cord injuries, including reduced cell death.[17] Estrogen also protects against several other types of induced nerve cell death, such as from various types of biologic stress.[18]

Blood flow to the brain is an obvious critical asset in avoiding disease. Estrogen exerts protective effects in the mitochondria of the brain's blood vessels, which is a likely mechanism for its known ability to increase blood flow to the brain, especially in the microcirculation. It binds to receptors found on the inside walls of blood vessels, stimulating the release of nitric oxide, an endogenous compound that dilates blood vessels.[19]

In the 21st century, most of the conveniences of modern life require the movement of electrons to establish a current of electrical activity. The movement of neurotransmitters is similarly central to the brain's electrical activity. At the point of a neuronal synapse, where an electrical current has to be transmitted from one cell to the next, estrogen increases levels of the neurotransmitters, serotonin, dopamine, and norepinephrine, as well as increasing the number of receptors for these chemicals to interact with. Estrogen bestows neuroprotective effects against oxidative stress, tissue damage from inadequate blood flow, and the damage caused by the notorious amyloid protein, a hallmark and likely trigger of Alzheimer's disease. Estrogen also stimulates growth and maintenance repair of neurons and the production of nerve growth factors.[20] Microscopic damage is less in female animals than in age-matched males after simulation of a stroke via localized loss of blood flow, and the source of this protection is linked to female reproductive steroids.[21] Estrogen also seems to sustain astrocytes and microglia, which helps protect against the advance of numerous neurodegenerative diseases.[22]

The amount of estrogen produced during a woman's life influences her eventual risk of developing Alzheimer's. That means that if a female menstruates earlier, goes through menopause later, and gives birth to more children, her risk of Alzheimer's will be decreased. Unfortunately, that life pattern will do the opposite for her risk for breast cancer. More specifically, having three or more children compared to having one child reduces a women's Alzheimer risk about 12%. Estrogen spikes in the third trimester of pregnancy,[23] prompting a surge in immune cells, such as regulatory T cells. Alzheimer's patients have fewer regulatory T cells, which increases vulnerability to inflammation.[24] Having menopause occur prior to age 45 increases the risk of having Alzheimer's by 28%. Furthermore, the hot flashes of menopause are also associated with impaired memory performance.[25]

Sex hormones, estrogen in particular, are also protective of the immune system because they act as antioxidants, scavenging and neutralizing free radicals that are triggers for many diseases and are part of the profile of tissue trauma.[26] This is particularly important for the brain because it has rather low DNA-repair capability. Mitochondria are the sub-cellular structures that function as a cell's power plant. Loss of estrogen impairs mitochondrial function, accelerates the decline of synaptic function and weakens defense mechanism against neuroinflammation.[27] Mitochondria are critical to maintaining cellular viability and preventing the death of neurons. Mitochondria in the cells of young females are better protected against the build-up of the toxic proteins that define Alzheimer's.

Estrogen receptors are widely distributed throughout the brain. In fact, the brain is both a source of and a destination for all the endogenously produced sex hormones—estrogen, progesterone, and testosterone.[28] Women who complain that their male partners have sex on the brain are actually correct, at least in the biochemical sense. Sex hormones, including testosterone, have antioxidant properties that enhance nerve function and promote neuron longevity. Both female sex hormones decline rather quickly after menopause. But in men, testosterone's decline occurs more gradually. In both sexes, neuron functional deterioration and risk of neurodegenerative diseases correspond to the loss of both male and female sex hormones.

Hormone replacement therapy is controversial because it has numerous effects on cancer and heart-disease risks. It has been shown to have a protective effect against neurodegenerative diseases, but only in a woman that starts it before or at the time of menopause. In fact, if started well after the onset of menopause, it may be harmful, including increasing the risk of Alzheimer's.[29] "The evidence suggests that estrogen strongly protects women's brains before the age of 50, but does so only moderately between the ages of 50 and 59, and perhaps becomes harmful at age 60 and after," according to Walter Rocca of the Mayo Clinic in Rochester, Minnesota.[30]

At the microscopic level, in animals, spine density and synapse numbers decrease as ovarian hormones are lost, but in the aged animal, estrogen replacement does not restore that micro anatomy.[31] Loss of testosterone has a similar effect.

Estrogen also can help reduce stroke damage by decreasing inflammation, reducing coagulation of white blood cells, and dilating cerebral vessels.[32] Microscopic damage after a simulated stroke in animals is less in females than in males and is linked to their reproductive hormones.[33]

A healthy management of fear is something everyone must master. Fear of public speaking, fear of bodily injury, fear of having to use the bathroom at the Maverick gas station in Buford, Wyoming. Estrogen appears to be protective against the fear response, and it therefore, helps the brain in avoiding Post Traumatic Stress Disorder (PTSD), like that which follows having no other choice but to use that bathroom in Buford, Wyoming. A single gene, *HDAC4*, has been discovered that is integral to a person's experience of fear. That gene becomes chemically altered (methylated) in PTSD patients compared to controls, and that methylation correlates with lower estradiol levels. Lower estradiol levels in women are associated with greater susceptibility to fear from PTSD.[34] Women who have experienced psychological trauma are more likely to have flashbacks in the mid-luteal phase of their menstrual cycle, when they are producing more progesterone and less estrogen.

From a metabolic standpoint, women's brains are about three years younger compared to men's brains of the same chronological age. As alluded to in Chapter 2, our brains require a lot of energy to operate, and that comes in the form of glucose (sugar). At early stages after birth, that fuel is provided by aerobic glycolysis (nonoxidative glucose use), which supports brain growth, maturation, and development. The leftover glucose is burned for enough energy for daily tasks of brain function for an infant or toddler, i.e., thinking, babbling, and analyzing how well applesauce works as a hair mousse. Normal aging decreases the brain's metabolic rate, and therefore energy requirements, and the use of aerobic glycolysis steadily drops, reaching very low amounts when people reach their seventh decade.[35]

Studying men and women from ages 20 to 82, researchers found that based on oxygen flow and glucose utilization, women's brains averaged three years younger than men's brains. This was even true among the youngest subjects in their 20s.[36] This may help explain why even older women, far past menopause, tend to score better than men of the same age on tests of reason, memory, and problem solving.

Corresponding to the gradual decline in energy requirements, cerebral blood flow gradually declines with age. After puberty, females start to demonstrate less decline in cerebral blood flow, especially in the temporal and parietal lobes.[37] However, by around age 65, women's blood flow advantage tends to disappear. In women, there is less loss of protein synthesis–related gene expression during aging,[38] evidence for less memory decline and less atrophy in the hippocampus in females as they age compared with males.[39]

During aerobic metabolism, when oxygen (O_2) enters the body it splits into two single oxygen atoms with unpaired electrons, and presto, you have free radicals—normal waste byproducts of the process. Electrons prefer to exist in pairs; this makes these atoms unstable, much like a divorced male on the rebound, so they seek out other compounds with whom they can, in today's parlance, "hook up," i.e., another compound from which they can borrow electrons causing a domino effect of electron stealing. Seeking out and attaching themselves to other compounds causes damage to cells and to critical proteins, including DNA.

Much like political radicals, free radicals don't become good citizens through counseling, but through the "justice" wrought by anti-oxidants. They scavenge free radicals and donate an electron without becoming destabilized themselves, creating a new, stable electron pair, stopping the domino effect of electron stealing. Reactive oxygen species (ROS) is another term for free radicals. During normal metabolism, there is a stable, low level of ROS balanced by anti-oxidants. But in the presence of environmental toxins, ROS can increase, significantly disrupting the normal balance. Oxidative stress is the cocktail party word for the biologic state where there are insufficient antioxidants to counterbalance the free radicals. Neurotoxicity can result in brain damage from the induction of oxidative stress.[40]

Unneutralized free radicals are responsible for the steady and continual deterioration of organisms from aging and are the triggers for a long list of chronic diseases. Oxidative stress plays a prominent role in the age-related toxicity that results in neurodegeneration. One of the relevant actions of estrogen is its ability to donate an electron to neutralize free radicals. Damage to mitochondrial DNA from oxidative stress is much higher in males than females.[41]

Acting in a role largely as the polar opposite of estrogen, testosterone may enhance neurotoxicity.[42] For example, the neurotoxicity of the mercury-based vaccine additive, thimerosal (see Chapter 4), is enhanced when exposure to testosterone is added and it is mitigated by exposure to estrogens.[43]

GHRELIN

Ghrelin (not to be confused with gremlin) is commonly referred to as the "hunger hormone," which undoubtedly was a dominant stimulus for our ancestor hunter/gathers in their search for food. Technically it's a peptide (smaller molecule than a protein) consisting of 28 amino acids, and it is released primarily from an empty stomach but also in small amounts from the pancreas, kidney, pituitary gland, small intestine, placenta, ovary, and testes—I guess that's for whenever your testicles get hungry. If given to humans, ghrelin provokes an increase in food intake by about one third, which means that when you are trying to lose weight, don't ask for extra ghrelin on your pizza.

Ghrelin also has receptors in the pituitary gland and plays a role in the release of insulin and in cardiovascular homeostasis. Ghrelin levels increase when someone tries to restrict their diet, making losing weight all the harder. It can also act as an anti-depressant, stimulating nerves in the hippocampus.[44] Ghrelin triggers the production of BBFL (brain's best friend for life), brain-derived neurotropic factor (BDNF). More about that shortly.

Ghrelin levels are closely tied to sex hormones. Young women have three times as much ghrelin as young men,[45] but those levels decrease with age; not so with men. Estrogen creates a reinforcing feedback loop with ghrelin: the more estrogen, the more ghrelin. The interaction of estrogen and ghrelin gives the female another biochemical brain boost unavailable to the male.

> WARNING! The following paragraphs contain industrial-strength science. If you feel dizzy or faint while reading, grab a copy of People magazine and move quickly to an open window.

PROGESTERONE

$C_{21}H_{30}O_2$ — Progesterone

$C_{19}H_{28}O_2$ — Testosterone

Estrogen and progesterone are both primarily produced by the female ovaries, but they are also produced at other sites, including in men's adrenal glands and testicles. They are very different from each other in both chemical construction and in function. Progesterone is a precursor to testosterone, and in chemical structure, it is closer to testosterone than to estrogen.

Like estrogen, progesterone also has neuroprotective properties.[46] Progesterone protects brain tissue during fetal development and also after brain trauma.[47] Progesterone heals and protects injured brain tissue, and that is essentially what environmental contaminants such as air pollution do—they disrupt and injure brain tissue, even leaving in their wake what amounts to scar tissue. This neuroprotective effect is probably mediated by biological mechanisms similar to those of estrogen.[48] Like estrogen, progesterone likely inhibits the expression of genes responsible for releasing inflammatory cytokines, thereby reducing the harmful brain swelling associated with so many types of brain injuries, including pathologies such as strokes.[49] Progesterone also activates genes that inhibit the more controlled type of cell death, apoptosis, which helps prevent spread of the damage beyond the site of direct injury, preserving nerve cells and brain tissue.[50]

Similar to estrogen,[51] progesterone is effective in reducing brain swelling after injury, a critical part of the therapeutic strategy.[52] It was even effective if administration was delayed for a day after the injury.[53] Brain edema (swelling) can be an ominous development in such injuries because it impairs blood flow to the brain and contributes to the death of neurons. With traumatic brain injury, even brain cells at a distance from the original site of trauma are at risk of dying because they have long axons that may connect to the injured areas, a process called retrograde degeneration. Progesterone likely reduces that process after injury.

Normally, the mortality rate in patients with severe brain injury is about 30%. One study using progesterone treatment cut the mortality rate to 13%.[54] Based on animal research, human trials of intravenous administration of progesterone after brain injury showed clinical improvement in brain function and decreased incidence in mortality one month, three months, and up to six months afterwards.[55] Other human studies have not shown any benefit.[56] A recent meta-analysis, however, found that the survival rates and neurologic benefits of progesterone in brain trauma were significant at 3 months after injury, but not at 6 months after.[57] But many researchers felt like the differences in study designs make it harder to document the benefits in humans.

There are now about 100 papers showing evidence of the efficacy of progesterone in improving survival and neurologic outcomes with brain injury[58] My favorite of these is a study where researchers caused head injuries to female mice, then stimulated their cervixes, which increases progesterone production.[59] Those mice had less brain swelling and better brain performance afterwards. I want to know what kind of person applies for the job of mouse cervix stimulator? Congressman Matt Gaetz?

Progesterone limits tissue damage in brain trauma, stroke, diabetic neuropathies, and other types of neuropathologies in humans and other species. More specifically, research indicates that it helps rebuild the BBB and is associated with a dose-related reduction in brain swelling, inflammation, and cell death.[60] Progesterone has also been shown to be protective in animal studies of spinal cord injuries.[61]

Estrogen and progesterone serve as general neurotrophic molecules that stabilize nerve function, support the health and viability of nerve cells, and can be protective against the death of nerve cells from a variety of causes.[62] The types of clinical situations in which research has shown these hormones to be beneficial in both animals and humans include brain and spinal cord trauma, experiments that simulate a stroke by interruption of blood flow to both the entire brain and localized areas, and experimentally induced autoimmune encephalitis.

The mechanism of action of estrogen and progesterone presumably involves receptors for both compounds in the brain. Both estrogen and progesterone are lipophilic (fat soluble)—they pass through the blood-brain barrier, enter the brain cells by passive diffusion, and bind to those receptor sites, some of which are in the nucleus of the cell. The binding of these hormones to their receptors' sites flips the associated genes to an on position, and that enhances the release of neuroprotective proteins.

More specifically, these female hormones stimulate a cascade of warm and fuzzy brain goodness, my non–medical dictionary term for neurite outgrowth, sprouting of neurons, synaptogenesis (creates more synapses), an increase in the level of the neurotransmitter acetylcholine, increased density of N-methyl-D-aspartate receptors, and higher expression of neurotropic factors, including nerve growth factor.[63] Most of these effects are long term, but other effects on genes more specific to prevention of cell death, likely have immediate, short term benefits.[64]

Here's a brilliant idea for all you football fans. You have likely heard some alarming things about CTE being widespread in football. It's very clear that if you tried to dream up something with the goal of making your brain look like swiss cheese, you'd be hard pressed to come up with something worse than football. Ok, boxing. Ok, ultimate fighting. Ok, a part-time job as a woodpecker, or any other substance pecker. No one has improved their brain function by playing football, boxing, or perhaps even playing soccer, with all the microtrauma from headers. Given how much better women survive and heal from brain injuries, the NFL should replace all the men on their teams with women. At least the amount they are paying out in CTE lawsuits would decrease. And I have no doubt Beyonce could play quarterback in her sleep and make Tom Brady look like a chump.

On the subject of sleep, men and women also differ in their response to a much different type of sleep—anesthesia. Women require more intravenous anesthetic drugs in order to achieve the same depth of anesthesia, and they emerge more quickly from anesthesia than men.[65] The problem of awareness during surgery and anesthesia, periodically sensationalized by the media, is more likely to occur in women.[66] Women also have more pain after surgery and generally more difficult postoperative courses, with more nausea, shivering, and overall prolonged time to feel well afterwards.[67] Female hormones likely play a role in this difference between the sexes, highlighted further by the significant difference between menstruating and postmenopausal females. Increased progesterone during pregnancy, likely contributes to decreased anesthetic requirements during C-sections. There are receptors in the brain for estrogen and progesterone, which probably act as gatekeepers, allowing increased excitability of both the brain and spinal cord in females.

GLUTAMATE

Glutamate is one of the most prevalent excitatory neurotransmitters in the brain, and it is not exactly an asset. Many acute and chronic neurological disorders, such as brain trauma, stroke, intracerebral hemorrhage, meningitis, brain hypoxia, and malignant glioma tumors are associated with pathologically elevated glutamate levels in the fluid that surrounds the brain and spinal cord. Chronic excitotoxicity, i.e., overstimulation, leads to the death of neurons and is thought to play a role in other neurodegenerative diseases, including ALS, Alzheimer's disease, and Huntington's disease. So, if you live in, say, Memphis, and have never had to risk "excitotoxicity" over your city's NBA championship prospects, you can take consolation in knowing that you are averting neuronal death.

Any substance that decreases glutamate could be protective against a large group of brain insults. Enter the menstrual cycle. The rise of estrogen and progesterone in the first half of the menstrual cycle, peaking just prior to ovulation, is associated with a significant reduction in blood levels of glutamate and its adverse effects.[68] Overall, females are less susceptible to glutamate excitotoxicity.[69]

Anesthesia for brain surgery increases blood levels of glutamate. Scavenging glutamate from the blood seems to improve intraoperative neurologic outcomes.[70] But women have lower baseline blood levels of glutamate during such operations.[71]

BRAIN-DERIVED NEUROTROPHIC FACTOR (BDNF)

For those of you needing a part time job and are thinking about brain surgery, the next eight paragraphs are recommended before you pick up a scalpel.

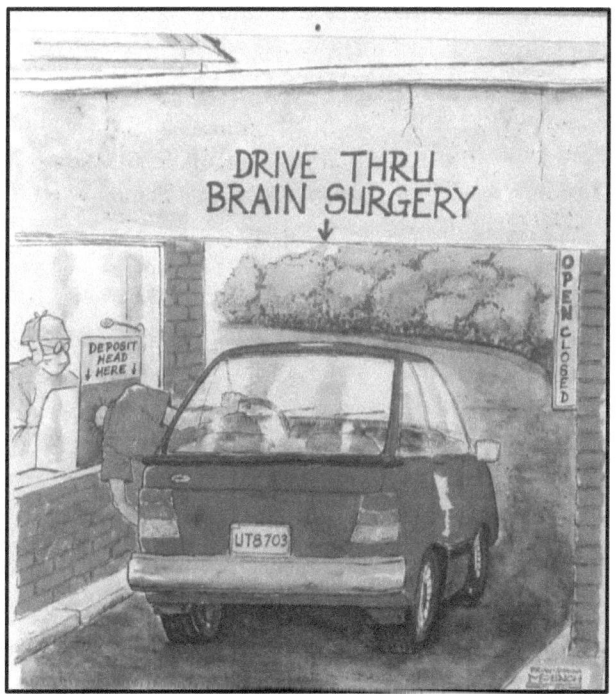

The BDNF gene provides instructions for making an important brain and intestine protein. Think of it as Miracle-Gro fertilizer for the brain. BDNF is probably the most important of several brain proteins, or neurotrophins, and is involved in virtually every kind of neuronal activity. It's almost this simple. Neurons that receive enough BDNF survive, while those that don't get enough are chewed up by the microglia.

Female Hormones—The Great Brain Protectors

It is thought that the supply of BDNF is not overly abundant and that neurons must actually competent for it.[72] I mentioned Darwin at the beginning of this book. The neurons that take the most advantage of BDNF have the upper hand in the brain's competition of survival of the fittest. This protein also promotes creation, maturation, and healthy maintenance of nerves wherever they are located in the brain. BDNF plays an important role in dendritic branching and in maintaining synapses. You can also think of it as the brain's personal handyman repair service. BDNF helps synapses adapt over time in response to experience, a key process important for learning and memory. BDNF also stimulates the chemical transmitters that propagate nerve impulses.[73] It is found in regions of the brain that control eating, drinking, and body weight. Its presence in these areas suggests that the protein likely contributes to the management of these essential, visceral functions.

BDNF is not unique to humans. It is found in many species throughout the animal kingdom. In fact, it was first isolated from a pig brain. Lower than normal levels of BDNF in either the blood or cerebrospinal fluid correlates with the susceptibility to, and the prognosis of, numerous common neurologic diseases—Alzheimer's, Parkinson's, and Huntington's diseases, Rett Syndrome, multiple sclerosis, and ALS.[74]

Higher levels of BDNF are likely to be important for maximizing cognitive abilities and maintaining mental health. Relative deprivation of BDNF may also contribute to numerous psychiatric disorders.[75] Stress decreases BDNF expression in several parts of the brain, and BDNF deprivation is associated with depression. Numerous things can raise levels of BDNF, many of them related to optimal personal lifestyle and habits. Exercise, intermittent fasting, limited caloric intake,[76] curcumin, green tea, omega 3 fatty acids, grapes (and wine), dark chocolate, pistachios, blueberries, peanuts, sunlight, vitamin D, and social interaction have all been shown to increase levels of BDNF. (More about diet and the brain in Chapter 9.)[77]

There is some variability among mammals as to which gender has a BDNF advantage. Female rats have more BDNF than males,[78] but male mice have more than females. If you are a human and would like more BDNF in your pre-frontal cortex, it helps to be a female.[79] Among females, levels of BDNF fluctuate with the menstrual cycle, rising and falling in concert with estrogen levels.[80] Decreasing estrogen by removing ovaries dramatically decreases BDNF, and supplemental estrogen afterwards can at least partially restore BDNF levels.[81] In lab animals, stress-inducing events decrease BDNF in males but increase BDNF in females.[82] Some researchers postulate that estrogen and BDNF function synergistically.[83]

Women have higher blood levels of BDNF than men.[84] Furthermore, various maneuvers that decrease testosterone increase BDNF reactivity. Menstruating women have higher levels than postmenopausal women.[85] Even short-term estrogen replacement increases BDNF levels.[86] In the BDNF sweepstakes, all is not lost for males because testosterone can be locally converted into estrogen by enzymes residing in specific brain areas that happen to regulate BDNF as well.[87]

Females have more cellular receptors for BDNF than males, and these receptors trigger apoptosis, the less destructive form of cell death. The brains of male mice, on the other hand, have fewer of these receptors, the scarcity of which causes neurons in the male brain to undergo the more violent type of cell death marked by bursting or disintegration of the cell, called necrosis, and that process can spread the damage and free radicals to neighboring cells. This may partially account for the significantly higher rates of birth injury–caused cerebral palsy among males.

Playing perfectly into the hands of anyone looking for jokes about male brain activity being detoured through their penises is a great deal of research that shows that significant BDNF activity in the male is routed (wasted?) toward the nerves that supply the male gonads.[88] Other species demonstrate a similar connection. In male songbirds, testosterone levels peak in the spring in anticipation of breeding opportunities, and that coincides with increased BDNF activity, again supporting the brain/gonad connection in males.[89] This is evidence that it isn't just male homo sapiens whose thought processes are too often dominated by the control centers positioned between their legs.

BRAIN AGING

Some things improve with age, such as wine, gouda cheese, and manure; but perhaps not our politicians, despite their sharing many manure-like characteristics. In 2024, if one were to judge the most important issue facing our country in the run up to the election, based on how many news stories were launched about the issue, you would conclude that saving American democracy, saving humanity from the climate crisis, preventing Voldemort Putin from feasting on our allies in Europe and starting a nuclear catastrophe, were not among them. Instead, you would think that the age of our presidential candidates was the only thing that mattered. Let's talk about the aging brain.

One thing that does not get better with age is gene expression. Loss of gene expression that stimulates protein synthesis is an important driver of brain aging. Female hormones help preserve that gene expression. Overall, between the ages of 20 and 90, the number of neurons in the average human brain decreases less than 10%.[90] Likewise, the number of synapses is relatively well maintained. But the brains of men and women age differently. To be blunt, the brains of women age more gracefully than men. In men, brains atrophy more as they age, especially in the critical frontal and temporal lobes.[91] Through changes in the expression of genes, different parts of the brain age at different rates, especially by the sixth and seventh decades. On average, across all brain regions, men showed three times more gene changes than women.[92] Furthermore, a higher percentage of gene changes were down-regulated (shut off) in men compared to women. This pattern of gene changes in men translates broadly into a decreased capacity for energy production and less production and transportation of proteins. More specifically, this means a decreased ability to remove dead cells and less capacity to replace them.

In both sexes, those genes that were up-regulated (turned on) by aging were more likely to be genes involved in inflammation and immune activation. This is consistent with growing evidence that in the brain, as in other organs, chronic inflammation is central to aging.

The most significant change in the male brain occurs as they reach their 60s and 70s, but it usually remains relatively stable at age 80 and beyond. All the hand wringing about Biden's age should apply to most of the members of Congress and it would certainly apply to Trump. In contrast, the most significant changes occur in women in their 70s and 80s. This pattern of age progression with gene expression is similar to the clinical pattern of age-related dementia in the two sexes. Men's risk of dementia plateaus after the mid 80s, whereas women's risk continues linearity with age. (See Chapter 7.)

INFLAMMATORY CONDITIONS

In animals and humans, the prognosis for females afflicted with a variety of acute inflammatory conditions, including those caused by infections and the catabolic and inflammatory state caused by surgical procedures, is better than for males.[93] For example, males are at higher risk than females for developing meningitis and encephalitis from West Nile Virus,[94] and Eastern Equine Encephalitis.[95] In contrast, that gender advantage is reversed for chronic inflammatory conditions of autoimmune disorders such as cystic fibrosis, severe asthma, lupus, arthritis, and chronic obstructive pulmonary disease. The inflammatory process is simply different for women than for men.[96]

Inflammation is a double-edged sword. In acute circumstances, the ability to mount an inflammatory response is an essential asset, almost certainly one of the reasons that women have almost double the survival rate of men in serious COVID infections. But when inflammation becomes chronic, inflammation can cause serious tissue destruction and can become the cause of disease rather than the cure. Put another way, a robust immune system is important to good health. But an overactive immune system can be a one-way ticket to real trouble. The immune and inflammatory responses are likely influenced by hormones. Animal studies indicate that females demonstrate less brain inflammation than males when exposed to xenobiotics and brain trauma.[97]

STROKES

Strokes, also known as "brain attacks," are the third leading cause of death for both sexes. Women in their 20s and 30s have a higher incidence of strokes than men,[98] probably related to pregnancy, birth control pills, and a higher incidence of migraines with significant visual disturbances and other aura.[99]

After their 30s, however, women have a lower incidence of strokes compared to men for the next several decades. Nonetheless, after menopause, women's advantage is largely lost, and by the early 80s, women are again the victims of stroke much more often than men.[100] There is also a geographic stroke belt, an area from Virginia down to Florida and west to Texas that has America's highest rates of morbidity and death from stroke.

Experimental studies suggest that administered estrogen can protect the brain from stroke damage[101] in both male and female animals.[102] One likely mechanism is that estrogen seems to preserve blood flow in brain areas downstream of where a blood vessel is occluded. Animal studies clearly show that males are more susceptible to brain damage from strokes.[103] Brain cell death caused by a stroke follows a different mechanism for each sex, related to the activation of different enzymes. This suggests that research into brain protection in strokes should involve different medications depending on the sex of the patient.

Clinical studies on strokes throw a bit of a curveball in the narrative of estrogen's being brain protective. Estrogen-producing women have a lower incidence of stroke than age-matched males or menopausal women, and women survive strokes at higher rates than men, but they have greater disability.[104] There is a suspicion among researchers that this is a reflection of inferior treatment for women once they are admitted to the hospital, as well as higher rates of less adequate treatment of the pre-existing risk factors before the stroke happens.

On average, women are also four years older when they have their first stroke than men are.[105] They are more often in worse pre-existing health and suffer more severe strokes compared to men. Social factors are also likely to be at play because, for example, more women live alone and are less financially secure than men. Women also fare worse than men after a heart attack, heart surgery, and angioplasties.[106] In the pediatric population, strokes occur more often in boys, and they have worse outcomes.[107]

I have a patient that has a pea-sized bulge (called a diverticulum) in his aorta, which is the garden hose–sized artery that carries blood from the heart to the entire body. This diverticulum is right next to the origin of smaller, critical arteries providing blood supply to the brain and spinal cord. He faces the dilemma of two poor choices. If he opts for a repair of his aorta (either through entering a smaller, distal artery and threading an innertube retrograde to close off the diverticulum or having his chest cracked for essentially open-heart surgery), he risks damaging the blood supply to the brain or the spinal cord. The end result could be a stroke, paralysis, or both. If he opts to avoid those risks, he leaves himself at risk for an aortic rupture, and virtually guaranteed sudden death. The patient is probably at higher risk for a more catastrophic outcome simply because he is a male. That patient is me.

Almost regardless of the type of brain insult—trauma, heavy metals, environmental toxins, stroke, and the aging process—the female hormones are the great brain protectors

> Complete tech support is available for this book. For "Who the hell wrote this?," press one. For "Who can I sue?," press two. For "This caused my divorce, you bastards," press three. For "This caused my divorce, thank you," send us money and press four.

Female Hormones—The Great Brain Protectors

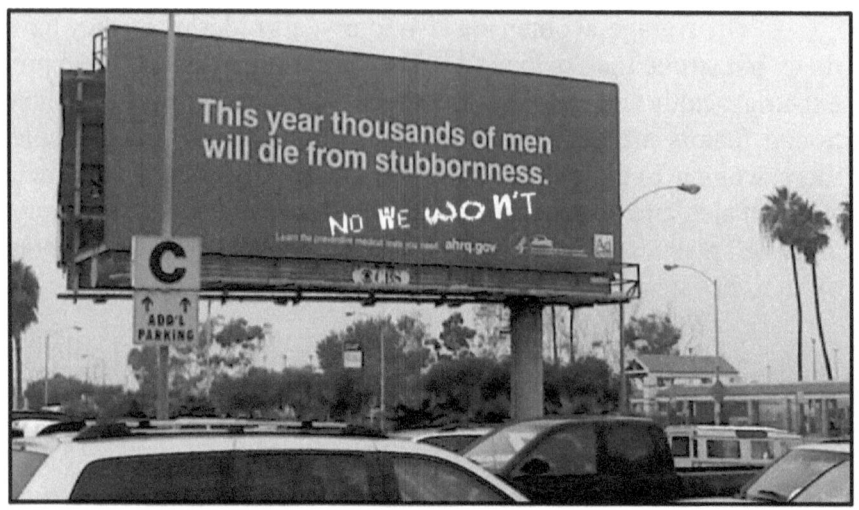

Winner of the 2020 Pultizer Prize for Billboard Graffiti

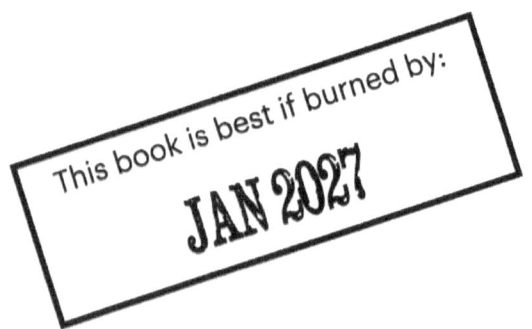

Chapter 7

THE ALZHEIMER PARADOX-THE MALES STRIKE BACK

> "The brain is an amazing organ. It starts working in a mother's womb and doesn't stop working till you get elected to Congress."
>
> —Senator John N. Kennedy, R-Louisiana, adapting a quote from the poet Robert Frost

> "Just like Jesus said, 'The poor will always be with us....'There's a group of people that just don't want health care and aren't going to take care of themselves."
>
> —Representative Roger Marshall, R-Kansas, decrying Obamacare

> "I think it was great at the time when families were united—even though we had slavery—they cared for one another....Our families were strong; our country had a direction."
>
> —Roy Moore, alleged pedophile and ousted ex-judge who lost the Alabama Senate race waxing nostalgic over America's golden age of slavery

In high school, I had a friend who was the quintessential '60s high school glamour girl: pretty, popular, a cheerleader. She had the physical attributes of a femme fatale but was a genuinely sweet, kind, and unassuming person. My wife allowed me to play the role of her date at our 30-year high school reunion because she trusted her implicitly not to make anything untoward of it. She was diagnosed with Alzheimer's at age 65. Within a couple of years, she went from being a beautiful, vibrant woman to being bedridden, unable to communicate or feed herself, and unable to do anything but generate a blank stare. She died at age 70, seemingly robbed of everything that had made her human.

After they reach middle age, adults fear Alzheimer's more than any other disease, including cancer. More specifically, twice as many Americans fear losing their mental capability as fear losing their physical capability.[1]

Everything I have written so far, I am about to seemingly contradict in discussing the Alzheimer's Paradox. But read carefully, because the devil, and my premise, is in the details. Alzheimer's causes progressive cognitive deterioration and 80% of cases of dementia. Microscopically, its hallmark features are deposits of beta-amyloid proteins and neurofibrillary tangles made up of abnormally phosphorylated tau protein in the cerebral cortex and subcortical gray matter. That leads to a shrinking of brain matter, including loss of neurons and synapses. On gross examination, these brains appear excessively shriveled up.

The diagnosis is made only from the symptoms, because there are no blood tests or imaging studies that are definitive for the disease. Although the symptoms and pathology are well known, the actual cause of Alzheimer's is still not understood. There is significant individual variability in Alzheimer's pathology, and in the progression, symptoms, and overall clinical course. That variability suggests it is likely that there are multiple causes and pathways to the disease.[2]

Alzheimer's is the fifth leading cause of death for women and the eighth leading cause of death for men.[3] In 2017, Alzheimer's cost the American healthcare system $259 billion. By 2050, it is projected to cost a staggering $1.1 trillion dollars per year.[3] Alzheimer's is a disease process that starts about 20 years before it becomes clinically apparent and a diagnosis is made.[4] Losing a sense of smell is an early sign of both Alzheimer's and Parkinson's disease. Two thirds of Alzheimer's patients are women, and the age of onset is typically earlier in women than men, starting in the late 50s and early 60s, and their decline in cognitive function happens twice as fast as in men.[5] Another way to look at it is that at age 45, a man has a one in ten chance of eventually developing Alzheimer's;

a woman of the same age has a one in five chance. Advanced age is the strongest risk factor for Alzheimer's, and there are more women at older ages, when the development of Alzheimer's is most likely. However, female longevity does not wholly explain the higher frequency and increased lifetime risk for women.[2]

Confounding the sex differences in Alzheimer's is that women have a higher risk of diabetic complications than men, including coronary heart disease, heart attacks, and depression, all of which are risk factors for Alzheimer's. High blood pressure, high cholesterol, and diabetes in middle age increase the risk of Alzheimer's later on in both sexes, but they increase the risk more for women than men.[6] Midlife depression increases the risk of later Alzheimer's by 70%.[7] As early as puberty, females have about twice the risk of depression as men,[8] and that vulnerability increases with menopause.[9]

Perhaps it is not surprising that at every stage of life, depression is associated with impaired cognition and memory, given that these mood and memory functions originate in the same areas of the brain. For women, a past history of depression nearly doubles the risk of Alzheimer's.[10] Correlating with depression is volume loss of brain mass in the hippocampus and prefrontal areas.[11] Low socioeconomic status, low education attainment, and marginal employment history are all risks for Alzheimer's in both women and men. But those underlying risk factors are more common for women,[12] although the educational attainment of younger women, on average, is becoming greater than for men of comparable age, as alluded to earlier in the book. Along with improved occupational opportunities, this may explain why rates of dementia are declining more for women than for men.[13]

Physical activity at midlife and beyond is associated with reduced Alzheimer's risk,[14] and women exercise less than men.[15] Marital status affects Alzheimer's risk. Men who have never married or are widowed have a greater risk compared to single or never-married women.[16] Marital status is also an important element in the prevalence of depression and happiness. Recall that the happiest cohort in modern society are single, childless women, and they also live longer. Ouch!

During our awake state, we accumulate toxic beta amyloid proteins, and during sleep, the "intra-cerebral" clean-up crew arrives and clears them out. Poor or fragmented sleep increases the risk of eventually developing Alzheimer's because the clean up crew can't do its job.[17] Sleep and circadian rhythm disturbances are common among all patients that develop Alzheimer's.

Hypertensive pregnancy disorders (HPD) are increasing in frequency for at least two reasons—an increasing rate of obesity and later-age pregnancies. Women with a history of HPD suffer from more brain atrophy and more white matter hyperintensities (see Chapter 5) decades after their pregnancies.[18] Even with the same amount of Alzheimer's plaques in the brain, men with Alzheimer's have fewer cognitive and memory deficits than women with the disease. How can that be?

Estrogen helps the brain utilize blood glucose. When estrogen drops at menopause, lab animals then turn to ketones for brain energy. You've heard of the "Keto diet," the daily, 18-hour-fasting approach to weight loss? That's close to what's going on in the post-menopausal female brain. Astrocyte brain cells produce ketones from fatty acids. To facilitate this energy production process, a microscopic version of cannibalism takes place inside a woman's brain. To create fatty acids, the post-menopausal female brain cells will actually start eating myelin (the protective coating of axons) from nearby neurons, for a source of fuel.[19] I'm pretty sure that's against the Geneva Convention. Post-menopausal women average a drop of one standard deviation in the volume of their white matter on MRI scans, and the areas most affected are those that correspond to the regions first clinically impacted in Alzheimer's.[20]

Adults over 70 years of age, of both sexes, experience greater decline in cognition, functionality, and brain volume after general anesthesia than would be expected from continued aging.[21] This is especially true if they are already experiencing pre-operative cognitive loss. But women decline more than men, at a faster rate, and they decline even more if they have to undergo multiple surgeries.[22] It is unfortunate that this issue is seldom addressed in a pre-operative visit between a patient and her physicians.

Researchers at the Neurobiology Lab for Brain Aging and Mental Health, Transfaculty Research Platform Molecular and Cognitive Neuroscience, University of Basel, Switzerland, said, "In [Alzheimer's] patients, women showed more dramatic losses of steroid sex hormones as compared to men with [Alzheimer's], and these losses paralleled Alzheimer's-related cognitive decline and accumulation of amyloid-ß."[23]

A woman who has a hysterectomy increases her risk of eventually suffering from Alzheimer's. I can virtually guarantee that women are not having that discussion with their gynecologist when they consider having a hysterectomy. If she has one ovary removed with the hysterectomy, that increases her risk further, and if she has both ovaries removed at the time, that increases her risk even more—140% over women who had none of those gynecological surgeries.[24]

If a woman manages to avoid Alzheimer's by the age of 65, she'll have a one in five chance of developing it during the remainder of her life[25] compared to the one in 11 chance for men. Once women hit their 60s, they'll be twice as likely to develop Alzheimer's disease as they are to develop breast cancer. Post-menopausal women accumulate more amyloid than men but can also develop more tau (abnormal protein) and have worse symptoms even for the same amount of amyloid. Carriers of the notorious Alzheimer's gene, *APOE4,* are at twice the risk if they are women, but for men the gene barely increases the risk at all. Women with mild memory impairments deteriorate at much faster rates than men in both cognitive and functional abilities.

Estrogen acts as a natural anti-depressant.[26] Nonetheless, women are more susceptible to depression, and recall that depression is also a significant risk factor for acquiring Alzheimer's. Woman are even more susceptible after menopause.

Through chemical transformation, both men and women make estrogen out of testosterone. But it may be counterintuitive that men make approximately twice as much estrogen as post-menopausal women.[27] Until recently, researchers focused on how the presence or absence of estrogen affects women and how testosterone decline affects men. But that is starting to change. The middle-aged abdominal spread in men may be due as much to a loss of estrogen as it is a loss of testosterone.

Estrogen loss in both women and men accelerates aging of the brain. In men, a small amount of testosterone is converted by enzymes into estrogen, and that is the primary source of estradiol in men. Because testicular secretion of testosterone never completely stops, at least among men who still have their testicles (few in Congress), serum estrogen levels are higher in elderly males than in postmenopausal women. More estrogen in elderly males compared to women of comparable age probably explains the Alzheimer's paradox. But that confirmation research is still waiting.

Hormone replacement therapy (controversial for many reasons) instituted after menopause does not appear to be brain protective in women. (See Chapter 6). Brand new research published just before this book was finished showed another twist in the differences between men and women with Alzheimer's. While post-menopausal women have a greater risk for Alzheimer's than men, paradoxically, women live longer than men once they get Alzheimer's, even after the estrogen benefit has long faded. No one seems to have an explanation for that yet.

A gene that exists only on the X chromosome, *KDM6A*, gives women additional protection. Malfunctioning of this gene causes Kabuki syndrome, associated with developmental delay and intellectual disability, anywhere from mild to severe. Women with two X chromosomes compared to a man's single X chromosome have two copies of this gene that produce a protective protein. A particularly active version of the *KDM6A* gene is present in 13% of women and in 7% of men. Having two X chromosomes gives women a better chance of this gene variant, with some women even having two copies of the gene. Women, in general, have more of the KDM6A protein in their brain than men do. The protective effect of this gene found only on the X chromosome was also confirmed in mice.[28]

Throughout most of human life, the male brain is simply a more fragile organ, more sensitive to almost all insults, from trauma, disease, and environmental toxins, and less able to repair the damage. Unfortunately, our government and society have done virtually nothing to address this sobering reality.

P.S. There's one way men are more responsible than women. Half of all women are guilty of applying make up while driving. Around 450,000 vehicle accidents are caused every year by women "beautifying" themselves while driving.

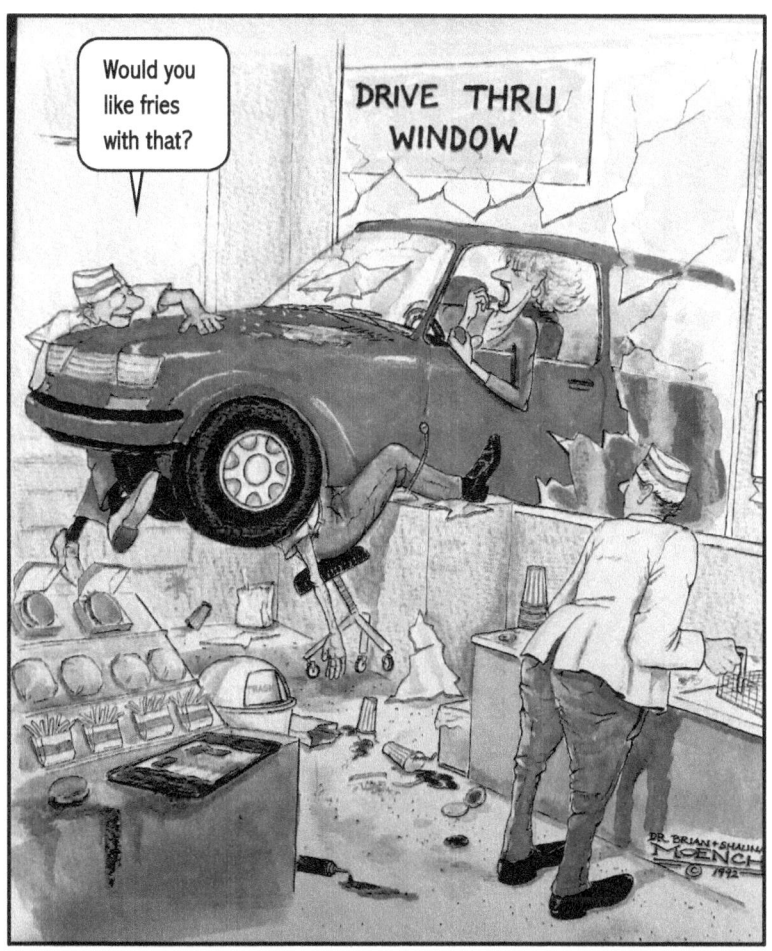

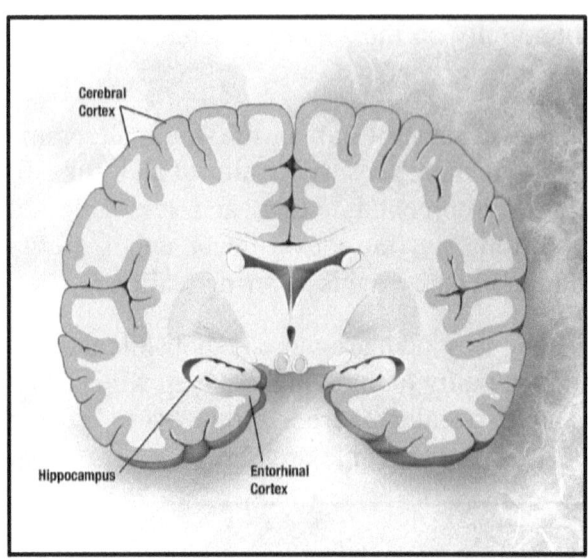

Normal brain, frontal plane

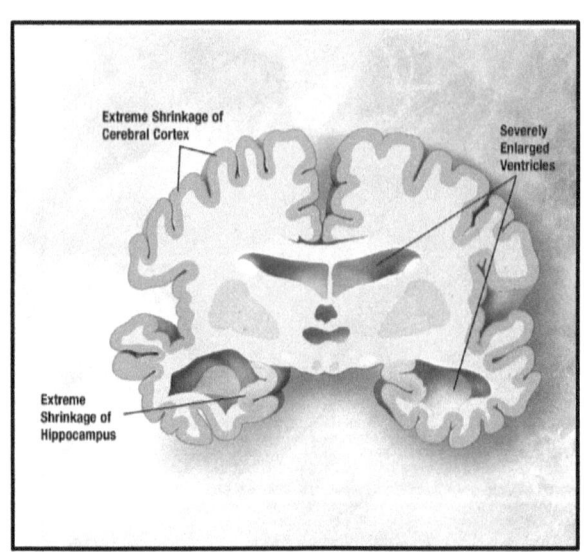

Alzheimer's brain, frontal plane

Chapter 8

AUTISM: A MALE PANDEMIC

"The Great Flood is an example of climate change. And that certainly wasn't because mankind overdeveloped hydrocarbon energy."

—Texas Representative (R) Joe Barton

"I guess I'm gonna fade into Bolivian"

—Mike Tyson, former heavy weight boxing champion

"I've been on food stamps and welfare. Anybody help me out? No."

—Craig T. Nelson, actor in the TV Show *Coach*

In 1943, Leo Kanner first used the term "infantile autism" to characterize children who were withdrawn and unable to socialize with their peers. Autism is just the most conspicuous of an entire spectrum of brain disorders that are now far too common. There are no biologic indicators of the disorder, and the diagnosis depends solely on the presence of a range of behaviors.

Autism is often thought of as a single isolated entity, a debilitating malfunction of the brain. In fact, it is a heterogeneous spectrum of brain disorders, ranging from mild to severe, characterized by deficits in managing social interactions and communication capability, often punctuated by repetitive, non-productive behavior and restricted interests. It is typically manifested in childhood and continues into adolescence and adulthood. But even as a spectrum rather than a single entity, it is only the most prominent member of a very large fraternity of brain disorders, many of which have strong environmental connections and a significant gender bias.

Autism—A Male Pandemic

Autism is the extreme manifestation of an inability to process social stimuli and construct appropriate responsive language. It is 4 to 5 times more common in boys than girls. Some studies found even higher ratios. Moreover, while autism is assumed to involve behavioral, language, and perhaps cognitive deficits, it is usually much more than that, including seizures, mood disorders, gastrointestinal diseases, hormonal imbalances, obesity, and sleep disorders. The 2015 economic cost of autism has been estimated to be $162-$367 billion per year.[2]

Autism is increasing in frequency in the U.S. at an alarming rate. Even if some of the increase relates to an expanded definition of the disorder and better awareness and identification of afflicted patients, consider this trend. The autism rate in the U.S. in the late 1980s was 3.3 in 10,000.[3] In 2007, it was 1 in 150. In 2009, it was 1 in 100. In 2012, it was 1 in 88. In 2014, it was 1 in 68. In 2018 it was 1 in 59. If this rate of increase were to continue, by 2025 it will be 1:2, i.e., 50%. That would be preposterous, but it speaks to how sharply the rate is increasing. The CDC says that since the 2012 estimate that 1 in 88 children were identified with autism, the criteria used to diagnose, treat, and provide services have not changed, but the rate has increased another 30%. As I write this, among children aged 3-17 years in the U.S., one in 40 has been diagnosed with autism,[1] the highest rate in the world. Twenty-seven studies from 18 different countries representing five continents have found that the rate of autism has been increasing over time in every region evaluated.[5]

Although autism carries a unique and alarming stigma, and it can be profoundly life altering, it is only one point on the wide spectrum of childhood and developmental disorders of the brain that have a strong connection to environmental neurotoxins mentioned elsewhere in this book. Although autism is touched on in some of the other chapters, it deserves its own special emphasis.

Formal diagnostic criteria for autism did not exist prior to the publication of the third edition of Diagnostic and Statistical Manual of Mental Disorders (DSM-III; American Psychiatric Association [APA]) in 1980. Any diagnoses made prior to this publication were not based on any standard criteria. Since 1980, official criteria evolved and were expanded throughout the subsequent versions of DSM (APA, 1987, 1994, 2000 [DSM IV-TR]) up until its latest revision, the DSM-5, May 2013, in which the definition of autism has been changed.[6]

There are a few modifying factors that may contribute a small artifact to the alarming increase in the number of children diagnosed with autism. A child with both intellectual disability and autism is now more likely to be diagnosed with autism than in the past.[7] But hand wringing over that element of statistical uncertainty seems irrelevant, because in both cases, important brain dysfunction is being identified and only serves to compel us to find contributing factors to both.

Improved neonatal care for premature infants also plays a minor role in the numbers of people with autism. As survival of very premature and low birthweight infants improves, those survivors will have a significantly increased risk for neurodevelopmental disorders, including autism, compared to the rest of the population.[8]

Carrying on the long American tradition of downplaying risks to the public, several skeptical groups and individuals have emerged, working hard to minimize what the overwhelming body of evidence suggests is an alarming epidemic. *Spectrum* magazine is one example; they seem particularly committed to the idea. *Spectrum* makes the argument that the increase in those case numbers is primarily an artifact of more prevalent diagnoses rather than a more prevalent disease. They publish an article every year with that theme.[9] They point to the fact that in 1991, the U.S. Department of Education ruled that a diagnosis of autism qualifies a child for special education services, which incentivized parents to seek the diagnosis. In 2006, the American Academy of Pediatrics recommended that all children be screened for autism at 18 months and 24 months. The earlier the diagnosis, the more intervention and the better the outcome. Despite that, the age at which most children are diagnosed with the disorder has changed very little. For the last decade it has remained around age 4 1/2, which would seem to undercut the argument that it's just today's parents being more motivated to find answers, clinicians being more attuned to the disease, and everyone more eager to join the bandwagon.[10]

Higher socioeconomic status and access to good medical care increases the rate of diagnoses. This explanation was offered for why white children were once diagnosed with autism at higher rates than blacks. That has now changed; the rates of diagnoses are now equal in both, which, oddly, is being heralded as a good thing, presumably as a reflection of more racial equality for diagnostic visits. But the rates in Latinos still lag behind. Sceptics also point to parents' having children at an older age now as increasing the autism risk.

It seems difficult to fathom that these minor explanations can wipe away what otherwise appears to be an increase in the disease of 7,500% in slightly more than 30 years. To begin with, were parents 40 years ago more oblivious to their children's inability to communicate than they are now? Doubtful. The idea that parents of 40 years ago were less aware of a child that was struggling to communicate and was not developing appropriately for his or her age would be hard to explain. Yes, the words, "autism," "Asperger's," and the acronym "ASD" maybe more part of the lexicon now, and there are autism support groups that parents can join, but it defies reason that children with these deficits would somehow slip under the rug 40 years ago but not now. My wife and I were parents of young children 40 years ago, well connected to other parents of young children. We were all as attuned to the intellectual and social development of our children as any parents are now.

If autism was always really that prevalent and we're just diagnosing it better, where are all the adults with autism that everyone failed to recognize when they were children 40 years ago? Children today are less likely to be raised exclusively by a stay-at-home mother, more likely to be raised, in part, by a care giver or in a day care center. So, for parents of today to be more attuned to their child's development than parents of a few decades ago seems hard to rationalize.

If, according to the "it's not really increasing" theory, and the incidence of autism has actually been stable for decades, that would mean that one in every 40 adult Americans has autism—over 8 million people. In 2015, there were not 8 million people in America with autism; there were fewer than half that, 3.5 million diagnosed cases.[11] It seems doubtful there are 4.5 million cases of undiagnosed autism hiding in a barn somewhere in this country. If all homeless people in America, all prison inmates, and all state mental hospital residents had autism, that still wouldn't add up to 4.5 million more cases. Furthermore, if sociological and diagnostic trends characteristic of America were the explanation, that does not explain the increased rates in other countries, albeit not as dramatic as in the U.S.

Focusing on whether the autism epidemic is increasing is also missing the heart of the issue. Regardless of whether the number diagnosed is dramatically increasing, there is an epidemic of autism and other developmental disorders, even if the rate is stable. It is an unparalleled public health emergency that millions of people are debilitated by a serious functional brain disorder that persists throughout their lifetime, hindering their enjoyment of life, limiting or eliminating their career potential, largely refractory to interventions, financially and emotionally burdening family members, and costing society billions of dollars in lost wages and care costs.

If the rise in the prevalence of autism is more real than artifact, what are the possible causes? A specific cause with reasonable certainty is only found in about 10-12% of autism cases.[12] Regarding the others, there is a substantial body of research to provide some clues. Maternal dietary and nutritional deficiencies in folate and vitamin D are possible causes. Gestational diabetes during pregnancy increases the risk about 60%.[13] Obesity during pregnancy doubles the risk.[14] Given the population trends in obesity and type II diabetes, this could play a role. Infections like influenza and rubella increase the risk of autism 100-200%. But there is much more to the story.

Autism—A Male Pandemic

Autism's much higher prevalence among boys than girls is likely related to a defect in the single male X chromosome contributing to antioxidant deficiency. But there is no such thing as a de novo genetic disease epidemic because genes don't change that quickly. So, the alarming rise in autism must be the result of increased environmental exposures that exploit these genetic defects.

A recent Stanford University study examining 192 pairs of twins, where one twin was autistic and one was not, found that genetics account for 38% of the risk of autism, and environmental factors account for 62%.[15] Suggesting an environmental and genetic tag team are other studies showing that mothers of autistic children and autistic children themselves have a high rate of a genetic deficiency in the production of glutathione (see Chapter 6), an antioxidant and the body's primary means of detoxifying heavy metals.[16]

The list of autism's environmental suspects is long and comes from many different studies that show higher rates of autism with greater exposure of the pregnant mother to flame retardants, plasticizers such as BPA, endocrine disruptors in personal care products, heavy metals in air pollution, mercury, pharmaceuticals such as anti-depressants, and pesticides.[17]

Analyzing concentrations of environmental toxins in air, water, and soil is of limited value in determining health hazards because exposures among a human population can vary widely. Hair analysis in individuals, however, is considered an important, reliable biomarker and is very helpful in assessing heavy metal exposure. Migration of metals from body tissues to hair is a route of excretion, and a destination where those metals can accumulate. Concentrations of metals in hair generally reflect the mean level in the human body, providing a biological window to an individual's or even an entire population's exposure to heavy metals.

A study of children in Egypt found that compared to controls, autistic children had higher levels of mercury, lead, and aluminum in their hair.[18] High levels of toxic metals in children are strongly correlated with the severity of autism.[19] Typical urban air pollution from fossil fuel extraction, processing and combustion, and wood burning is one of the important delivery mechanisms for some of the toxins found to be contributors to autism. (See Chapter 5).[20] That should be of particular concern to states like Utah and New Jersey, because Utah has had the highest rates of autism of any state in the country until being recently eclipsed by New Jersey.[21]

Given the heavy preponderance of autism in boys, it would seem logical that if air pollution is an autism risk factor, air pollution neurotoxicity would be found preferentially in males. Indeed, that is the case. Women pregnant with a boy, breathing air pollution even at a level 50% lower than the EPA's official safe threshold, were found to have an about 20% increase in their risk of delivering a baby with autism.[22] Furthermore, pregnant mothers who took extra folic acid, which helps increase glutathione production, offset the increased risk of their newborn eventually being diagnosed with autism that comes with air pollution exposure.[23]

The human intestine is home to an astounding quantity and an enormous variety of bacteria and other microorganisms, referred to as the human microbiome. There are roughly the same number of bacteria in our GI tracts as human cells in the body, around 40 trillion,[24] and that includes about 2,000 different bacteria species.[25] Recently, the connection between the GI tract and the brain has been shown by evidence that the "trillions of bacteria, viruses, archaea, and eukaryotes that make up the gut microbiome" are altered in a wide range of neurologic disorders—including autism, depression, and Parkinson's.[26] This increasing recognition within the medical community that there is a strong connection between the brain and the GI tract has prompted some to call the GI tract our second brain. For men, it may be the third brain, after the one in the skull and the other one well known to dangle between their legs.

There is a two-way signaling connection between the GI tract and the brain.[27] Because of that, disruptions of the normal bacterial population of the intestines can have neurologic consequences. Altered gut bacteria have been found in a variety of neurodevelopmental and neurodegenerative conditions. In December 2019, the journal *Neurotoxicology* had an entire issue devoted to this subject.[28] Neurons in both the brain and the intestines are affected in autism. There is a consistent pattern of bowel inflammation in a high proportion of children with autism.[29] In fact, as many as 90% of autism patients have abnormal GI symptoms. There appear to be the same kinds of genetic mutations involved in both.[30]

While autism rates in the U.S. have climbed dramatically, rates in Europe have remained closer to flat for the last decade, and that is with the backdrop of air pollution probably being slightly worse in Europe than in much of the United States. Their clean air standards are less strict than those in the U.S., and more Europeans still smoke cigarettes. But they have better protective laws regarding chemical exposures.

Recent estimates of autism in European countries range from 1 in 5,000 in Germany to 1 in 700 in Portugal. So, what are Americans doing to harm themselves and their children's brains that Europeans aren't, besides watching Fox News and *New Jersey Housewives*? No one knows for sure, but there are at least two possible reasons for Americans' being more at risk. One is the massive use and steady increase in GMOs in our food supply, and the concomitant upsurge in pesticide and herbicide use. (See Chapter 5.) Another is the fluoridation of community water supplies. (See Chapter 4).

In more than 60 developed countries worldwide, there are significant restrictions or outright bans on the production and sale of GMOs. In the U.S., federal agencies have approved the GMO/pesticide industrial agriculture system, with safety assumed solely on the basis of studies conducted by the same corporations that created them and profit directly from their sale.

At a June 12, 2013, autism conference in Edinburgh, Scotland, Dr. Martha Herbert, pediatric neurologist, expert on autism from Harvard Medical School and author of *Autism Revolution*, explained her conclusion that the culprit is an environmental toxin in autistic children that interferes with nutrient absorption from the intestines. Humans only absorb nutrients courtesy of the bacteria in our gut, which is disrupted by glyphosate, the most common herbicide used with GMOs. Because glyphosate is a chelating agent, binding minerals such as cobalt, zinc, manganese, calcium, molybdenum, and sulfate, it obstructs the absorption of essential nutrients.

The neonatal period is, simultaneously, a critical window of development for microbes to inhabit the infant gut as well as a window for rapid brain growth and development. In the early 2000s, animal studies showed that both beneficial and adverse manipulation of the bacterial content of the GI tract was associated with changes in neurological development of the animals.[31]

Relevant to the observation that autism is at least four to five times more common in boys than girls, researchers found that manipulating the intestinal microbiome resulted in altered levels of the neurotransmitter serotonin in male mice but not in their female counterparts.[32] Other studies show that altering the gut microbiome impairs a person's ability to excrete other known neurotoxicants, like mercury, arsenic, and nicotine.

Several studies show that the gut microbiome is abnormal in children with poor neurological development, and others show a wide range of abnormal GI symptoms among people with autism. Moreover, changes in the gut bacterial flora are associated with changes in the symptoms of autism.[33]

Strong circumstantial evidence suggests that by altering the microbiome of the gut, Bt-toxins from GMOs and the pesticides used in concert with them, could be causing microscopic leaking in the intestinal walls of newborns, facilitating the absorption of incompletely digested foods and toxins into the blood. That, in turn, triggers systemic inflammation, precipitating autoimmune diseases and food allergies. Furthermore, since the BBB is not developed in newborns, toxins in the blood may migrate into brain tissue itself, interfering with normal brain development. This is a very plausible biological pathway for autism. The brains and cerebrospinal fluid of autism patients consistently show a marked inflammatory process.[34]

A connection between the GI tract and the brain has recently been strengthened by other new research. Symptoms of gastrointestinal problems are also common in other neurologic diseases like Parkinson's. Eighty to 90% of Parkinson's patients have GI complaints, especially constipation, but also including delayed gastric emptying, dysphagia (difficulty swallowing), and excessive saliva. Patients with autism, Parkinson's, Alzheimer's, and multiple sclerosis all have a high incidence of an abnormal bacterial population in their GI tract.[35]

Not surgprisingly, antibiotic administration alters the bacterial population of the GI tract. Pregnant mothers who are given antibiotics for whatever reason have a 10% increased risk of having their children diagnosed with autism after birth.[36] Other studies of prenatal and postnatal antibiotic exposure have been somewhat inconsistent. However, a meta-analysis of these studies published in 2019 did show a significant relationship between early life antibiotic exposure and autism, especially prenatal antibiotics.[37]

There is a significant relationship between people who have had appendectomies and the incidence of Parkinson's. Contradicting previous smaller studies, in an analysis of the records of over 62 million people, patients who had had appendectomies had triple the risk for developing Parkinson's at some point afterwards, regardless of race, age, or gender, although men had a higher rate than women.[38]

The protein alpha-synuclein, previously mentioned, is found in nerves that innervate the intestines of patients early in the disease course of patients with Parkinson's. Alpha-synuclein contributes to neuron death in Parkinson's in several different ways, primarily by forming toxic aggregates such as Lewy bodies, the protein clumps that develop inside neurons, characteristic of Parkinson's and some dementias. A severe form of early onset Parkinson's has been linked to a gene that helps produce alpha-synuclein. These Lewy bodies accumulate in the lower brain stem that controls GI function and in the nerves that line the GI tract—the enteric nervous system. These Lewy bodies are present in the GI tract many years before the appearance of the classic motor/muscular components of tremors, slowness, and stiffness.

Amplifying the brain/gut connection is the fact that patients with inflammatory bowel diseases, such as Crohn's and ulcerative colitis, have an increased risk of eventually developing Parkinson's, and patients with autism have higher rates of inflammatory bowel disease.[39]

PESTICIDES AND "BEE AUTISM"

There are more connections between autism and pesticides. To explore that further, it's helpful to look into what is happening with the world's bee population. On a recent front page of *The Salt Lake Tribune*, a frightening, oversized headline read, "Highest rate in the nation, 1 in 32 Utah boys has autism." Less well publicized, another national story ran the same day: "New pesticides linked to bee population collapse." If you eat food and hope to do so a few years from now, this should be even more frightening. A common denominator may underlie both stories.

Recall that during the critical first three months of gestation, a human embryo adds 250,000 brain cells per minute, reaching about 100 billion by the fifth month. Furthermore, the creation of neurons and communication pathways is nearly complete by birth, and then it drops off rapidly. Very little neuron creation continues into adulthood, with the exception of a few specific locations.[40]

There is no chemical elixir that improves this biological miracle, but thousands of toxic substances can cross the placenta and impair that process, leaving brain cells stressed, inflamed, less well developed, fewer in number, and with fewer anatomic connections with each other. The opportunity to make up for the resulting deficits later on is almost non-existent. All combined, when such a child reaches adulthood, he/she will suffer a wide range of neurologic deficits.

To protect fetal development, doctors have long advised women during pregnancy to avoid any unnecessary consumption of drugs or chemicals. They should also be advising them to never listen to *Black Sabbath's Christmas Album* for the same reason. As mentioned before, the average newborn has, at a minimum, over 200 different chemicals and heavy metals contaminating its blood when it takes its first breath, with 158 of them known to be toxic to the brain. With the tens of thousands of untested chemicals permeating our environment, 100 times more than two generations ago, it is little wonder that rates of autism, attention deficit, and behavioral disorders are so prevalent and are on the rise.

How does this relate to disappearing bees and your ability to put "food on your family," in the immortal words of President George W. Bush? Numerous studies show that the rapid rise in the use of insecticides is likely responsible for the mass disappearance of bee populations.[41]

In May 2014, a study that should be regarded by regulators as the definitive answer was published by the Harvard School of Public Health in the "Bulletin of Insectology." It showed that bees exposed to neonicotinoids at commonly found doses showed a fatality rate of 50%, with the deaths showing all the characteristics of Colony Collapse Disorder. Furthermore, in the control hives, only one of six colonies were lost, and that was due to a parasitic fungus. But in that hive, the dead bees remained in the hive. Despite the fact that virtually all the colonies were infected with pathogens, those that collapsed and those that didn't, only those exposed to the pesticides had abandoned their hives. The authors stated, "It is striking and perplexing to observe the empty neonicotinoid-treated colonies because honey bees normally do not abandon their hives during the winter. This observation may suggest the impairment of honey bee neurological functions, specifically memory, cognition, or behavior, as the results from the chronic sub-lethal neonicotinoid exposure."[42]

Researchers from Royal Holloway University of London fitted bumble bees with tiny radio frequency tags, similar to those used by courier firms to track parcels, (and I guess the kind James Bond uses when he wants to know if international bumblebee villains are trying to kill him), and found that neonicotinoid pesticides (neonics) affected their choice of flowers to visit and impaired their ability to forage and gather pollen.[43]

Scientists affiliated with the Task Force on Systemic Pesticides (a global group of 29 independent scientists) completed a full analysis of all the available literature as of 2014, involving 800 peer-reviewed reports, and stated, "The evidence is clear that neonics pose a serious risk of harm to honey bees and other pollinators. In the case of acute effects alone, some neonics are at least 5,000 to 10,000 times more toxic to bees than DDT." But focusing on only acute effects conceals their true impact. As mentioned earlier, the breakdown products (metabolites) of neonics are often as toxic or more toxic than the original active ingredients.

Recall that neonics are systemic pesticides; they permeate the entire plant. The review emphasized that the classic measurements used to assess the toxicity of a pesticide (short-term lab toxicity results), only scratch the surface for systemic pesticides. The combination of persistence over months or years and solubility in water has led to large-scale contamination of, and accumulation in, soils and sediments, ground and surface water, and treated and non-treated vegetation. They concluded that neonics pose a serious risk to honeybees and other pollinators, such as butterflies, and to a wide range of other invertebrates, such as earthworms and vertebrates, including birds.

I recently provided anesthesia for a professional beekeeper who had hundreds of hives. I asked him what he thought was the cause of bee colony collapse disorder. Without hesitation, he said pesticides. The nervous system of insects is the intended target of these insecticides. They disrupt the bees homing behavior and their ability to return to the hive. "Bee Autism" is a perfect description of what these pesticides do to bees. Because about 90% of native plants require pollinators to survive, most of the world's food chain hangs in the balance.

But let's get back to humans for a moment. You might be thinking insects are different than humans, right? Human and insect nerve cells share the same basic biologic infrastructure. Chemicals that interrupt electrical impulses in insect nerves will do the same to humans. But humans are much bigger than insects, and the doses to humans are miniscule, right? At around seven weeks after conception the human brain starts to develop in earnest, but the embryo is still only about a half inch long, smaller than a honey bee.

Based on size alone there is every reason to believe that pesticides could wreak havoc with the developing brain. But human embryos aren't out in corn fields being sprayed with insecticides and herbicides, are they? Recall that we mentioned in a previous chapter that a recent study showed that every human tested, including urban dwellers who had no direct contact with any stage of crop or livestock agriculture, had the world's most popular pesticide, Roundup, detectable in their urine at concentrations between five and twenty times the level considered safe for drinking water.[44]

Glyphosate (Roundup) is a potent endocrine disruptor (see Chapter 5), meaning it can interfere with the production, release, transport, metabolism, or elimination of the body's natural hormones, which are the most potent biologic substances known to science. Fetuses and infants are particularly at risk, as any disruption of endocrine systems can affect brain development.

Research published in the *New England Journal of Medicine* [45] compared brain autopsies of autistic children who had died from unrelated causes to brain autopsies of children without autism. The brains from autistic patients demonstrated abnormal patches of disorganized neurons disrupting the usual distinct layers in the brain's cortex. The primary implication of the research is that the abnormalities almost certainly had to have occurred in utero, during key, short, developmental windows between 19- and 30-weeks' gestation. Brief exposure in utero is likely to have lasting consequences to brain development. Even more important than the dose of a toxin is the timing of exposure, i.e., during critical developmental windows, and the presence or absence of other facilitators or synergistic toxins.

As noted earlier, there is obvious genetic variability in susceptibility to autism among individuals. That autistic genetic profile may have deep evolutionary roots,[46] because a subset of genes found in "antisocial" bees share molecular similarity with a subset of genes in humans that have autism. This group of genes can affect how well bees become integrated into a hive.

Through ineptitude, ignorance, apathy, and corruption, we are allowing the same handful of chemical companies that are wiping out pollinators critical to our food supply to also threaten the intellectual potential of our children.

Several authors point to a number of studies implicating exposure to fluoride and aluminum, and the possibility of synergism between the two, in increasing the risk of autism. It is worth noting that a lower incidence of autism is found in European countries that banned fluoridated water (See Chapter 4).[47] In contrast, a high rate of autism has been found in countries that add fluoride to municipal water or have areas with endemic fluorosis.[48]

Low levels of glutathione, coupled with high production of another chemical, homocysteine, increase the chance of a mother's having a child with autism to one in three, according to Dr. Jim Adams, director of Arizona State University's Autism/Asperger's Research Program. Abnormally low production of glutathione is well established in plasma, immune cells, and brains of children with autism.[49] Fluoride can reduce the cellular concentrations of glutathione, precipitate oxidative stress, and increase the sensitivity of neurons and astrocytes to chemical excitation and ultimately, cell death. That, in turn, leads to neuroinflammation and the release of chemicals that interfere with the flow of blood through microscopic blood vessels in the brain. Indeed, inflammation is a common but not universal biochemical feature of the brains and the cerebrospinal fluid of autistic individuals of any age.[50]

The human pineal gland is best known for regulating melatonin, and therefore, it plays a role in helping to establish healthy sleep patterns. But melatonin also regulates mitochondrial metabolism, and therefore, is essential to a nerve cell's energy pathway. It plays a role in digestion, a functioning immune system, and is an antioxidant. Fluoride's inhibitory effect on melatonin may be an explanation for the gastrointestinal symptoms, brain inflammation, and immune disorders common to patients with autism.

Sleep problems, insomnia in particular, plague 50-80% of patients with autism. Fluoride accumulates in the pineal gland which can interfere with the release of melatonin from the blood. Over half of patients with autism have abnormally low plasma levels of melatonin.[51] A few studies have correlated melatonin levels with the severity of autism.[52]

Oxytocin, the prosocial, nurturing neuropeptide mentioned in Chapter 2, that is more abundant in women, has recently been studied for its potential benefit in patients with autism. There is early evidence that it may, indeed, provide amelioration of some of the symptoms and behaviors associated with the disease. Adult patients with autism were given a month's worth of daily intranasal oxytocin or a placebo. In the oxytocin treatment group, there was less reported repetitive behavior, diminished feelings of social avoidance, and higher levels of energy and vigor compared to the placebo group. The effects lasted a month after treatment, and some effects persisted a year after treatment.[53] That women have higher levels of oxytocin than men also suggests another reason why females are less afflicted by the disorder.

With alarming and still rising rates of autism and behavioral disorders in the U.S., public health officials and politicians should be running around with their hair on fire in a frantic effort to find out exactly what is happening, why, and most importantly, how to stop it. However, the current American aversion to holding powerful industries accountable for anything makes it virtually certain that regulatory agencies will continue to turn a blind eye to most, if not all of the likely environmental triggers of autism.

Chapter 9
We Must Put More Women in Charge

"It's time for the human race to enter the solar system!"

——Former Vice President, Dan Quayle

"I think there is a world market for maybe five computers."

—IBM Chairman Thomas Watson, 1943

"Television won't be able to hold onto any market it captures after the first six months. People will soon get tired of staring at a plywood box every night."

—Daryl Zanuck, cofounder of 20th Century Fox

If men are left with more brain damage from the gauntlet of environmental toxins that both sexes are exposed to, what can be done to help protect them? Let's first review what won't protect them and how to save some money in the process.

"NO" ON NOOTROPICS

With all the talk about computer generated AI, artificial intelligence, threatening to destroy the human race, another type of artificial intelligence is threatening to empty the wallets of the human race. You may not realize that a large and profitable industry thinks you are spending far too little of your hard earned (or inherited, or stolen) cash on "Nootropics." What are those? you ask. Nootropics is the hundred-dollar word for brain cleaner among those who are "supplementarily enhanced," and "hundred-dollar" because you can spend that much money or more every month on your nootropics. And if you don't know what the word "supplementarily enhanced," means then you are undoubtedly supplementarily deficient, which only means you've saved yourself a lot of money by not becoming supplementarily enhanced. For that hundred dollars you can get an entire smorgasbord of things that sound like they could really frighten away stupidity.

In just one pill you can get "Alpha GPC, Lion's Mane Extract, Centrophenoxine, Bacopa Monnieri, Tyrosine, Phosphatidylserine, Ginkgo Biloboa Extract, L-Theanine, Rhondiola Rosea Extract, Taurine, Huperzine–A, apoaequorin, purified water and hypromellose." I was a little skeptical until I read that I could also get "purified water" at no extra charge (I'm not kidding), rather than your usual polluted water I suppose. And you can get this potpourri of brain rocket booster goodness all rolled into one with names like *Focus Factor, Einstein, Brain Booster, Neuriva, Ultimate Omega, Genius Mushrooms, Cognium, Basis,* and *Grass-fed Beef Brain* (I did not make that up).

"You might take something for your heart… your joints… your digestion. So why wouldn't you take something for the most important part of you… your brain?... With an ingredient originally found in jellyfish!" It "improves memory and supports healthy brain function, sharper mind, clearer thinking." "Healthier brain, better life!"

If you watch TV for more than five minutes a month you have undoubtedly been bombarded with ads like this one for Prevagen, whose main ingredient (apoaequorin) was found in jellyfish. No doubt that prompts some questions like, "Well, I already eat tons of jellyfish. I must be a genius!" or, "Just how many Nobel Prize winners have been jellyfish?" And, "If jellyfish are so smart, why are they letting humans suck out their intelligence?" All good questions to ask. That someone is exercising sufficiently poor judgement to waste their money on Prevagen is proof that Prevagen isn't working for them.

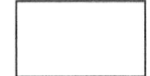

Group photo of all the jellyfish Nobel Prize Winners

In filing a lawsuit against the makers of Prevagen, former New York Attorney General Eric Schneiderman must have asked himself those same questions before he said, "The marketing for Prevagen is a clear-cut fraud, from the label on the bottle to the ads airing across the country. It's particularly unacceptable that this company has targeted vulnerable citizens like seniors in its advertising for a product that costs more than a week's groceries but provides none of the health benefits that it claims."[1]

In 2012, the Federal Trade Commission and the New York Attorney General filed suit charging the makers of Prevagen, Quincy Bioscience, with false advertising. They filed suit again in 2017 for "making false and unsubstantiated claims that the product improves memory, provides cognitive benefits, and is 'clinically shown' to work."[2] Quincy's "too good to be true" claims rested on one study that initially didn't show any cognitive or memory benefit beyond that of a placebo. Quincy then paid for 30 retrospective re-analyses of the data (a practice known as "data dredging," a classic technique for elevating false positive findings to the status of a proven claim), and then contended that within a few subgroups there was some memory improvement. But in yet another sad commentary on the weakness and inadequacies of government agencies, and the slow grinding of the wheels of justice, as of 2024, the lawsuit had not been settled, and the Prevagen advertising continues.

Just about everyone would like to be smarter than they are (except a certain former President, who is already endowed with maximal human intelligence, evidenced by his being able to recite, "person, woman, man, camera, TV," all at one time, and in some kind of order (You just can't improve on perfection). The demand for brain supplements comes from over 70 million baby boomers living in America but also from college students, corporate CEOs, scientists, and millions of other people that find occasional use for their brains. A recent survey of adults over age 50 discovered that one in four take some kind of over-the-counter supplement for brain health.[3]

Americans from both sides of the cultural spectrum are easy targets for supplement manufacturers. Too many Americans believe that their government protects them from dangerous or worthless products, including drugs and supplements. They are not aware that government agencies, in this case the FDA, simply don't function that way. That is thanks in large part to the Dietary Supplement Health and Education Act (DSHEA) of 1994, which treated supplements more as food than as drugs, and relieves manufacturers from the burden of proving to the FDA that their products actually work. They can make all kinds of wonderful claims as long as they keep them vague. That's why TV ads for these supplements, like those for Prevagen, consist of feel-good personal testimonials but include no actual data or facts from scientific studies.

My home state of Utah is the mecca of the dietary supplement industry. The formalized turning of a blind eye to oversight of the industry is thanks in large part to the influence of the former senior senator from Utah, Orrin Hatch, the principal author of the DSHEA. Hatch cultivated an intimate relationship with the industry, with a lot of mutual back scratching, such as sponsoring very favorable legislation and killing unfavorable legislation from colleagues. The relationship also included hundreds of thousands of dollars in campaign contributions and inserting multiple family and staff members into lucrative industry and lobbying jobs.[4]

Thanks to Hatch, here are the current, rather absurd FDA rules. "Supplement makers can make general claims about connections between their supplement and the body's structure and function. For example, a vitamin maker touting calcium in a product can say it's good for bone health—although calcium supplements may offer little or nothing for most people with healthy bones...."[5] "Supplement makers cannot claim their product treats or prevents a particular disease. That disclaimer, which may seem to contradict marketing promises, must appear on every package. So, commercials suggesting that a supplement can reverse or slow Alzheimer's disease, or any dementia, are perilously close to running afoul of the rules on marketing supplements."[5]

Manufacturers of these supplements can keep one toe in the legal bucket and avoid an FDA slap on the wrist by using phrases like "laboratory tested," "clinically proven," and "maintains good brain health." Those are science-ish kinds of words, right? Yes, and that is the language of a 21st century snake oil salesman.

Paradoxically, on the other side of the cultural divide, we have millions of Americans for whom distrust of government, doctors, scientists, authority figures, experts, pharmaceutical companies, and every other non-Facebook source of information has never been higher. That crippled the nation's ability to control the COVID pandemic, and has thrown nearly half the country into the fog of a fact free world. Those are also exactly the kind of people that succumb to the allure of non-scientific persuasion and therefore supplements.

Ginkgo biloba is one of the best-selling supplements that seniors take in hopes of dodging the bullet of Alzheimer's. The label makes this claim: "Supports healthy brain function and mental alertness," followed by a small asterisk. On the back side of the label, after the asterisk, is this disclaimer: "This statement has not been evaluated by the Food and Drug

Administration. This product is not intended to diagnose, prevent or cure any disease."

Not only do most of these nutritional supplements fail to provide proven health benefits, they sometimes include dangerous ingredients, in some cases intentionally and in other cases unintentionally. These include ingredients and contaminants like ephedrine, which can cause life-threatening rapid heart rate and dangerous high blood pressure, and anabolic steroids and lead. The General Accounting Office issued a report in 2010 that found trace amounts of lead in 37 of 40 products tested.[6] Over a 2-year span, 2,292 cases of serious illness related to supplements, including 33 that were fatal, were reported, according to federal records.[4]

American adults are particularly easy targets for sales pitches for brain supplements, because, as I mentioned before, they fear Alzheimer's more than any other disease:[7] more than heart disease, cancer, or whatever other diseases are caused by all the drugs advertised on TV. In fairness, it should be noted that so far, no medication made by our altruistic friends in the pharmaceutical industry has been found to be helpful either, including drugs that supposedly reduce levels of amyloid in the brain.[8]

Allow me a short detour into the world of the latest and hottest supplement dead ends. An emerging star of the supplement industry is *Basis*, the work of Leonard Guarente, the head of MIT's aging center, and famous Harvard University geneticist David Sinclair. Sinclair was listed in *Time Magazine's* 100 most influential people in 2014 and their 50 most influential people in health care in 2018 for his research in aging. He recently announced that he had shaved more than two decades off his biological age.[9] He boasted that he achieved this remarkable fountain of youth metamorphosis by "ingesting a molecule his own research found improved the health and lengthened the life span of mice. Sinclair now boasts online that he has the lung capacity, cholesterol, and blood pressure of a young adult and the heart rate of an athlete."[10] Actually he doesn't. He claimed a heart rate of 57, which shows he doesn't know what the heart rate of a fit athlete would be. Mine is 50, and I'm hardly an exceptional athlete, even for my advanced age, and Sinclair is only 51 years old.

Fountain of youth scams have been around since Adam and Eve were scammed by the serpent in the Garden of Eden. Alexander the Great searched for the fountain of youth in the 4th century AD. The Japanese have had for centuries, and still do, myths about springs with magic healing powers and restoration of youthful vigor. The legendary 16th century Spanish explorer Juan Ponce de Leon, spent years searching for the fountain of youth in Florida. The Fountain of Youth Archaeological Park is the oldest attraction in Florida.

For centuries life extending magic elixirs have been the province of literal snake oil salesmen and charlatans. In recent years a dose of science and research was stirred into these pots of quackery giving us dehydroepiandrosterone (DHEA), human growth hormone, testosterone for men, and hormone replacement therapy (HRT) for women, all of which had their day in the sun as the next fountain of youth, and all of which turned out to be leaking faucets of youth.

To his credit, Sinclair is well respected as a scientist. But other scientists cringe about what they see as the personality, if not the motivations of an undaunted salesmen. A decade ago Sinclair unveiled resveratrol as the triumph of aging prevention research, but the sun set on that one after about five years. Sinclair's book, *Lifespan: Why We Age—and Why We Don't Have To,* reached 11 on the *New York Times* best seller list in only a week after publication. Sinclair's reputation allowed him to form no less than 17 companies, including a fertility company, based on his research.

Sinclair is part of an all-star cast in a company, Elysium Health, and *Basis* was their original product. The scientific foundation for *Basis* is research in mice that showed it could improve longevity.[11] The company managed to assemble an advisory board of 35 scientists with stellar reputations, including eight Nobel Prize winners, like Thomas C. Südhof, a Stanford University neurophysiologist who won the 2013 Nobel Prize in Physiology or Medicine. That's eight more Nobel Prize winners than helped write this book. But before you get Nobel Prize heart palpitations, let's take a look at missteps of some of the world's greatest scientific minds when they stepped out of their area of expertise.

After establishing critical laws of physics, in the latter part of his life, Sir Isaac Newton began to study the architecture of the Temple of Solomon based on its description in the Bible. A religious fanatic, he began obsessing about the angles in the structure, and sketched detailed drawings of it. Then he began to claim he could predict the future. By the way, he predicted a second coming of Christ would usher in the apocalypse by 2060.[12] I'd put my money on the climate crisis beating him to it.

The Greek philosopher and mathematician Pythagoras invented the triangle (actually he just fathered the Pythagorean theorem allowing us to measure the length of a side of a right triangle). When straying from triangles, he envisioned how humans could write messages on the moon's surface by writing in human blood on a mirror and reflecting it to the sky.[13]

William Herschel, the 18th century astronomer who discovered Uranus, Oberon, and Titania, also thought the sun was a planet, covered with clouds that rained, and it was inhabited by aliens with big heads.[14]

The father of molecular biology, Linus Pauling, the only two-time winner of the Nobel Prize (chemistry and peace), in his later years became convinced Vitamin C cured everything, including cancer. Ironically, Pauling ultimately died of untreated prostate cancer. His mega Vitamin C consumption may have even hastened his death.

The inventions of Nikola Tesla in circuits and electricity became the foundation the electricity infrastructure of modern civilization. Tesla also believed he had invented a death ray that could cut the earth in half, but would also somehow prevent all future wars. He tried to market it to the governments of several countries.[15]

Then there's Elon Musk, the engineering "genius" that founded Tesla, PayPal, online banking companies, SpaceX, Starlink, Open AI, Neuralink, and others. He's become a modern-day Lex Luthor maniac.

Advisory boards usually don't do much beyond having their names on brochures. I've been on a university honors college advisory board, and all I did on it was become a target for more donation solicitations. That there are superstars on Elysium Health's advisory board is not a reason to fill your swimming pool with *Basis*, hoarding it in anticipation of Newton's 2060 apocalypse. Elysium claims that *Basis* gives you a veritable smorgasbord of miraculous, age-defying ingredients—well, two anyway. Just 2 capsules contain 250 mg of Nicotinamide Riboside, and 50 mg of Pterostilbene (distilled from stilbenes of pterodactyls, I suppose). Impressive. The more well-known name for Elysium's secret miracle ingredient, Nicotinamide Riboside, is simply Vitamin B3. In fact, it is just one of the three forms of Vit B3 (the others being niacin and nicotinamide). Nicotinamide Riboside is slightly better at converting itself into nicotinamide adenine dinucleotide (NAD^+) than the other forms of vitamin B3. This is an important cofactor vital to all living cells, so you do need it.

But just because you need oxygen doesn't mean that breathing extra oxygen will do anything for you (unless you have significant lung disease and are unable to deliver sufficient oxygen to your blood). In fact, breathing a higher percentage of oxygen than what exists in the atmosphere, 21%, will be toxic to normal lungs over time. Retrolental fibroplasia is an eye disease of babies born prematurely, caused by the oxygen therapy they require because of their immature lung development. In severe cases, it can cause blindness.

If you buy a Lamborghini that can go 140 mph, that's great, except if you drive it that fast, you're likely to get killed or kill someone else. You've merely wasted a lot money on a feature you can't use that is potentially dangerous. Likewise, spending a lot of money on more NAD^+ is also pointless. There is no evidence that increasing NAD^+ levels accomplishes anything. In fact, excess Vit. B3 in the form of niacin, was found in a 2024 study to cause inflammation and damage blood vessels. The authors of the study advised against niacin supplements.[110]

Pterostilbene, the other ingredient in *Basis*, is a powerful antioxidant. But that doesn't mean taking extra antioxidants beyond what is available in a healthy diet makes you any healthier.

Another red flag is that Elysium gets their ingredients from another fountain of youth supplier, ChromaDex. "ChromaDex normally supplies its ingredients to about a dozen consumer brands under the NIAGEN trademark but had worked out a special deal with Elysium so the startup did not have to mention where its ingredients came from," according to TC Sessions.[16] ChromaDex actually sued Elysium in 2016 for nonpayment of their bills. ChromaDex sells its own ingredients to consumers under the brand name TRU NIAGEN. So, if any of this actually works, why not just go straight to the manufacturer and eliminate the middleman?

Basis can be yours for a mere $50 a month, typical for fountains of youth sold to people drinking from fountains of gullibility. Coincidently, Sinclair has a major financial stake in the success of *Basis*. Peer-reviewed scientific research has not proven that *Basis* works on humans. When a manufacturer only cites their own in-house research, you should maintain a stratospheric-level of suspicion. As an article in Kaiser Health News said, "Discerning hype from reality in the longevity field has become tougher than ever as reputable scientists such as Sinclair and pre-eminent institutions like Harvard align themselves with promising but unproven interventions—and at times promote and profit from them." [17]

Jeff Flier, a former Harvard Medical School dean, who has publicly expressed his skepticism about these kinds of products, said there is so much financial reward that the inventors and the institutions they are associated with seem to be willing to cut major corners in establishing verifiable efficacy. "If you say you're a terrific scientist and you have a treatment for aging, it gets a lot of attention. There is financial incentive and inducement to overpromise before all the research is in," said Flier.[17]

"The sale of nutritional supplements of unproven clinical benefit is commonplace," said Stephen O'Rahilly, the director of Cambridge's Metabolic Research Laboratories that withdrew from a financial arrangement with Elysium. "What is unusual in this case is the extent to which institutions and individuals from the highest levels of the academy have been co-opted to provide scientific credibility for a product whose benefits to human health are unproven."[17] Felipe Sierra, the Director of the Division of Aging Biology at the National Institute on aging at the NIH said, "The bottom line is I don't try any of these things. Why don't I? Because I'm not a mouse."[10]

It turns out *Basis* isn't all you need. Elysium has discovered that you also need a back-up miracle. Just in case you've still got some money left in your pocket, you need a brain supplement called *Matter*. Apparently, Facebook's algorithms have concluded my brain needs real help. About ten times each day, an ad pops up on my Facebook page pitching *Matter*. It's "clinically proven" (where have we heard that before?), and it comes to you in partnership with Oxford, Cambridge, and Harvard Universities. It turns out Dr. Frankenstein's supercharging brain electrodes are nothing compared to a whiff of *Matter*.

There are too many unproven brain health supplements to address in this book—*Ageless Brain, Ideal Brain, Dynamic Brain, Neuro-Peak, Qualia Mind, Instant ATT, Focus Pep, Genius Consciousness*, just to name a few that you can buy right now, and coming soon I'm sure, *Albert Einstein's Ground Up Toe Nail Clippings Extract (it won't do anything for your brain, but it will give you Einstein's hair)*. But a few more deserve mention. In April 2019, playing a role more protective of consumers than the FDA has played, the Federal Trade Commission (FTC) settled its charges against the sellers of Geniux, Xcel, EVO, and Ion-Z. "With an aging population, it is more important than ever that advertisers have solid evidence to back up their claims about memory and cognitive health benefits," said Andrew Smith, Director of the FTC's Bureau of Consumer Protection. "Moreover, the FTC will hold companies accountable when they deceptively design their ads to look like news articles and fabricate celebrity endorsements and consumer testimonials."[18]

The dietary supplement industry is primarily unregulated, essentially a back alley, free-for-all bazaar of more than 90,000 products. The $20-$60 that many seniors spend every month on minerals, herbal mixtures, nutraceuticals, and/or amino acids supposedly for brain health really adds up. Supplement industry sales have reached about $40 billion every year; nearly $6 billion of that is spent on brain supplements, and almost all of it is money flushed down the toilet, literally, because almost all of it just makes your urine more expensive.

In another corner of Harvard University, hopefully next door to the office of anti-aging huckster Dr. Sinclair, comes this advice from Harvard Medical School. "Don't buy into brain health supplements."[111]

A recent poll found that half of Americans regularly take some form of vitamins, especially multivitamins, and 25% of adults over 50 take a brain supplement. And in only a fraction of those consumers do those vitamins do anything for their overall health or their brains. At the same time, other recent polls also show declining trust in traditional institutions of expertise, including mainstream medicine, which likely contributes to the supplement craze for patients seeking to treat symptoms themselves or thinking that their internet access has turned them into highly qualified physicians. Righteous indignation at the profiteering of the pharmaceutical industry drives other people to turn to supplements. But they are usually also turning a blind eye to the unproven efficacy of the supplement industry, perhaps because they mistakenly believe they are "natural medicines."

The research is now overwhelming that, rather than being the holy grail of health and longevity, for people that have a healthy diet, manufactured vitamins in pills and the myriad of supplements sold over the counter provide no benefit other than sustaining enormous profits for the supplement industry.[19] Furthermore, a test by ConsumerLab found that nearly half of vitamin supplements didn't contain what their labels claimed. In addition, they have fillers and dyes containing exactly the kinds of ingredients that many health-conscious consumers go to great lengths to avoid in their diet, like hydrogenated fats, oils, and even magnesium silicate, i.e., talc, which behaves like asbestos. Far too many people take vitamins and over-the-counter supplements with the rationale that antioxidants are a good thing, and you can never have too much of a good thing. But that is not the case with vitamins, and in some cases, too much is dangerous, like that 140 mph Lamborghini.

The Great Brain Robbery –Brian Moench

Even if you could achieve an over population of antioxidants within your cells, you would likely regret it. Free radicals (think Bernie Sanders), the target of antioxidants, aren't always the biologic villains they are routinely made out to be, just like antioxidants aren't always mythical superheroes. Both of them can reverse their assigned roles. Free radicals actually prevent cells from growing and dividing indefinitely, i.e., starting a cancer. Several studies of antioxidant supplements showed modest increases in cancer among those people that faithfully took supplements. They also play a role for the immune system in killing off invaders, like viruses and bacteria. Likewise, when an antioxidant such as vitamin C "takes a hit for the team" and accepts an election from a free radical, neutralizing it, the vitamin C now becomes itself weaponized as a free radical. In that role, it now is capable of wiping out beneficial proteins and damaging cells, including their DNA. The biochemistry of cellular metabolism is much more complex than just good guys (antioxidants) versus bad guys (free radicals).

Fat-soluble vitamins, such as A, D, E, and K, are readily stored in the body and are now well recognized as being capable of accumulating to levels that are counterproductive or even dangerous. Furthermore, numerous studies have shown that when antioxidants are ingested in pill form rather than consumed naturally from the food on your plate, they fail to protect memory or slow cognitive decline, and fail to provide any other health benefit. The Johns Hopkins Bulletin is one of many that throw cold water on a routine practice of vitamin supplements.[20] They highlight a study of 450,000 people that found multivitamins didn't reduce the risk of heart disease or cancer. Another study that followed nearly 6,000 men for 12 years found that vitamins did not provide any measurable benefit in preventing cognitive decline. In another study of over 1,700 heart-attack patients that were observed for 55 months, researchers found that taking multivitamins did not reduce heart attacks, surgery, or risk of death.

There are a few notable exceptions. People with a diet deficient in vitamins A, C, D, B6, or B12 can benefit by taking a quality supplement, as can people who have difficulty with absorption, like those with Crohn's or celiac disease. Pregnant women should take a daily folic acid supplement of 400 mcgs to help prevent birth defects. There is some research that suggests a combination of vitamin C, vitamin E, carotenoids, zinc, and copper can reduce the progression of age related macular degeneration.

What about omega-3 fatty acids? Dr. Donald Trump might think that injecting a dead fish along with the disinfectant he thought might ward off COVID would help ward off stupidity. Eating a dead fish would be much better. Omega-3 fatty acids likely have anti-inflammatory and antioxidant properties and help maintain cell membranes. As such, they have a good chance of helping prevent age-related loss of brain function.[21]

There are eleven different types of omega-3 fatty acids, but three types are the most relevant to discuss. Eicosapentaenoic acid (EPA) and docosahexaenoic acid (DHA) are found in oily fish, primarily salmon. Alpha-linolenic acid (ALA) is found in vegetables like Brussels sprouts, spinach, and kale, vegetable oils like canola or soybean, nuts (especially walnuts), and seeds (such as flaxseeds and pumpkin seeds). The human body is able to convert only a small amount of ALA into EPA or DHA.

There is limited research addressing the possible brain benefit of eating oily fish on a regular basis, but a few studies are encouraging. According to the Harvard School of Public Health, "An analysis of 20 studies involving hundreds of thousands of participants indicates that eating approximately one to two 3-ounce servings of fatty fish a week—salmon, herring, mackerel, anchovies, or sardines—reduces the risk of dying from heart disease by 36 percent."[22] But just as with vitamins and supplements, taking fish oil pills has not been proven to have much effect. You would have to take a small glass of fish oil every day in order to get enough to help your brain. On the upside, your fish breath would also help you avoid catching COVID from someone in a crowded bar and would make you more attractive to fish, in case you are still thinking about trying that *Shape of Water* thing.

For the average person, for virtually all the remaining supplements, especially multivitamins, there is no scientific evidence to support their use. Brain supplements will not be able to rescue men from consequences of their environmental exposures.

TRAINING AND HACKING YOUR BRAIN

Supplements are not the only pseudo brain boosters people waste a lot of money on. Hundreds of "brain training" programs and games are available to purchase and download. These programs lure consumers who are hoping to improve mental capability and the performance of personal and work-related everyday tasks. Commercial cognitive training has mushroomed into a nearly $2 billion industry despite the fact none of it has been shown to produce any measurable improvement in brain function in most people.[23]

The Great Brain Robbery –Brian Moench

The FTC ruled against the company behind one of the most well-known brain training programs, *Lumosity,* for an advertising campaign making unsubstantiated claims about improving cognition and school performance, protecting against Alzheimer's disease, and even treating ADHD. At best, these brain games may make you better at the games in these programs, and if you enjoy those exercises, that in itself may be somewhat beneficial. Anything that elevates mood is good for your brain. But for most people, that doesn't translate into improved overall concentration, mental acuity, or increased work productivity. That is not to say that challenging your brain with new skills, hobbies, practices, or even new travel doesn't help (more about that shortly). But unless you are New York Times and NPR puzzlemaster Will Shortz, who structured his own for-real master's degree in Enigmatology (you had no idea there was such a thing), and designs games for a living, brain game programs do not apparently improve your brain for any practical, non-Lumosity tasks.

I mentioned in the prologue that in the 1950s, my father was the first to incorporate electroshock therapy in a psychiatric practice in the state of Utah. He actually made his own ECT machine. ECT has a serious role to play in the treatment of severe depression. Probably inspired by the efficacy of ECT treatments in reducing depression, a fad called transcranial direct-current stimulation (tDCS), i.e., low-current electrical brain stimulation, is spreading, thanks to the internet and Facebook. It's being lauded as if it were an electrical brain supplement that improves memory, creativity, attention span, and even athletic performance. Thousands of research papers have been published in the last decade that include the term, "tDCS," which refers to the emission of a weak electrical current, usually between two electrodes attached to the forehead.

It's certainly true that the brain runs on electricity. Those tiny electrical charges send signals across the synapses that bridge neurons together. Learning occurs because the synapses involved "learn" to fire more readily, and tDCS supposedly enhances that process. The small current used in tDCS—one to two milliamps—is not enough to trigger neurotransmitters to cross synapses, but the theory is that tDCS makes learning more efficient. Some studies suggest it can enhance learning tasks and improve reaction times.

This "brain hacking" movement has morphed into "do-it-yourself" tDCS, not unlike sticking your finger in a light socket. You can waste anywhere from $20 to $700 for a kit that includes essentially wires, adhesive pads, and a 9-volt battery. There is no shortage of "how to" advice on the internet from armchair experts who can show you how to zap yourself to brilliance, fortune, and a spot in the starting five of the Los Angeles Lakers.

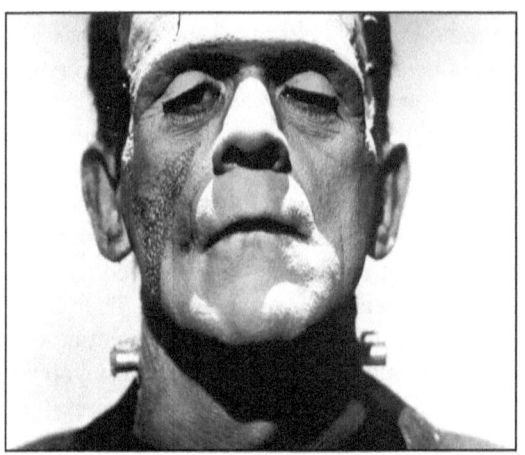

Note the world's first attempt at tDCS didn't go so well because, as you can see, Dr. Frankenstein put the electrodes in the wrong place.

Michael D. Fox, MD, PhD, assistant professor at Harvard Medical School, and associate director of the Berenson-Allen Center for Noninvasive Brain Stimulation at Beth Israel Deaconess Medical Center, Boston, Massachusetts, was one of 43 scientists that endorsed an open letter in the journal *Annals of Neurology* advising against this do-it-yourself brain hacking.[24] He explained, "There is so little that we understand about what happens with transcranial brain stimulation....The effects reported in scientific papers are usually small after being averaged across many different subjects. Effects in a single subject are highly variable, and in some people, it can have an adverse effect on cognitive function."[25] It is, at best, premature to believe that tDCS holds the key to making anyone's brain a fire hydrant of brilliance, a ticket to glory in the world of sports, or a horror movie star. An in-depth review of this practice is beyond the scope of this book, but suffice it to say that it is controversial and remains a curiosity and a research tool at best.

Hyperbaric oxygen therapy (HBOT) has been used for many years to help wound healing that can be compromised by various disorders. A hyperbaric chamber achieves higher-than-normal atmospheric press while delivering 100% oxygen to a patient, which in turn, delivers more oxygen to the wounded or abnormal tissues compromised by poor blood flow. It is helpful and is approved by the FDA for healing necrotizing infections, decompression sickness, diabetes-related wounds, and even radiation burns. It has been used with some success in improving outcomes for patients with traumatic brain injuries (See Chapter 6). HBOT has also been overused in some clinics that promise such things as preventing or curing cancer, even though there is little if any evidence that it works for those diseases.

There is some research to support using HBOT to improve memory in patients who have had strokes, and even the rather fantastical claim that it works years after the stroke.[26] It is still controversial, because most other studies show that it must be initiated in such a short time frame after the stroke that patients are still too unstable to be placed in a hyperbaric chamber, and the benefit may not last. It has not become standard treatment for stroke rehabilitation or to minimize stroke damage.

An intriguing new study from July 2020 found that HBOT could also help reverse some of the characteristics of age-related mental decline, in particular, executive functioning, attention, and processing speed, via improvement in microscopic cerebral blood flow,[27] but many more studies will have to be done before HBOT could be considered a practical means of suspending or reversing age-related mental decline.

If you're a man and have waded through what could be a depressing, even maddening book to this point, you deserve to have it end on a more positive note. If you're a female, you haven't had to wade through the book because you already knew it all. In either case, don't give up, because the light at the end of this tunnel is not the headlight of an oncoming train, it's the police, because this book was banned in Florida.

YOUR BRAIN IS WHAT YOU EAT

While supplements, training programs, and brain hacking are not likely helpful, a healthy diet certainly is. I had a relative who was so obsessed about eating the perfect diet she thought each critical organ required a different diet. It was almost like her left kidney was vegan and her right kidney needed Atkins low carb. But the rest of us are in luck, because a Mediterranean diet, the same one that is most beneficial to your heart, blood vessels, and all your other favorite organs, is also the most beneficial to your brain. It improves cerebral blood flow, increases neuroplasticity, reduces inflammation, and improves intraneural communication.

One study on diet and brain health typifies many others. Researchers followed 960 people for 4.7 years who ate just 1.3 extra servings of green, leafy vegetables each day. They had cognition scores 7.5 years younger than those with the least-healthy diet scores.[28] Over the course of six years, elderly people who ate more flavanols (antioxidants in fruits and vegetables) were 48% less likely to develop dementia.[29]

On the flip side, the same foods you know are bad for your heart, weight, and waistline, including fried food, fast food, high-fat food, high-sugar food, processed meals (anything made with partially hydrogenated oil), cured or processed meats, refined carbs, frozen pizza, ice cream, chips, candy, soda (including diet soda), fruit juice, alcohol, etc.—in other words, the Super Bowl Diet—increase systemic inflammation, harming all critical organs, especially the brain.

You know the drill on what kind of diet you should be adopting. A primarily plant-based diet—fresh fruits and vegetables, whole grains, and legumes, i.e., a diet where you get your protein from as many non-meat sources as possible. The Harvard Medical School newsletter[30] and numerous other expert sources provide a researched guide of what foods are best for brain health. Here is a short list:

- Wild salmon, flaxseeds, avocados, and walnuts are good sources of omega 3s. Avocados may also help reduce blood pressure.[31]
- Other nuts and seeds, such as almonds, cashews, Brazil nuts, hazel nuts, and sunflower seeds are good sources of omega-3s, fatty acids, and vitamin E.[32]
- Peanuts, which are legumes, are an excellent source of vitamin E, the antioxidant resveratrol, and unsaturated fats.[33]
- Dark chocolate contains cacao flavonoids, which are important antioxidants that can penetrate and accumulate in the hippocampus.[34]
- Berries are another good source of flavonoids, especially the dark and brilliantly colored ones like strawberries, blackberries, blueberries, currants, and mulberries.[35]
- Whole grains, including brown rice, barley, bulgur wheat, and oatmeal, and whole-grain breads are all good sources of vitamin E.[36]
- Tea and coffee contain caffeine's antioxidants and may provide more than short-term benefit by increasing brain entropy, allowing enhanced processing of information. Obviously, caffeine's downside is that it can become addictive.[37]
- Eggs are a good source of vitamins B-6, B-12, and folic acid, which may help prevent brain atrophy.[38]
- Broccoli, kale, and Brussels sprouts are rich in glucosinolates (drop that term on someone at your next dinner party). When metabolized, these compounds produce isothiocyanates (an even better term to impress others with),

which may reduce oxidative stress and lower the risk of neurodegenerative diseases.[39]
- Soy contains polyphenols called isoflavones, including daidzein and genistein, that suppress neurotoxins.[40]
- Tomatoes contain the anti-inflammatory lycopene, especially in their skin. For that reason, smaller cherry tomatoes are the best.
- Turmeric is a potent anti-inflammatory spice.
- Spinach is high in vitamin K. There is growing interest in the role this important vitamin plays in the proliferation, differentiation, and survival of brain cells.[41]
- Pomegranates contain 21 compounds called polyphenols and urolithins, which have antioxidant properties.[42]

So rather than challenge the world record for hot dog eating, 75 in ten minutes by perennial champion Joey Chestnut, I suggest you go after the world record for wild salmon eating—4,157 in 30 minutes currently held by this guy.

EXERCISE: PUT YOUR LEGS ON THE TREADMILL, NOT YOUR BRAIN

You have likely heard the aphorism that you should think of your brain as you would a muscle, and that exercising your brain helps maintain its health. Actually, no. Your brain doesn't have a single muscle fiber in it. It turns out, if you want to improve or maintain your brain function, rather than trying to find a way to put your brain on a treadmill, put your legs on a treadmill instead.

Different functions of the brain peak at difference ages on average. Information processing peaks just after you leave high school, around the age of 18 or 19. Short-term memory peaks when you are around age 25 and starts to decline when you are around age 35. Visual short-term memory peaks in your early 30s. Your ability to recognize someone else's emotions peaks in the fourth or fifth decade of life. Vocabulary normally doesn't peak until a person's late 60s or early 70s.

Physical exercise enlarges the hippocampus and prefrontal cortex, areas of the brain associated with memory, task management, coordination, planning, and execution. These two areas are particularly vulnerable to neurodegeneration and cognitive loss from aging. Contrary to all the sales pitches for penis-enlargement scams, bigger isn't always better. (Men learn this after having tried all those scams). But when it comes to the hippocampus, bigger is actually better. Enlargement means these parts of the brain are functioning faster and more efficiently.

I mentioned in Chapter 7 the stimulation of BDNF by exercise. The runners' anti-depressant high that you have likely heard about and resolved to never experience, is also associated with increasing neurogenesis in the hippocampus.[43] But other proteins such as insulin-like growth factor-I and fibroblast growth factor may also contribute to the exercise-induced enhancement of the growth of new synapses in many important cortical areas of the brain.[44] Not only does physical exercise stimulate the growth of new neurons, but it improves plasticity of the neurons, which is their ability to adapt and perform in response to a stimulus.

Exercise immediately increases the release of the neurotransmitters dopamine, serotonin (the runners' high neurotransmitters), and norepinephrine, which facilitate interneuronal communication. Clinically, the result is an increased attention span, enhanced ability to focus, and improved reaction time, lasting at least two hours after the exercise session ends.

Anxiety damages the brain by increasing levels of the stress hormone cortisol and epinephrine, a hormone synthesized in the adrenal glands from the amino acid, tyrosine. The effect is to raise blood pressure and heart rate, increase the strength of heart contractions, raise the blood pressure and ultimately the blood supply to the major muscle groups. This provides enhanced energy in the face of danger, i.e., the "fight or flight response," which is the domain of the sympathetic nervous system. However, long-term release of these stress chemicals narrows arteries, reduces blood flow, impairs the pumping mechanics of the heart, and is a contributing factor to a long list of chronic adult diseases, including those of the brain.

Stress impairs memory and complex thinking. People who are plagued by chronic stress and anxiety are nearly 50% more likely to develop dementia later in their life.[45] In fact, anxiety and dementia enhance each other, creating a vicious, downward cycle. The advance of neurodegenerative diseases disrupts neural pathways that mediate the stress response, producing more depression, anxiety, insomnia and malaise.[46]

Exercise helps people handle stress better, decreasing the release of cortisol. The hippocampus of a couch potato consists of younger, inexperienced, or untrained neurons. More immature neurons are more excitable and are stimulated more by stress, making the response to the stress more damaging.

Researchers Rachel Mitchell and Veena Kumari make the case that the shape of a person's brain is associated with certain personality traits and mental illnesses, like neuroticism.[47] Cortisol can trigger changes in brain shape and the degree of folding. Both exercise and the triggering of the sympathetic nervous system release the same batch of hormones and neurotransmitters as chronic neuroticism and anxiety. But exercise prompts the growth of specific neurons that release GABA neurotransmitters, dubbed as the anti-anxiety molecules. GABA neurotransmitters are thought to act as a stabilizing force, preventing other neurons from firing in excess. This becomes manifest clinically in that those who exercise more are biologically better able to appropriately control their emotional responses to stress.

Telomeres are repeating sequences of DNA at the ends of chromosomes that function much like the end caps of shoelaces: they act to prevent the ends of chromosomes from fraying, unraveling, fusing with other chromosomes, and from being misidentified as a double break in the chromosome that would trigger a repair cascade. The name was coined by Nobel Prize winner in genetics Hermann J. Muller (see also Chapter 5), from the Greek for "end" (telos) and "part" (meros).

Telomere length can fluctuate over time but generally steadily decreases with aging, and this contributes to deterioration of cell and organ health. Furthermore, every time a cell divides, it loses a little telomere length, which is one of the reasons none of us lives forever. Telomere length is associated with longevity at the cellular level, and therefore, the organism level. Paradoxically, many cancer cells have shorter than normal telomeres but are still able to continuously replicate.

Things that shorten telomere length shorten life expectancy. Various environmental contaminants, for example, air pollution, shorten telomere length. Exercise and physical activity increase the length of telomeres, slowing the aging process.[48] Endurance and intensity training have been found to be superior to strength and weight training for maintaining telomeres, but athletes across the board are more likely to have increased telomere length.[49]

One study estimated that the difference in telomere aging between individuals who exercised and those who were sedentary was a whopping 9 years' worth of normal aging.[50] To qualify as a member of the exercise cohort, a woman had to do an equivalent of jogging for 30 minutes five days each week, and a man for 40 minutes five days each week. Compared to a sedentary lifestyle, low or moderate exercise only improved telomere length the equivalent of 2 years.

Telomere preservation via exercise is probably mediated by an increase in the enzyme telomerase reverse transcriptase, a critical protein necessary to maintain telomere stability and to synthesize new telomere DNA to somewhat offset the shortening that normally occurs during cellular division and DNA replication. There is some evidence that adoption of a healthy lifestyle, exercise, and a good diet can not only slow telomere loss but reverse it. A single 45-minute jog spiked telomerase activity for several hours afterwards. After six months of exercising at that level for 3 times each week, participants saw a 3-4% increase in telomere length.[49] If you are interested in your telomere length, a finger stick blood test and an $89 at-home DNA kit can tell you how old your cells are.

Researchers recently discovered that a hormone called irisin is produced during exercise. They initially determined that it plays a role in energy metabolism. More recent research found that irisin may also stimulate neuronal growth in the hippocampus, which, if you recall from earlier in this chapter, is a region critical for learning and memory. And if you don't recall that from earlier in this chapter, then you need my Deluxe Tiger Hippocampus Nectar for only $19.99, which I should have mentioned earlier in this chapter.

Irisin may help protect neurons and synapses well enough to prevent Alzheimer's.[51] We know that irisin is reduced in the hippocampus of patients with Alzheimer's, and that healthy centenarians have unusually high levels.[52] The temporary increase in irisin after exercise is stronger in lean women compared to men, implying some sort of catalysis between estradiol and irisin.[53] Researchers have seen clinical evidence for quite some time that physical exercise helps maintain brain function. More recently, they have found in virtually all age groups—children, healthy middle-aged adults, and in the elderly—exercise is associated with a larger hippocampus and better cognition.[54] Cardiorespiratory fitness has likewise been associated with empirical changes in brain gray matter volume,[55] which also correlates with better cognitive function in later life.

Resting-state functional connectivity (RSFC) describes patterns of intrinsic activity of the brain when no specific tasks place demands on neuronal firing; for example, on Sunday morning or when someone is watching *The Real Housewives of Salt Lake City*. I take that back; intrinsic activity of the brain is flat lined when watching *The Real Housewives of Salt Lake City*. Assessing RSFC allows researchers to observe and quantify the impact of lifestyle influences like exercise habits on brain function. RSFC is diminished by the aging process, which reduces higher-order executive functioning.

Despite the greater increase in irisin in women after exercise, there is some evidence that the brain's benefits from physical fitness are more pronounced in men than women.[56] Cardiovascular fitness improves RSFC in older adults. Elderly men but not elderly women show consistent association between physical fitness and indicators of RSFC.[57]

Instead of supplements, regular exercise has a lot more to offer in fighting off aging of the brain, quite possibly helping men even more than it helps women. Beyond better physical fitness and a better diet, what else can society do to help end the Great Brain Robbery, and close the gap between themselves and women on brain function?

MEDITATION, NOT MEDICATION

This is definitely in the category of leftovers in the buffet of what men can do to help their brains. In Chapter 2, I addressed the importance of adequate sleep. Think of meditation as a form of wakeful sleepiness, or sleepful wakiness, or simply a politically correct term for too lazy to fix dinner. But whatever it is, it is probably good for your brain. Meditation thickens the pre-frontal cortex and other areas in the front part of the brain, and can slow, stall, or even reverse the cortical thinning from aging.[58] Harmful stress hormones, such as cortisol are decreased, and beneficial hormones like serotonin are increased. Compared to non-meditator slackers, meditators have more gyrification (See Chapter 3).

Meditation decreases stress, and correspondingly, the density of the amygdala. (Recall from Chapter 3 that the amygdala is the brain structure associated with the fight or flight response).[59] It can reduce cognitive rigidity (a PhD term for improving creativity)[59] and improve attention, decision-making ability[60] short-term memory, and increase the volume of the all-important hippocampus.[61]

Full disclosure: I was not a meditator before I wrote this book, and my wife says my personality makes me probably the worst candidate ever to succeed at meditation. To prove her wrong, I entered the Buddhist Monk XXX Ultimate Cage Match Meditation Tournament. I'm undefeated, having won every match by a knockout.

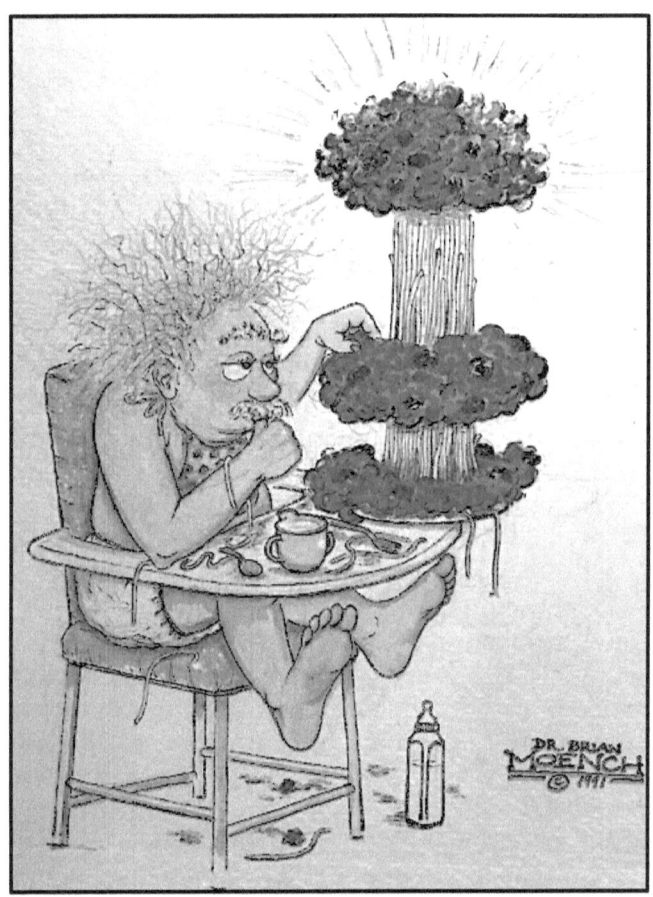

Baby Einstein plays with his food

ELIMINATE THE NEUROTOXINS IN A JAR

If we are going to make men more intelligent, we'll have to start when they are young, really young, like right out of the chute. It's hard to convince newborns and infants to exercise more (trust me, I've tried), so we should take a hard look at what we are feeding America's babies. From mercury-contaminated HFCS to cadmium-contaminated sewage spread on farmland (see Chapter 4), the cumulative impact on our food supply is staggering, especially for babies.

A nonprofit organization, Healthy Babies Bright Futures (HBBF), released a report in 2019, "What's in my baby food," that found that 95% of baby food tested was contaminated with heavy metals known to be neurotoxic, including the worst of the worst, arsenic and lead.[62] Of 168 samples of baby food from 61 different brands, detectable levels of lead were found in 94%, arsenic was found in 73%, cadmium in 75%, and mercury in 32%. One in four baby foods contained all four heavy metals—lead, mercury, arsenic, and cadmium. There are essentially no government regulations limiting the concentrations of these contaminants in our food, even baby food. Organic brands have fewer toxins but are not entirely pristine either.

Fifteen foods account for half the risk. The most heavily contaminated are rice-based foods—infant rice cereal, rice dishes, and rice-based snacks, which are high in inorganic arsenic, the most toxic form, and are the most likely to be contaminated with all four heavy metals.

Researchers estimate that across the country, 11 million IQ points are lost among American children because of the lead and arsenic in their food from birth to age 24 months.[62] Bear in mind this doesn't address other neurotoxins, in-utero exposure, exposure after two years, or any other source other than diet. These researchers believe that the amount of arsenic in baby food is responsible for four times as much neurotoxicity as lead contamination. Some of these baby foods were also tested for perchlorate, another neurotoxin mentioned in Chapter 5, and found to be positive.

It is tempting to minimize the findings because the concentrations are small. But this analysis did not address other known chemical and metal contaminants in our food supply, like pesticides, phthalates, aluminum, and many others. And don't forget that if each jar of baby food is contaminated, then children will be absorbing essentially neurotoxins not just occasionally, but several times a day, during the most crucial stages of brain developmental in their lives after birth.

A recent Congressional report was released with even more damning evidence of heavy metals in baby food.[108] Internal testing from four companies that manufacture baby food revealed alarming results.

Perhaps even more concerning, three companies refused to response to this Congressional subcommittee to compile this report, basically concealing the concentrations of contaminants in their products. Those companies were Walmart, Campbell's, and Sprout Organic Foods.

A 100-ppb limit for arsenic is the only FDA regulation of toxins in baby food, and numerous experts have called even that limit far too lax. But among four companies (Nurture, Gerber's, Earth's Best Organic, and Beech-Nut) their own testing yielded results like this for arsenic: 25% of Nurture's products exceeded the 100-ppb limit, Earth's Best Organic included ingredients with up to 309 ppb, and Beech-Nut included ingredients with up to 913 ppb of arsenic. The tests also mirrored those done by HBBF in finding high levels of lead, cadmium, and mercury. All four of those brands also had levels of lead that exceeded the EPA's standard for the amount of lead allowed in water, 15 ppb. "Nurture sold Happy Baby products testing as high as 641 ppb for lead, Beech-Nut used ingredients with as much as 886.9 ppb lead and Hain [parent company for Earth's Best Organic] used ingredients with as much as 352 ppb lead."[109] Levels of cadmium in all four companies' products exceeded the FDA's standard of 5 ppb. Only one company routinely tested for mercury. "The test results of baby foods [showed] results up to 91 times the arsenic level, up to 177 times the lead level, up to 69 times the cadmium level, and up to 5 times the mercury level.... Internal company standards permit dangerously high levels of toxic heavy metals, and documents revealed the manufacturers have often sold foods that exceeded those levels." [109]

No doubt, if parents prepared these foods themselves from scratch with raw ingredients, they might also find disturbing results because of the contamination of our farmland from things like biosolids (municipal sewage), as mentioned in Chapter 4. But that is no comfort or excuse; it just expands the alarm.

For parents of young infants, there are several take-home messages about what not to take home when you're at a grocery store. Rice-based foods should be eliminated because of the high contamination with all these metals, especially arsenic. Testing by other groups have found high levels of arsenic in oat-based cereals as well, like Cheerios. (Recall that Cheerios alo contains alarmingly high concentrations of pesticides.) It is best to avoid teething biscuits, which also often contain heavy metals. Fruit juices like pear, grape, and especially apple, often contain heavy metals, as do root vegetables like carrots and sweet potatoes. These are all best avoided for infants and toddlers. We hope that "organic" baby food has less pesticide contamination. As beneficial as that is, clearly that alone does not mean that all is well with what's inside the jar.

Aggressively addressing the shocking contamination of the nation's baby food should be considered a national emergency. But inherent in this exposé is an indictment of our entire food supply, for if this kind of contamination is rampant in baby food, you can assume something similar or worse is in the food supply for everyone else.

PUT WOMEN IN CHARGE

In December 2019, former President Barack Obama opined that he was "absolutely confident that for two years, if every nation on earth was run by women, you would see a significant improvement across the board on just about everything."[63] My only disagreement with that statement is, why for only two years? I don't think Obama was making that statement flippantly or in jest, because the research, history, and empirical evidence suggests he's right.

Beyond improving individual and parental behavior, we are not going to save the brains of men unless we change society at large. And the key to that small task is putting more women in charge of businesses, government, and public policy. Women experience life from a different vantage point than men; they think of problems and solutions differently. Women make businesses more profitable, government more responsive to constituents, and communities healthier. They are more family oriented. Women are better at communicating through listening, encouraging diversity and dialogue, and seeking cooperation and consensus. Women are more likely to be intergenerationally oriented, more concerned about the needs, challenges, and predicaments of future generations.

Despite current popular pressure to minimize or deny all differences between the sexes, even anatomic differences, research demonstrates that men's and women's basic personality traits differ, generally, in important ways that could pay large dividends if extrapolated to nationwide public policy and cultural norms. That females think and act differently from males when placed in positions of broad responsibility could have transformative influence on society at large.

The brain's reward structure, called the corpus striatum, has dense neuronal connections to the cerebral cortex. Through the release of dopamine, the feel-good neurotransmitter, the striatum orchestrates behavior that stimulates reward and steers away from punishment.

Neuroimaging studies show that pro-social behavior delivers a higher level of "feel good" reward for females than for males. In experimental situations of money sharing, researchers found significant discrepancies in what stimulated the striatum of men versus women.[64] Women were more endogenously rewarded by sharing than were men.

In a subsequent experiment, chemically blocking the release of dopamine resulted in more selfish behavior in women but less selfish behavior in men. Lead author Alexander Soutschek said, "These results demonstrate that the brains of women and men also process generosity differently at the pharmacological level."[65] While this difference was demonstrated to be biologic, it does not necessarily settle the chicken and egg argument. Which comes first, the behavior or the biochemistry? I don't think it actually matters; the end result is the same—women are more altruistic than men.

In an article in Psychology Today, *Are Men More Helpful, Altruistic, or Chivalrous Than Women?,* David Schmidt details key differences in how males and females behave toward others. Even as children and adolescents, females are more giving than males. Regardless of nationality or culture, women value benevolence and universalism (understanding, appreciation, tolerance, and protection for the general welfare and nature) more than men.[66] In contrast, behavior that is more self-centered, achievement-oriented, and power accumulative is biochemically rewarded in the brains of males. Counterintuitively this dichotomy is even more pronounced in Scandinavian culture, where there is substantial gender equality in sociopolitical, health, and employment opportunities (where both sexes are freer to pursue behavior they care about and less confined to stereotypical gender behavior). This suggests it is born more of biological or evolutionary processing than of sociologic bias or training, or of women's being more culturally committed to their role in reproduction, child care, and nurturing.

In just about every study of this ever done, women are more willing to give to charities and causes championing the common good. The National Altruism Study of 2002 found that women surpass men in "prosociality," i.e., in altruistic values, behaviors, and empathy.[67] Women are more likely to give to charities for medical research, animal rescue, and disaster relief.[68] Among married and single people, women, on average, donate more to these types of charities than the average man.[69]

A report in the New York Times notes, "among high-net-worth individuals in America, women gave nearly twice as much as men did."[107]

The Great Brain Robbery –Brian Moench

The article points out how, among our country's wealthiest citizens, like Jeff Bezos, Bill Gates, Steve Jobs, and Mark Zuckerberg, it has been their spouses or ex-spouses that have turned those massive fortunes into serious sources of philanthropy.

Even as older infants, females are better at recognizing facial expressions as representative of another person's emotions and feelings.[70] Most studies show women are more empathetic than men.[71] More women in charge means more empathy and altruism in the public sphere, and that means more concern about environmental neurotoxins.

Across all ages, women conduct themselves with more benevolence-related character strengths like kindness, love, and gratitude.[72] Women consider morality to be more caring oriented, and men consider morality to be more justice oriented.[73] Even though in recent history women have been able to pursue higher-paying and higher-status careers, they are still statistically more likely to choose people-oriented jobs, such as sociology, teaching, nursing, and real estate.[74] Even the other factors that enter into those choices, like bearing and caring for children, greater schedule flexibility, and a less demanding workload are a reflection of more people-oriented priorities, rather than financial, status, or materialism pursuits.

Women's personality traits in general include greater willingness to cooperate with others and less anti-social behavior, such as narcissism, Machiavellianism (the end justifies the means), and frankly, less psychopathy than men.[75] In economic activity, women are more likely than men to be altruistic if acting quickly on impulse, but their altruism dissipates when given more time to analyze and reflect on their decision.[76] In honesty experiments, compared to men, women were less likely to be dishonest if it would bring harm to another person.[77]

In one area of prosocial behavior, men are more likely to help strangers, such as picking up a hitchhiker, or helping someone in need in a subway. However, that comes with a huge qualifier. It seems that men's behavior even in these situations is more selfishly motivated, i.e., to impress onlookers,[78] and in the case of hitchhikers, men are less likely to feel physically vulnerable.

The first female physician in the country was Elizabeth Blackwell, who was admitted to Geneva Medical College in 1847 as a result of a unanimous vote of the students. The students voted for her as a prank on their faculty, which had rejected her application, just like more than a dozen other medical schools had.[106] One of the first female graduates of the University of Utah Medical School in the 1950s was my grandmother. Thankfully, things are much different now for women in medicine. As of 2019, slightly more than half of all medical students are women, and we should all welcome that trend.

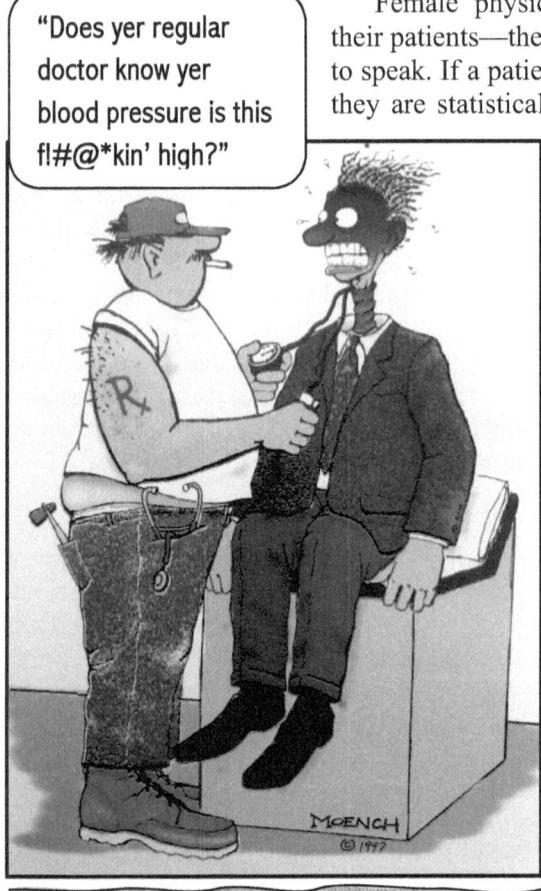

Female physicians take better care of their patients—they are "health's angels," so to speak. If a patient's physician is a female, they are statistically more likely to survive and less likely to require re-hospitalizations for serious illnesses, according to a study by the Harvard School of Public Health.[79] It isn't just that female physicians are more empathetic. They tend to be a little bit better at sticking to the evidence and doing the things that are known to work better, according to Dr. Ashish Jha, who directed the study.[80] Researchers reviewed records of over 1.5 million elderly Medicare patients requiring hospitalization for medical reasons over four years. The statistical outcome differences between the two genders of physicians were small, but in the aggregate, the difference is significant. They concluded that if all patients had female physicians, 32,000 lives would be saved every year. It should be noted that in this respect, the capitalistic nature of American medicine is not helping the situation. Female physicians are paid less for their better outcomes.

Another study of more than 580,000 heart patients followed for nearly 20 years found that mortality rates for both men and women were lower if their physician was a female. Women who were treated by male physicians had the highest mortality rate.[81] Previous studies found that female physicians communicate better with their patients, are more encouraging and reassuring, and spent 10% more time with patients than male physicians.[82] In another study, female primary care physicians waited an average of three minutes before interrupting a patient, compared to male doctors who waited an average of 47 seconds.[83] The women I know are hardly surprised at the findings of this study. My wife says she doesn't have to interrupt me after 3 minutes because I never talk.

Two years after appointing a female CEO, companies saw improved momentum in their stock prices. Companies with female chief financial officers (CFOs) were also perceived as less risky bets by investors and were more profitable. Looking across an entire 17-year period, the study found that companies with female CFOs generated a combined $1.8 trillion more in gross profits than their sector averages. For example, one of the firms with a female CFO generated $208.6 million in gross profits in a given quarter. That was nearly $33 million more than the $175.7 million average gross profit for other companies in the same sector.[84] Companies that have more women on their boards have superior financial performance.

A survey of more than 600 board directors found that women are "more likely [than men] to consider the rights of others and to take a cooperative approach to decision-making."[85] This becomes a springboard to better financial performance for their companies. "Women seem to be predisposed to be more inquisitive and to see more possible solutions." Fortune 500 corporate boards with high numbers of females achieve a 53% higher return on equity, a 66% higher return on invested capital, and a 42% higher return on sales.[86] Having just one woman on a corporate board reduces the risk of bankruptcy by 20%.[87]

Therese Huston, interviewed in Forbes Magazine, addressed important myths of the behavior of men and women in business.[87] She said, consistent with the evidence cited earlier in this book, that the business stereotypes of women's becoming emotional and falling apart under stress and men's remaining calm and impervious to the stress have been demonstrated to be not just false, but inverted. When stressed, men become laser focused on rewards when their heart rates and cortisol levels are elevated, even if the chances of reward are small. Under stress, men are more prone to more and bigger gambles. When women are under stress, showing high cortisol levels, they become more cautious and risk aware.

Men are more likely to approach their careers inwardly focused as lone rangers, with their financial compensation as the focus of their lives. Women are more likely to view their work and careers holistically, as an integrated but not dominant part of their lives. Women view leadership differently from men, emphasizing sharing of information and collaboration with other employees and achievement of group goals.

Research also shows that women don't rely on intuition rather than data any more than men do. In fact, 12 of 32 studies showed women were more likely to stick to the evidence in making business decisions. None of the other 20 studies showed men to have an advantage in adhering to the empirical data.[88]

Many animals are able to cooperate to achieve a common goal, like defending their territories, hunting prey, or staying warm. Chimpanzees are able to cooperate to the point of sharing different tasks with different tools. Nonetheless, one of the most significant differences between humans and other apes is the degree to which they are able to cooperate to achieve a common purpose. That seems to also be a difference between men and women. Women have done better than men leading countries in their response to the coronavirus pandemic. A study of 194 countries found that the governments in the 19 countries that were led by women, including Germany, New Zealand, Taiwan, and Finland, communicated better with their constituents, locked down faster, and saw far lower fatality rates.[89]

Women govern differently from men on issues far beyond pandemic control. In the U.S., they are more likely to work in Congress in a bipartisan and collaborative manner. An analysis of 1,824 bills introduced in the House between 1973 and 2014 showed that women sponsor bills in social benefit areas such as civil rights, health care, and education more than men do.[90] Male members of Congress are more likely to sponsor more "masculine bills" like those related to energy, agriculture, and macroeconomics.[91] An examination of State of the State speeches from 2006 to 2008 found that female governors included more focus on social welfare issues than their male counterparts.[92] Regardless of political party, women are less likely to vote for war or for capital punishment according to an analysis of 22 established democracies from 1970 to

2000.[93] Michael Genovese, the director of the Institute for Leadership Studies at Loyola Marymount University, studies gender and leadership. He says, "Women share their power more; men guard their power."[94]

Most politicians are attorneys, of course. By examining the rates at which male attorneys faced disciplinary actions compared to female attorneys, researchers concluded that female attorneys are about half as likely to engage in unethical behavior.[95] Ethical behavior is a key indicator of the likelihood of that politician's working for legislation that prioritizes protection of the common good. Being a male, I'm partial to the assumption that protecting male brain development and function is a common good.

Women raise over half of the food in the world. Most often they are the primary caretakers of their own families. Women are more likely than men to prioritize spending their available money to the direct benefit of their families, including clean water, more nutritious foods, school fees for children, and health care.[96] The more political power women have, the healthier communities throughout the world become.[97] One study found that when women control the household budget, there was a 20% increase in childhood survival rates.[97] According to the UN Food and Agriculture Organization, women farmers given equal access to resources, education, financing, and land rights, could increase the yields on their farms by 20- to-30%.[97] When a woman is in charge, farms use less pesticides.[98]

More and more, social science research is finding that women care better for the environment than men do. Women score higher on tests that reveal how much a person values altruism, personal responsibility, and empathy. Moreover, women see environmentalism as important to protecting themselves and their families. Women are less likely than men to support environmental spending cuts and are less sympathetic to business profits when it comes to environmental regulation. They also have "more positive feelings about environmental activists and are concerned about environmental risks to health, especially locally."[99] Research by the Organization for Economic Cooperation and Development found that women are more likely to buy environmentally responsible and organic foods, more likely to recycle, and are more committed to energy conservation. Other research found women are willing to pay more to protect the environment, including accepting higher income taxes and taxes on gasoline prices.

A headline in *the Guardian,* February 2020, read, "The eco gender gap: why is saving the planet seen as women's work?"[100] The article details how most environmentally friendly products target women. You might say that women are still seen as care givers, even when it comes to the planet. "Research suggests that women have higher levels of socialization to care about others and be socially responsible, which then leads them to care about environmental problems and be willing to adopt environmental behaviours," says Rachel Howell, a lecturer in sustainable development (a subject that is, she notes, studied overwhelmingly by women at undergraduate level) at the University of Edinburgh.[100]

Unfortunately, environmental responsibility and femininity are associated with one another in the minds of both men and women, which plays a role in men not taking responsibility. One study from researchers at Penn State found that men could be dissuaded from using a reusable shopping bag, recycling, or any number of environmentally friendly behaviors, including adopting a vegetarian diet, for fear of being perceived as gay or feminine.[101] Another study in the *Journal of Consumer Research* found that men are perversely motivated to avoid environmentally friendly behavior as a means of demonstrating their masculinity.[102]

For years, studies of attitudes about nuclear power have shown a significant difference between men and women. Most polls show that more than 70% of men favor nuclear power, while only around 40% of women do.[103] It has been a common assumption that is because women don't understand the technology as well as men. However, that doesn't turn out to be the case. It is somewhat because women are more environmentally conscious, but even more, it is because women and men assess risk differently. Women are less likely to support virtually any type of project that carries a risk to their local community, including quarries, landfills, power plants, gas pipelines, oil drilling, even wind farms, power transmission lines, and especially, nuclear power plants.[104]

But among non-whites, that gender gap disappears. So, the real divide is between white men and everyone else. Researchers that surveyed the issue said, "White males...on average...perceived risks as much smaller and much more acceptable than did other people."[104] Recall the Dunning Kruger Effect from earlier in the book. It's like, "Hold my beer, and watch me build a nuclear power plant."

White males worry less about risk in the world overall, including things like nuclear power, the climate crisis, industrial pollution, and environmental contamination, because they are more likely to be in positions of power and influence to create, control, and benefit from this kind of risky and detrimental activity. On the other hand, women and non-white men may see the world as more dangerous because they are further down the line, or nowhere in the line of beneficiaries, and because they have less power and control over the situation.[104]

The average single male in the United States is responsible for more carbon dioxide emissions than his female counterpart, primarily related to the type of vehicle he drives. In Europe, surveys found similar differences. Men eat more meat than women, another means by which they have a greater impact on greenhouse gases. A Gallup poll found that women have greater scientific knowledge of the climate crisis than men, and women also express slightly greater concern about this threat. Environmental protection is one of the reasons why women are drifting away from the Republican Party to the Democratic Party. Another study found that men preferred arguments about the climate crisis that emphasized science and business considerations, as opposed to ethics and environmental justice.[105]

CONCLUSION

The human brain, the wrinkled, unattractive, three-pound glob of spongy tissue posted above our shoulders and stuck between our ears, is the greatest evolutionary organic asset in the billions of years of existence in the known universe. It is the only reason why we stand at the apex of the biological world. But we have done a stunningly poor job of protecting our most precious resource. We are literally changing and diminishing who humans are, rendering us all less than what we should be, less able to engage in individual, communal, and global problem solving, less able to pursue our career aspirations, or create rewarding relationships. Throughout most of the course of human life, the male brain is, by nature, more fragile than our female counterparts' brains and more sensitive to almost all internal and external threats.

The information in this book can feel overwhelming and depressing. We have paid a heavy price for the conveniences of modern civilization. We have littered our environment, our homes, our most personal space, our bodies, and especially our brains with a seemingly endless array of environmental contaminants. Many of them are toxic specifically to the brain. We have allowed government and business far too much latitude in exposing us to chemicals and pollution that were known to be dangerous and deadly.

But we should not feel hopeless or helpless. There are easy things we can all do personally that will help and that do not necessitate wholesale disruption or constraint of our lifestyle. Some will require reconsidering society's value system as well as our own. On a community, state, or national scale, you can get engaged in one of the many organizations working for local ordinances, legislation, and improved public policy on environmental protection, climate mitigation, reformation of industrial agriculture, and corporate accountability. You can vote for and work to elect politicians who understand that protection of public health must always be prioritized over corporate profit.

The neurotoxins I was exposed to during my own fetal development and childhood in the 1950s, were largely unknown by the public, but at least some of them were known by my father. When my own children were at the same stage of vulnerability, in the 1970s and 1980s, little more was known about the increasingly pervasive spread of these heavy metals and toxic chemicals. Fortunately, when my granddaughter was at the same critical stage of brain development in the 2000s, enough medical research was starting to emerge that I could help orchestrate a little safer environment for her.

In 2024 and beyond, it is my hope that this book can get into enough hands to, in some small way, help arrest the "silent pandemic of neurotoxicity." Every child deserves to have their potential in life protected and uncompromised from of the failures of governments. Historically it has been men who have controlled the levers of power that have allowed this pandemic to flourish and spread. But men are less than adequately equipped with the personality traits, emotional impulses, and thought processes necessary to lead the political and societal transformation that will be required. It will probably be up to women to save men from themselves and bring an end to The Great Brain Robbery.

About the Author

Dr. Brian Moench is a physician in private practice and a former junior faculty member of Harvard Medical School. His environmental expertise includes a former adjunct faculty position at the University of Utah Honors College teaching public health and the environment. He gave the first ever lecture on environmental neurotoxins to medical students at the University of Utah Medical School in 2020.

He was nominated by President Obama and was a finalist for the award, Champion of Change, for his work on public health and the climate crisis in 2013. He is the president and co-founder of Utah Physicians for a Healthy Environment (UPHE). Since 2007, UPHE has become the largest civic organization of medical professionals in the Western U.S. who are actively engaged in many environmental battles throughout the country and Western Canada.

Dr. Moench has had about 145 Op Eds published in newspapers throughout the country, has appeared on national television, on MSNBC and Fox Business Channel, to discuss the relationship between neonatal deaths and pollution from fracking. He has been quoted in national newspapers (when newspapers used to be a thing), appears regularly on local television and radio programs in Utah discussing the health consequences of air pollution, and is well recognized by the Utah public as an expert on air pollution and health. He gives dozens of lectures each year on numerous issues related to environmental contamination. He has testified as an expert witness in environmental lawsuits.

On a lighter note, Dr. Moench grew up the child of extensive brainwashing and corruption by *MAD Magazine*. Still under its formative influence as an adult, he became the creator and founder of a company that produced humorous greeting cards, *In Your Face Cards*, which sold 35 million cards over 11 years, a few of which have reproduced in this book. CNN did a personal profile on him in the late 1990s highlighting his idiosyncratic mix of careers as a physician, humorous cartoonist, and creator of *In Your Face Cards*. A few of those cartoons are included in this book.

Dr. Moench's family thinks his first name should have been Sisyphus because he is forever rolling the boulder of saving the world uphill. To that effort, he persists in being a thorn in the side of state and federal government, industrial polluters, oil and gas drillers, wood burners, climate deniers, amoral politicians, purveyors of "fake news," and perpetrators of corporate malfeasance.

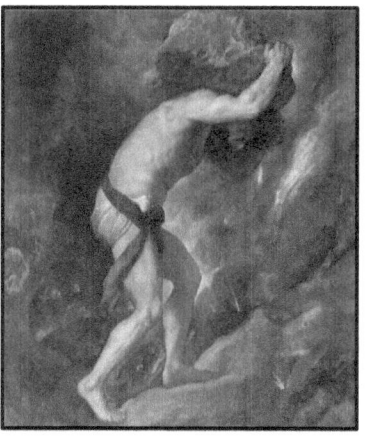

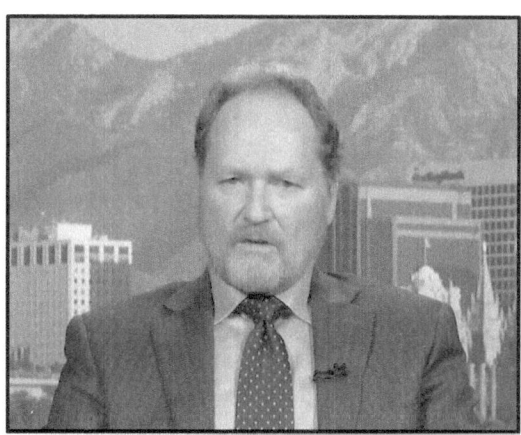

Dr. Moench as he appeared on MSNBC to discuss the association of neonatal deaths and pollution from fracking.

We Must Put More Women in Charge

Appendix

Organophosphates

An ingredient in naled, trichlorfon, was found in a study to cause severely reduced brain weight in test animals exposed.[1] In keeping with their potential to mimic or interfere with human hormones, exposure to OPs is a risk factor for acquiring hormone-related cancers, i.e. including breast, thyroid, ovary and lymphoma.[2] Recall that dichlorvos is classified as a group C carcinogen by the EPA. Exposure during pregnancy or childhood is linked to an increased incidence of brain tumors and leukemia.[3,4] Researchers found an association between exposure to dichlorvos saturated "no-pest" strips during pregnancy and childhood and the incidence of three types of childhood cancer: leukemias, brain tumors, and lymphoma.[5] A Missouri Department of Health study found similar results for childhood brain cancer.[6]

Pesticides attack the immune system. Both pyrethroids and organophosphates have been found to specifically inhibit a critical enzyme in white blood cells, and impair the growth and survival of those cells.[7,8] A World Resources Institute's report entitled "Pesticides and the Immune System: The Public Health Risks,"[9] concludes that immunosuppression by pesticides can provoke allergies, autoimmune disorders such as lupus, and cancer. It may also lead to increased susceptibility to viral infections (like COVID and WNV) and bacterial infections. The immunosuppressive effects of pesticides will be raised again later in discussing whether pesticide spraying decreases the public health risk of West Nile Virus.

Animal studies have found that naled causes anemia, and birth defects in laboratory animals.[10] Labels on naled acknowledge it is a "severe" eye irritant, and "causes eye damage" and is "corrosive" to skin.[11]

The commercial preparation of naled, Dibrom, contains other ingredients that according to US pesticide law can be classified as "inert," but are hardly benign. They include the aromatic hydrocarbons naphthalene and 1,2,4- trimethylbenzene. Naphthalene is a toxin classified by the EPA as a possible human carcinogen, and causes neurologic disorders and anemia in newborns. 1,2,4- trimethylbenzene is a tissue irritant and depresses brain function.

Naled has been banned in the European Union. A popular mosquito industry talking point claims that the EU didn't actually ban naled, rather that the manufacturer didn't apply for re-licensure for economic reasons. That claim is easily disproved. Official EU states in no uncertain terms that naled represented an "unacceptable risk" to human health and the environment, and that naled was to be removed from all European markets, Nov. 1, 2012.[12]

Naled defenders claim its degradation is extremely rapid, i.e. 30 minutes. Growing research contradicts that claim. But naled's half-life is almost irrelevant because it primarily degrades into another organophosphate, dichlorvos, which is about as toxic as naled with a much longer half-life. In various types of water, dichlorvos can last up to 6 months. In soil it can last more than two weeks. Dichlorvos was banned in the EU in 1998, and also banned in many other countries, including Sri Lanka, Cambodia, and Bangladesh, not exactly known for robust environmental protection. Dichlorvos is the pesticide used in "no pest strips." The EPA rates dichlorvos as a class C carcinogen, "possible cause of cancer" which is a worse rating than naled.

The commercial preparations of naled also contain other ingredients that are listed as "inert," but are not benign. They include the naphthalene, and 1,2,4- trimethylbenzene. Naphthalene is a toxin classified by the EPA as a possible human carcinogen, and causes neurologic disorders and anemia in newborns. 1,2,4- trimethylbenzene is a tissue irritant and depresses brain function. Low concentrations of naled claimed by mosquito districts to be "safe," also need to be viewed in this context: chlorpyrifos, a pesticide in the same category as naled, causes brain damage in humans at the lowest possible detectable dose. That's why the EPA recently banned 90% of uses for chlorpyrifos. A recent study found that naled joined chlorpyrifos in being the most neurotoxic of 30 organophophates.[13]

Another study found that small droplets of naled (the size produced by the ultra-low volume sprayers were about four times more acutely toxic than larger droplets.[14] There are numerous studies in animals showing that naled at low dose exposures causes a wide variety of adverse health outcomes, including diseases of the nervous, circulatory, reproductive, and immune systems. OPs are associated with lower sperm counts and poor sperm quality.[15] They are endocrine disruptors. As with other neurotoxins, one of the mechanisms of endocrine disruption and therefore impact on brain development by OPs is inhibition of thyroid hormone production.[16] Other clinical outcomes associated with pre-natal OP pesticide exposure include abnormal primitive reflexes in newborns; mental and motor delays among preschoolers; and decreases in working and visual memory, processing speed, verbal comprehension, perceptual reasoning, and IQ among elementary school–age children. Prenatal exposures are also associated with elevated risks for symptoms or diagnoses of attention-deficit/hyperactivity disorder (ADHD) and autism spectrum disorder (ASD).[17]

The Great Brain Robbery –Brian Moench

Other systematic reviews and multiple epidemiologic studies have linked OP exposures during fetal development with poorer cognitive, behavioral, and social development in children.[18]

In one review, adverse effects of OP pesticide exposure on neurodevelopment were seen in all but one of the 27 studies evaluated; the strongest associations occurred following prenatal exposures,[19] but it has also been found with post-natal exposure as well.[19] Another study showed that young mammals, including humans, may be at risk of impaired neurological development from organophosphate pesticides, even at low, commonly encountered environmental levels.[20]

More specific studies are worth mentioning. A meta-analysis by researchers at University College London found chronic, low-level exposure to organophosphate pesticides causes permanent damage to cognition, including information processing and working memory.[21] Urinary levels of organophosphate metabolites in pregnant mothers were measured, then the children they gave birth to were tested at age 7. Children from those mothers who were in the highest 20% of exposure, showed an average IQ deficit of a stunning 7 points.[22]

The relationship between biomarkers of organophosphate exposure in pregnant mothers and neurologic tests at one year, two years, and 6-9 years, showed that more prenatal exposure caused a loss of perceptual reasoning as early as one year of age, and continued through childhood.[23] Prenatal exposure to organophosphates was associated with delayed mental milestones in 2 year olds.[24] In another study prenatal exposure to organophosphates was associated with decreased non-verbal IQ measured at age 6.[25] The US Congress produced a report back in 1990 that showed an organophosphate pesticide, in this case malathion, can damage the nervous system after just one exposure.[26]

A higher likelihood of an ASD diagnosis was observed for children born to women residing within 1.5 km of OP pesticide applications on agricultural fields.[27] Living in a residence close to an agricultural site with OP use during fetal development was associated with a reduction in seven-year old children's IQs.[28] Risks for impaired neurodevelopment increased in children of farmworkers who experience higher exposures to OP.[29] Higher OP pesticide metabolite levels in the urine of pregnant mothers were associated with ASD traits in adolescence in those children.[30]

Some children are genetically more susceptible to organophosphates. Children with genetic disadvantages that reduce capacity to detoxify OP pesticides have higher rates of neurodevelopmental disorders.[31] Prenatal exposure to one of the most potent OPs, chlorpyrifos, has also been shown to have an association with decreases in brain volume in the areas responsible for attention, receptive language processing, social cognition, and regulation of inhibition.[34]

OP pesticides can interfere with brain development at levels previously thought to be safe or inconsequential, and through mechanisms other than the lethal mode of action for insects.[32] This is an indication of an additional, as yet undetermined mechanism of toxicity.[33] Consistent with human studies, experimental animal studies also confirm the toxicity of early-life OP pesticides on neurodevelopment, resulting in impaired motor activity, behavior, and cognition, even at doses below the known mechanism by which they kill.

References

Prologue

1. https://www.ieer.org/latest/iodnart.html.

2. Pars N. Environmental Factors Inducing Human Cancers. Iran J Public Healthv.41(11); 2012: Wu S, et al. Substantial contribution of extrinsic risk factors to cancer development. Nature, 2015; DOI: 10.1038/nature16166.

3. Wu S, et al. Substantial contribution of extrinsic risk factors to cancer development. Nature, 2015; DOI: 10.1038/nature16166.

4. http://www.ipsnews.net/2016/11/air-pollution-emerges-as-a-top-killer-globally-part-1/.

5. https://www.sciencemag.org/news/2017/01/brain-pollution-evidence-builds-dirty-air-causes-alzheimer-s-dementia.

6. https://www.health.harvard.edu/womens-health/toxic-beauty.

7. Bouatra S, et al. The Human Urine Metabolome. PLoS One. 2013; 8(9): e73076. Published online 2013 Sep 4. doi: 10.1371/journal.pone.

8. https://www.ewg.org/research/body-burden-pollution-newborns.

Introduction

1. https://www.dailymail.co.uk/news/article-512170/British-man-killed-Alps-sledging-mountainside-mattress.html.

2. Lendrem B, et al. The Darwin Awards: sex differences in idiotic behaviour BMJ 2014; 349:g7094.

3. Northcutt W. The Darwin Awards: The official Darwin Awards: 180 bizarre true stories of how dumb humans have met their maker. Orion, 2004.

4. Cooper K, et al. Who perceives they are smarter? Exploring the influence of student characteristics on student academic self-concept in physiology. Advances in Physiology Education, 2018; DOI: 10.1152/advan.00085.2017.

5. https://www.fastcompany.com/3030088/why-women-ceos-are-more-likely-to-be-forced-out.

6. Ernesto R, et al. The emergence of male leadership in competitive environments. Journal of Economic Behavior & Organization. Volume 83, Issue 1, June 2012, Pages 111-117.

References

7. Bian, L., Leslie, S.-J., & Cimpian, A. (2018). Evidence of bias against girls and women in contexts that emphasize intellectual ability. American Psychologist, 73(9), 1139–1153. https://doi.org/10.1037/amp0000427.

8. https://www.cnbc.com/2019/01/07/study-men-still-seen-as-smarter-than-women-get-intellectual-jobs.html.

9. https://www.forbes.com/sites/kathycaprino/2016/05/12/how-decision-making-is-different-between-men-and-women-and-why-it-matters-in-business/#7b326ab24dcd.

10. https://www.sciencedirect.com/science/article/pii/B9780123855220000056.

11. https://www.nytimes.com/interactive/2018/06/13/upshot/boys-girls-math-reading-tests.html.

Chapter One

1. O'Dea, R.E., Lagisz, M., Jennions, M.D. et al. Gender differences in individual variation in academic grades fail to fit expected patterns for STEM. Nat Commun 9, 3777 (2018).

2. Voyer D, Voyer S. Gender Differences in Scholastic Achievement: A Meta-Analysis. Psychological Bulletin, 2014, Vol. 140, No. 4, 1174–1204.

3. https://www.nationsreportcard.gov/tel.

4. https://cepa.stanford.edu/sites/default/files/wp18-13-v201806_0.pdf.

5. https://www.npr.org/templates/story/story.php?storyId=14175229.

6. https://www.scientificamerican.com/article/are-boys-better-than-girls-at-math/.

7. https://www.nytimes.com/interactive/2018/06/13/upshot/boys-girls-math-reading-tests.html.

8. https://nces.ed.gov/programs/digest/d16/tables/dt16_303.70.asp: https://nces.ed.gov/programs/coe/pdf/coe_ctr.pdf.

9. https://www.futurity.org/gender-stereotypes-surveys-2109502/.

10. Naglieri JA, Rojahn J. Gender differences in planning, attention, simultaneous, and successive (PASS) cognitive processes and achievement. J. Educ. Psychol. 2001; 93:430. doi: 10.1037/0022-0663.93.2.430.

11. Balart P, Oosterveen M. Females show more sustained performance during test-taking than males. Nat Commun. 2019;10(1):3798. Published 2019 Sep 3.

doi:10.1038/s41467-019-11691-y.

12. https://www.businessinsider.com/women-just-beat-men-in-worldwide-iq-tests-for-the-first-time-ever-2012-7.

13. https://www.pbs.org/newshour/economy/making-sense/analysis-how-poverty-can-drive-down-intelligence.

14. https://medicalxpress.com/news/2015-06-reveals-men.html.

15. Lundervold A.J., Wollschlager D., Wehling E. Age and sex related changes in episodic memory function in middle aged and older adults. Scand. J. Psychol. 2014; 55:225–232. doi: 10.1111/sjop.12114. [PMC free article] [PubMed] [CrossRef] [Google Scholar]; Sunderaraman P., Blumen H.M., DeMatteo D., Apa Z.L., Cosentino S. Task demand influences relationships among sex, clustering strategy, and recall: 16-word versus 9-word list learning tests. Cogn. Behav. Neurol. Off. J. Soc. Behav. Cogn. Neurol. 18. 2013; 26:78–84. doi: 10.1097/WNN.0b013e31829de450. [PMC free article] [PubMed] [CrossRef] [Google Scholar]; Herlitz A., Nilsson L.G., Backman L. Gender differences in episodic memory. Mem. Cogn. 1997; 25:801–811. doi: 10.3758/BF03211324. [PubMed] [CrossRef] [Google Scholar]; Davis P.J. Gender differences in autobiographical memory for childhood emotional experiences. J. Personal. Soc. Psychol. 1999; 76:498–510. doi: 10.1037/0022-3514.76.3.498. [PubMed] [CrossRef] [Google Scholar].

16. Herlitz A., Nilsson L.G., Backman L. Gender differences in episodic memory. Mem. Cogn. 1997;25:801–811. doi: 10.3758/BF03211324. [PubMed] [CrossRef] [Google Scholar]; Dixon R.A., Wahlin A., Maitland S.B., Hultsch D.F., Hertzog C., Backman L. Episodic memory change in late adulthood: Generalizability across samples and performance indices. Mem. Cogn. 2004; 32:768–778. doi: 10.3758/BF03195867. [PubMed] [CrossRef] [Google Scholar]; Herlitz A., Yonker J.E. Sex differences in episodic memory: The influence of intelligence. J. Clin. Exp. Neuropsychol. 2002; 24:107–114. doi: 10.1076/jcen.24.1.107.970. [PubMed] [CrossRef] [Google Scholar]: Heisz J.J., Pottruff M.M., Shore D.I. Females scan more than males: A potential mechanism for sex differences in recognition memory. Psychol. Sci. 2013; 24:1157–1163. doi: 10.1177/0956797612468281. [PubMed] [CrossRef] [Google Scholar]; Megreya A.M., Bindemann M., Havard C. Sex differences in unfamiliar face identification: Evidence from matching tasks. Acta Psychol. 2011; 137:83–89. doi: 10.1016/j.actpsy.2011.03.003. [PubMed] [CrossRef] [Google Scholar]; W., Choi J., Silverman I. Sexual dimorphism in spatial behaviors: Applications to route learning. Evol. Cogn. 1996; 2:165–171. [Google Scholar].

17. Seidlitz L., Diener E. Sex differences in the recall of affective experiences. J. Personal. Soc. Psychol. 1998; 74:262–271. doi: 10.1037/0022-3514.74.1.262. [PubMed] [CrossRef] [Google Scholar].

References

18. Eagly A, et al. Gender Stereotypes Have Changed: A Cross-Temporal Meta-Analysis of U.S. Public Opinion Polls From 1946 to 2018. American Psychologist, Vol. 75, No. 3, pp. 301–315.

19. https://www.ipr.northwestern.edu/news/2019/eagly-gender-stereotypes.html.

20. https://www.cdc.gov/mmwr/volumes/69/wr/mm6924e1.htm?s_cid=mm6924e1_w.

21. https://baltimore.cbslocal.com/2020/07/07/coronavirus-study-impacts-on-gender-latest-information/.

22. https://www.bop.gov/about/statistics/statistics_inmate_gender.jsp.

23. Choy, Olivia; Raine, Adrian; Venables, Peter H.; Farrington, David P. "Explaining the Gender Gap in Crime: The Role of Heart Rate," Criminology, 2017. doi: 10.1111/1745-9125.12138.

24. Ortiz J, Phil ARD. Heart Rate Level and Antisocial Behavior in Children and Adolescents: A Meta-Analysis. Journal of the American Academy of Child & Adolescent Psychiatry. Volume 43, Issue 2, February 2004, Pages 154-162.

25. https://www.washingtonpost.com/outlook/2020/06/18/women-police-officers-violence/.

26. https://theconversation.com/scientists-may-have-proven-women-are-better-at-multitasking-than-men-71877.

27. https://hbr.org/2019/06/research-women-score-higher-than-men-in-most-leadership-skills.

28. Proudfoot D, et al. A Gender Bias in the Attribution of Creativity: Archival and Experimental Evidence for the Perceived Association Between Masculinity and Creative Thinking. Volume: 26 issue: 11, page(s): 1751-1761.

29. https://www.rollingstone.com/pro/features/research-proves-female-artists-are-more-creative-than-men-962899/.

30. https://www.usnews.com/news/health-news/articles/2020-04-07/women-are-much-safer-drivers-than-men-british-study-finds; Aldred R, et al. How does mode of travel affect risks posed to other road users? An analysis of English road fatality data, incorporating gender and road type. Injury Prevention. http://dx.doi.org/10.1136/injuryprev-2019-043534.

31. https://www.cbsnews.com/news/men-vs-women-who-are-safer-drivers/.

32. https://www.fidelity.com/bin-

public/060_www_fidelity_com/documents/women-fit-money-study.pdf.

33. Terrell J. et al. Gender differences and bias in open source: pull request acceptance of women versus men. PeerJ Computer Science. May 1, 2017.

34. A few studies have found that brown-eyed people have an advantage in physical skills that depend on reaction time and accuracy or even in time-limited intelligence tests. That would make individuals with brown eyes make better hitters in baseball. On the other hand, blue-eyed people are more likely to think in a slower but more thorough way and are better at planning and strategy. That would make them better baseball pitchers.58 Although these studies have been done for 30 years, the evidence is still rather weak.

35. https://www.smithsonianmag.com/smart-news/genetic-study-shows-skin-color-just-skin-deep-180965261/.

36. Teng C, Belfer I. Correlation between eye color and pain phenotypes in healthy women. April 2014. Journal of Pain 15(4):S25.

37. Bassett J, M. Dabbs J. Eye color predicts alcohol use in two archival samples. September 2001. Personality and Individual Differences 31(4):535-539.

38 https://www.shakespearelives.org/poisons-potions/.

39. Tsukahara J, et al. The relationship between baseline pupil size and intelligence. Cogn Psychol. 2016 Dec; 91:109-123. doi: 10.1016/j.cogpsych.2016.10.001. Epub 2016 Nov 7.

40. https://owlcation.com/stem/Does-eye-color-indicate-intelligence-and-personality-traits.

41. Sargezeh BA, Tavakolia N, Daliri MR. Gender-based eye movement differences in passive indoor picture viewing: An eye-tracking study. Physiology & Behavior Volume 206, 1 July 2019, Pages 43-5.

42. Heisz J. J., Pattruff M. M., Shore D. I. Females scan more than males: A potential mechanism for sex differences in recognition memory. Psychological Science. 2013; 24:1–7.

43. Sammaknejad N, et al. Gender Classification Based on Eye Movements: A Processing Effect During Passive Face Viewing. Adv Cogn Psychol. 2017; 13(3): 232–240.

44. Oliveira-Pinto A, et al. Sexual Dimorphism in the Human Olfactory Bulb: Females Have More Neurons and Glial Cells than Males. PLoS ONE, 2014; 9 (11): e111733 DOI: 10.1371/journal.pone.0111733.

References

45. University of Copenhagen. "Girls Have Superior Sense Of Taste To Boys." ScienceDaily. ScienceDaily, 18 December 2008. www.sciencedaily.com/releases/2008/12/081216104035.

46. https://www.researchgate.net/publication.247205232_Differences_exist_in_the_eating_habits_of_university_men_and_women_at_fast-food_restaurants.

47. Indiana University. "Men Do Hear—But Differently Than Women, Brain Images Show." ScienceDaily. ScienceDaily, 29 November 2000. www.sciencedaily.com/releases/2000/11/001129075326.htm.

48. Zweig J, et al. Are Women Happier than Men? Evidence from the Gallup World Poll Journal of Happiness Studies. 2015, vol. 16, issue 2, 515-541.

49. https://blogs.worldbank.org/impactevaluations/are-women-really-happier-men-around-world-guest-post-mallory-montgomery.

50. https://www.jstor.org/stable/40220088?refreqid=excelsior%3A2aa2eff434deaeebeaa31eef0b0dfb51.

51. https://www.washingtonpost.com/news/wonk/wp/2016/03/18/why-smart-people-are-better-off-with-fewer-friends/.

52. Faragó T, et al. Dog growls express various contextual and affective content for human listeners. Royal Society Open Science. Published:17 May 2017https://doi.org/10.1098/rsos.

53. https://www.newsweek.com/marjorie-taylor-greene-jewish-space-laser-mockery-1565325.

54. https://www.cnn.com/2021/01/26/politics/marjorie-taylor-greene-democrats-violence/index.html.

55. https://www.nytimes.com/2020/09/10/opinion/qanon-women-conspiracy.html.

56. https://www.aei.org/articles/whats-going-on-with-republican-women/.

Chapter Two

1. https://www.scientificamerican.com/article/do-people-only-use-10-percent-of-their-brains/.

2. Sereno M, et al. The human cerebellum has almost 80% of the surface area of the neocortex. Proceedings of the National Academy of Sciences, 2020; 202002896.

3. https://www.news-medical.net/health/Hippocampus-Functions.aspx.

4. Kanai R, et al. Political Orientations Are Correlated with Brain Structure in Young Adults. Curr Biol. 2011 Apr 26; 21(8): 677–680.

5. https://www.brainfacts.org/thinking-sensing-and-behaving/aging/2019/how-the-brain-changes-with-age-083019.

6. Huttenlocher PR, de Courten C. The development of synapses in striate cortex of man. Hum Neurobiol. 1987; 6(1):1–9.

7. Konkel L. The Brain before Birth: Using fMRI to Explore the Secrets of Fetal Neurodevelopment. Environmental Health Perspectives, Vol. 126, No. 11, 20 November 2018.

8. Hilgetag CC, Barbas H. Developmental mechanics of the primate cerebral cortex. Anat Embryol (Berl) 2005; 210(5–6):411–417.

9. White T, et al. The Development of Gyrification in Childhood and Adolescence. Brain Cogn. 2010 Feb; 72(1): 36. Published online 2009 Nov 25. doi: 10.1016/j.bandc.2009.10.009.

10. Bartley AJ, Jones DW, Weinberger DR. Genetic variability of human brain size and cortical gyral patterns. Brain. 1997; 120(Pt 2):257–269.

11. Yujiang Wang et al. Universality in human cortical folding in health and disease. PNAS, October 2016 DOI: 10.1073/pnas.1610175113.

12. https://medium.com/thrive-global/the-human-brain-vs-computers-5880cb156541.

13. https://www.scientificamerican.com/article/thinking-hard-calories/.

15. https://www.cell.com/current-biology/pdf/S0960-9822(08)00800-2.pdf.

16. https://www.sciencedaily.com/releases/2017/10/171025105041.htm.

17. https://www.vice.com/en/article/wnnvdm/for-one-second-a-supercomputer-mimicked-the-human-brain.

18 https://www.scientificamerican.com/article/a-new-supercomputer-is-the-worlds-fastest-brain-mimicking-machine/.

19. https://bgr.com/2016/02/27/power-of-the-human-brain-vs-super-computer/.

20. https://med.stanford.edu/news/all-news/2010/11/new-imaging-method-developed-at-stanford-reveals-stunning-details-of-brain-connections.html.

21. Joel D, et al. "Analysis of Human Brain Structure Reveals that the Brain

References

"Types" Typical of Males Are Also Typical of Females, and Vice Versa." Frontiers in human neuroscience vol. 12 399. 18 Oct. 2018, doi:10.3389/fnhum.2018.00399.

22. https://www.sapiens.org/column/field-trips/neanderthal-brain/.

23. Kochiyama, T., Ogihara, N., Tanabe, H.C. et al. Reconstructing the Neanderthal brain using computational anatomy. Sci Rep 8, 6296 (2018). https://doi.org/10.1038/s41598-018-24331-0.

24. Xin J, Zhang Y, Tang Y, Yang Y. Brain Differences Between Men and Women: Evidence From Deep Learning. Front Neurosci. 2019; 13:185. Published 2019 Mar 8. doi:10.3389/fnins.2019.00185.

25. Luders E, Narr KL, Thompson PM, Rex DE, Jancke L, Steinmetz H, et al. Gender differences in cortical complexity. Nat Neurosci. 2004;7(8):799–800: https://f1000research.com/articles/4-88; Luders E, et al. Why Sex Matters: Brain Size Independent Differences in Gray Matter Distributions between Men and Women. Journal of Neuroscience 11 November 2009, 29 (45) 14265-14270.

26. Witelson SF, Glezer I, Kigar DL. J Neurosci. Women have greater density of neurons in posterior temporal cortex. 1995 May;15(5 Pt 1):3418-28. doi: 10.1523/JNEUROSCI.15-05-03418.1995.

27. "Sex on the brain." New Scientist. July 19, 2008.

28. Tan A, et al. The human hippocampus is not sexually-dimorphic: Meta-analysis of structural MRI volumes. NeuroImage. Published online August 31 2015 doi:10.1016/j.neuroimage.2015.08.050.

29. Karama S. et al. Positive association between cognitive ability and cortical thickness in a representative US sample of healthy 6 to 18 year-olds. Intelligence. Volume 37, Issue 2, March-April 2009, Pages 145-155.

30. https://www.sciencemag.org/news/2017/04/study-finds-some-significant-differences-brains-men-and-women.

31. https://www.biorxiv.org/content/10.1101/123729v3.

32. https://stanmed.stanford.edu/2017spring/how-mens-and-womens-brains-are-different.html; Shiino, A., Chen, Y., Tanigaki, K. et al. Sex-related difference in human white matter volumes studied: Inspection of the corpus callosum and other white matter by VBM. Sci Rep 7, 39818 (2017). https://doi.org/10.1038/srep39818.

33. Ingalhalikar M, et al. Sex differences in the structural connectome of the human brain. PNAS. PNAS January 14, 2014 111 (2) 823-828.

34. Ingalhalikar M, et al. Sex differences in the structural connectome of the human brain. PNAS. PNAS January 14, 2014 111 (2) 823-828; https://www.the-scientist.com/the-nutshell/male-and-female-brains-wired-differently-38304.

35. Amen D, et al. Gender-Based Cerebral Perfusion Differences in 46,034 Functional Neuroimaging Scans. Journal of Alzheimer's Disease, 2017; 1 DOI: 10.3233/JAD-170432.

36. Toussaint L, Webb J. Gender Differences in the Relationship Between Empathy and Forgiveness. J Soc Psychol. 2005 Dec; 145(6): 673–685.

37. Mestre M, et al. Are women more empathetic than men? A longitudinal study in adolescence. The Spanish Journal of Psychology, 12(1), 76–83.

38. Christov-Moore L, Iacoboni M. Sex differences in somatomotor representations of others' pain: a permutation-based analysis. Brain Structure and Function (2019) 224:937–947.

39. Kim, DW et al. Multimodal Analysis of Cell Types in a Hypothalamic Node Controlling Social Behavior. Cell, 179 (3). pp. 713-728. ISSN 0092-8674; https://www.caltech.edu/about/news/male-and-female-mice-have-different-brain-cells.

40. https://www.the-scientist.com/features/sex-differences-in-the-brain-34758.

41. http://sciencemission.com/site/index.php?page=news&type=view&id=immunology%2Fsex-difference-in-brain.

42. Hanamsagar, R. et al. Generation of a microglial developmental index in mice and in humans reveals a sex difference in maturation and immune reactivity. Glia 65, 1504–1520 (2017).

43. McCarthy MM. Sex differences in the developing brain as a source of inherent risk. Dialogues Clin Neurosci. 2016; 18(4):361–372.

44. Daneman R, and Prat A. The Blood–Brain Barrier. Cold Spring Harb Perspect Biol. 2015 Jan; 7(1): a020412.

45. Castellazzi, M., Morotti, A., Tamborino, C. et al. Increased age and male sex are independently associated with higher frequency of blood–cerebrospinal fluid barrier dysfunction using the albumin quotient. Fluids Barriers CNS 17, 14 (2020); https://doi.org/10.1186/s12987-020-0173-2; Torres L, Bynoe M. Influence of gender on blood brain barrier permeability and adenosine receptor signaling. The FASEB journal. 03 October 2018 https://doi.org/10.1096/fasebj.31.1_supplement.1042.3.

46. Shors TJ. A trip down memory lane about sex differences in the brain.

References

Philos Trans R Soc Lond B Biol Sci. 2016; 371(1688):20150124. [PMC free article] [PubMed] [Google Scholar].

47. Cimadevilla J, et al. Sex differences in the Morris water maze in young rats: temporal dimensions. Psicothema 2004. Vol. 16, no 4, pp. 611-614; Singh G, Singh V, Sobolewski M, Cory-Slechta DA, Schneider JS. Sex-Dependent Effects of Developmental Lead Exposure on the Brain. Front Genet. 2018; 9:89. Published 2018 Mar 16. doi:10.3389/fgene.2018.00089.

48. Fernández-Quezada D, et al. Male/female Differences in Radial Arm Water Maze Execution After Chronic Exposure to Noise. Noise Health. 2019 Jan-Feb; 21(98): 25–34. Published online 2020 Feb 19. doi: 10.4103/nah.NAH_23_19.

49. Vaccaro A, et al. Sleep Loss Can Cause Death through Accumulation of Reactive Oxygen Species in the Gut. Cell, 2020; DOI: 10.1016/j.cell.2020.04.049.

50. Wang Y, Yip T. Sleep Facilitates Coping: Moderated Mediation of Daily Sleep, Ethnic/Racial Discrimination, Stress Responses, and Adolescent Well-Being. Child Development, 2019; DOI: 10.1111/cdev.13324.

51. Virta JJ, Heikkila K, Perola M, Koskenvuo M, Raiha I, Rinne JO, et al. Midlife sleep characteristics associated with late life cognitive function. Sleep. 2013; 36:1533–41, 41A.

52. Carrier J, Land S, Buysse DJ, Kupfer DJ, Monk TH. The effects of age and gender on sleep EEG power spectral density in the middle years of life (ages 20–60 years old). Psychophysiology. 2001; 38:232–42.

53. Hisler G, Miller A, Krizan Z. 0276 Does Losing Sleep Unleash Anger? Sleep, 2020; 43 (Supplement_1): A105 DOI: 10.1093/sleep/zsaa056.274.

54. Scullin, MK, Rowatt W, Fergason K. 0193 Sleep Health Across Religions: A Consideration of Bidirectional Processes. Sleep, 2020; 43 (Supplement_1): A76 DOI: 10.1093/sleep/zsaa056.191.

55. Beccutia G, Pannaina S. Sleep and obesity. Curr Opin Clin Nutr Metab Care. 2011 Jul; 14(4): 402–412.

56. Nagai M, Hoshide S, Kario K. Sleep Duration as a Risk Factor for Cardiovascular Disease- a Review of the Recent Literature. Curr Cardiol Rev. 2010 Feb; 6(1): 54–61.

57. Y. Wei, G. P. Krishnan, M. Bazhenov. Synaptic Mechanisms of Memory Consolidation during Sleep Slow Oscillations. Journal of Neuroscience, 2016; 36 (15): 4231 DOI: 10.1523/JNEUROSCI.3648-15.2016.

58. https://www.sciencedaily.com/releases/2020/08/200804122233.htm.

59. González O, et al. Can sleep protect memories from catastrophic forgetting? eLife, 2020; 9 DOI: 10.7554/eLife.51005.

60. Winer J, et al. Sleep Disturbance Forecasts β-Amyloid Accumulation across Subsequent Years. Current Biology, 2020; DOI: 10.1016/j.cub.2020.08.017.

61. Bixler E, et al. Women sleep objectively better than men and the sleep of young women is more resilient to external stressors: effects of age and menopause. J Sleep Res. 2009 Jun; 18(2): 221–228.

62. Burgard S, and Ailshire J. Gender and Time for Sleep among U.S. Adults. Am Sociol Rev. 2013 Feb; 78(1): 51–69.

63. https://www.dailymail.co.uk/health/article-1246029/Who-REALLY-needs-sleep—men-women-One-Britains-leading-sleep-experts-says-answer.html.

64. Thomas M, Sing H, Belenky G, Holcomb H, Mayberg H, Dannals R, et al. Neural basis of alertness and cognitive performance impairments during sleepiness. I. Effects of 24 h of sleep deprivation on waking human regional brain activity. J Sleep Res. 2000; 9: 335–52. [PubMed] [Google Scholar]; McKenna BS, Dickinson DL, Orff HJ, Drummond SPA. The effects of one night of sleep deprivation on known-risk and ambiguous-risk decisions. J Sleep Res. 2007; 16: 245–252. [PubMed] [Google Scholar].

65. Trockel M, et al. Assessment of Physician Sleep and Wellness, Burnout, and Clinically Significant Medical Errors. JAMA Netw Open. 2020;3(12):e2028111. doi:10.1001/jamanetworkopen.2020.28111.

66. Tefft B. Acute sleep deprivation and culpable motor vehicle crash involvement. Sleep, 2018; DOI: 10.1093/sleep/zsy144.

67. Ferrara M, et al. Gender Differences in Sleep Deprivation Effects on Risk and Inequality Aversion: Evidence from an Economic Experiment. PLoS One. 2015; 10(3): e0120029.

Published online 2015 Mar 20. doi: 10.1371/journal.pone.0120029.

68. https://melmagazine.com/en-us/story/your-dreams-are-genderedish.

69. https://www.dailymail.co.uk/femail/article-2037152/Why-womens-dreams-wilder-mens-.html.

70. Wamsley E, et al. Dreaming of a Learning Task Is Associated with Enhanced Sleep-Dependent Memory Consolidation. Current Biology. volume 20, issue 9, P850-855.

71. Vgontzas AN, Zoumakis E, Bixler EO, Lin HM, Follett H, Kales A,

References

Chrousos GP. Adverse effects of modest sleep restriction on sleepiness, performance, and inflammatory cytokines. J. Clin. Endocrinol. Metab. 2004; 89:2119–2126.

72. Ma Y, et al. Association Between Sleep Duration and Cognitive Decline. JAMA Netw Open. 2020; 3(9):e2013573. doi:10.1001/jamanetworkopen.2020.13573.

73. Cardoso C, et al. Acute intranasal oxytocin improves positive self-perceptions of personality. Psychopharmacology (Berl). 2012 Apr; 220(4):741-9.

74. Cardoso C, et al. The effect of intranasal oxytocin on perceiving and understanding emotion on the Mayer-Salovey-Caruso Emotional Intelligence Test (MSCEIT). Emotion. 2014 Feb;14(1):43-50. doi: 10.1037/a0034314. Epub 2013 Nov 4.

75. Li T, et al. Intranasal oxytocin, but not vasopressin, augments neural responses to toddlers in human fathers. Hormones and Behavior, 2017; DOI: 10.1016/j.yhbeh.2017.01.006.

76. Scheele D, et al. Oxytocin enhances brain reward system responses in men viewing the face of their female partner. PNAS December 10, 2013 110 (50) 20308-20313; https://doi.org/10.1073/pnas.1314190110.

77. https://www.yalescientific.org/2017/07/oxytocin-not-just-for-women/.

78. Fisher TD, Moore ZT, Pittenger MJ. Sex on the brain?: an examination of frequency of sexual cognitions as a function of gender, erotophilia, and social desirability. J Sex Res. 2012;49(1):69-77. doi: 10.1080/00224499.2011.565429. Epub 2011 May 24. PMID: 21512948.

Chapter Three

1. https://www.tandfonline.com/doi/abs/10.3109/03014460.2013.807878.

2. Kandel E. R., Schwartz J. H., Jessell T. M. (2000). Principles of Neural Science, 4th Edn New York, McGraw-Hill, pp. 19–20.

3. Baccarelli A, Bollati V. Epigenetics and environmental chemicals. Curr Opin Pediatr. 2009 Apr; 21(2): 243–251.

4. Klosin A, et al. Transgenerational transmission of environmental information in C. elegans. Science. 21 Apr 2017: Vol. 356, Issue 6335, pp. 320-323.

5. McCarthy MM. Sex differences in the developing brain as a source of inherent risk. Dialogues Clin Neurosci. 2016; 18(4):361–372.

6. Werling DM., Parikshak NN., Geschwind DH. Gene expression in human brain implicates sexually dimorphic pathways in autism spectrum disorders. Nat Commun. 2016; 7:10717. [PMC free article] [PubMed] [Google Scholar].

7. https://www.genome.gov/about-genomics/fact-sheets/Y-Chromosome-facts.

8. Graves, J. A. M. Sex chromosome specialization and degeneration in mammals. Cell 124, 901–914 (2006).

9. Hughes, J. F. et al. Strict evolutionary conservation followed rapid gene loss on human and rhesus y chromosomes. Nature 483, 82–86 (2012).

10. https://www.theatlantic.com/science/archive/2019/12/men-lose-y-chromosomes-cells-they-age/603013/.

11. Wong, JYY, et al. Outdoor air pollution and mosaic loss of chromosome Y in older men from the Cardiovascular Health Study. Environment International. 116:239-247 ·April 2018.

12. https://www.psychologytoday.com/us/blog/the-scientific-fundamentalist/201104/why-are-older-parents-more-likely-have-daughters.

13. Dumanski et al. Mosaic loss of chromosome Y in blood is associated with Alzheimer's disease. American Journal of Human Genetics, 2016 DOI: 10.1016/j.ajhg.2016.05.014.

14. McCarthy MM. Sex differences in the developing brain as a source of inherent risk. Dialogues Clin Neurosci. 2016; 18(4):361–372.

15. O'Driscoll D, et al. Expression of X-linked Toll-like receptor 4 signaling genes in female vs. male neonates, Pediatric Research (2017). DOI: 10.1038/pr.2017.2.

16. https://www.scientificamerican.com/article/are-men-the-weaker-sex/.

17. https://www.scientificamerican.com/article/his-brain-her-brain-2012-10-23/.

18. Carpenter M, Nagell K, Tomasello M, Butterworth G, Moore C. Social cognition, joint attention, and communicative competence from 9 to 15 months of age. Monogr Soc Res Child Dev. 1998; 63:1–143. doi: 10.2307/1166214. [PubMed] [CrossRef] [Google Scholar]; Fenson L, Dale PS, Reznick S, Bates D, Thal DJ, Pethick SJ, et al. Variability in early communicative development. Monogr Soc Res Child Dev. 1994; 59:1–185. doi: 10.2307/1166093.

19. Özçalişkan Ş, Goldin-Meadow S. Sex differences in language first appear in gesture. Dev Sci. 2010; 13:752–60. doi: 10.1111/j.1467-7687.2009.00933.

References

20. Kovačević M, Kraljevic K, Cepanec M. Sex differences in lexical and grammatical development in Croatian. Proceedings from the First European Network Meeting on the Communicative Development Inventories; 2006 May 24-28; Dubrovnik, Croatia. Gävle: University of Gävle; 2007.

21. Lutchmaya S, Baron-Cohen S, Raggatt P. Foetal testosterone and eye contact in 12-month-old human infants. Infant Behav Dev. 2002; 25:327–35. doi: 10.1016/S0163-6383(02)00094-2; Knickmeyer R, Baron-Cohen S, Ragatt P, Taylor K. Foetal testosterone, social relationships, and restricted interests in children. J Child Psychol Psychiatry. 2005; 46:198–210. doi: 10.1111/j.1469-7610.2004.00349.x.

22. Auyeung B, Taylor K, Hackett G, Baron-Cohen S. Foetal testosterone and autistic traits in 18 to 24-month-old children. Mol Autism. 2010; 1:11. doi: 10.1186/2040-2392-1-11.

23. Quast A, Hesse V, Hain J, Wermke K. Baby babbling at five months linked to sex hormone levels in early infancy. Infant Behav Dev. 2016; 44:1–10. doi: 10.1016/j.infbeh.2016.04.002.

24. Hollier LP, Mattes E, Maybery MT, Keelan JA, Hickey M, Whitehouse AJ. The association between perinatal testosterone concentration and early vocabulary development: A prospective cohort study. Biol Psychol. 2013; 92:212–5. doi: 10.1016/j.biopsycho.2012.10.016.

25. Schaadt G, Hesse V, Friederici A. Sex hormones in early infancy seems to predict aspects of later language development. Brain Lang. 2015; 141:70–6. doi: 10.1016/j.bandl.2014.11.015.

26. Mehl M, et al. Are women really more talkative than men? Science. 2007 Jul 6;317(5834):82. doi: 10.1126/science.1139940;

27. Brysbaert M, Stevens M, Mandera P, Keuleers E. How many words do we know? Practical estimates of vocabulary size dependent on word definition, the degree of language input and the participant's age. Front Psychol. 2016; 7:1116. doi 10.3389/fpsyg.2016.01116.

28. Bowers M, Perez-Pouchoulen M, Edwards NS, Mccarthy MM. Foxp2 mediates sex differences in ultrasonic vocalization by rat pups and directs order of maternal retrieval. J Neurosci. 2013; 33:3276–83. doi: 10.1523/JNEUROSCI.0425-12.2013.

29. Kurth F, Jancke L, Luders E. The Sexual Dimorphism of Broca's Region: More Gray Matter in Female Brains in Brodmann Areas 44 and 45. J Neurosci Res. 2017 Jan 2; 95(1-2): 626–632. doi: 10.1002/jnr.23898.

30. https://www.npr.org/sections/health-shots/2018/07/23/630688342/might-sex-hormones-help-protect-women-from-alzheimer-s-after-all-maybe.

31. Verburg P, et al. Sexual Dimorphism in Adverse Pregnancy Outcomes - A Retrospective Australian Population Study 1981-2011. PLOS ONE, 2016; 11 (7): e0158807DOI: 10.1371/journal.pone.0158807.

32. https://www.medicaldaily.com/womb-makes-it-easy-being-girl-how-placenta-protects-girls-more-boys-285690.

33. Buckberry S, et al. Integrative transcriptome meta-analysis reveals widespread sex-biased gene expression at the human fetal–maternal interface. Molecular Human Reproduction, Volume 20, Issue 8, August 2014, Pages 810–819; Gong S, et al. Placental polyamine metabolism differs by fetal sex, fetal growth restriction, and preeclampsia. JCI Insight. 2018 Jul 12; 3(13):e120723. doi: 10.1172/jci.insight.120723.

34. Gualtieri T, Hicks R. An immunoreactive theory of selective male affliction. Behav Brain Sci. 1985; 8:427–441.

35. https://www.scientificamerican.com/article/are-men-the-weaker-sex/.

36. https://onlinelibrary.wiley.com/doi/pdf/10.1111/apa.14390.

37. McClendon E, et al. Transient Hypoxemia Disrupts Anatomical and Functional Maturation of Preterm Fetal Ovine CA1 Pyramidal Neurons. The Journal of Neuroscience, 2019; 1364-19 DOI: 10.1523/JNEUROSCI.1364-19.2019.

38 Mackey, E., Ayyadurai, S., Pohl, C.S. et al. Sexual dimorphism in the mast cell transcriptome and the pathophysiological responses to immunological and psychological stress. Biol Sex Differ 7, 60 (2016). https://doi.org/10.1186/s13293-016-0113-7.

39. https://www.jimmunol.org/content/198/7/2681.long.

40. Gaignard P., Savouroux S., Liere P., Pianos A., Thérond P., Schumacher M., et al. (2015). Effect of sex differences on brain mitochondrial function and its suppression by ovariectomy and in aged mice. Endocrinology 156 2893–2904; Harish G., Venkateshappa C., Mahadevan A., Pruthi N., Bharath M., Shankar S. (2013). Mitochondrial function in human brains is affected by pre- and post mortem factors. Neuropathol. Appl. Neurobiol. 39 298–315. 10.1111; Gaignard P., Savouroux S., Liere P., Pianos A., Thérond P., Schumacher M., et al. (2015). Effect of sex differences on brain mitochondrial function and its suppression by ovariectomy and in aged mice. Endocrinology 156 2893–2904. 10.1210/en.2014-1913.

41. Harish G., Venkateshappa C., Mahadevan A., Pruthi N., Bharath M., Shankar S. (2013). Mitochondrial function in human brains is affected by pre- and post mortem factors. Neuropathol. Appl. Neurobiol. 39 298–315. 10.1111.

42. Khalifa A. R., Abdel-Rahman E. A., Mahmoud A. M., Ali M. H., Noureldin M., Saber S. H., et al. (2017). Sex-specific differences in mitochondria biogenesis, morphology, respiratory function, and ROS homeostasis in young mouse heart and brain. Physiol. Rep. 5:e13125 10.14814/phy2.13125.

43. Schwarz J. M., Sholar P. W., Bilbo S. D. (2012). Sex differences in microglial colonization of the developing rat brain. J. Neurochem. 120 948–963. 10.1111/j.1471-4159.2011.07630.

44. Mohagheghi F., Khalaj L., Ahmadiani A., Rahmani B. (2013). Gemfibrozil pretreatment affecting antioxidant defense system and inflammatory, but not Nrf-2 signaling pathways resulted in female neuroprotection and male neurotoxicity in the rat models of global cerebral ischemia–reperfusion. Neurotox. Res. 23 225–237. 10.1007/s12640-012-9338-3.

45. Pitts M. W., Kremer P. M., Hashimoto A. C., Torres D. J., Byrns C. N., Williams C. S., et al. (2015). Competition between the brain and testes under selenium-compromised conditions: insight into sex differences in selenium metabolism and risk of neurodevelopmental disease. J. Neurosci. 35 15326–15338. 10.1523/jneurosci.2724-15.2015.

46. Gillies G. E., Pienaar I. S., Vohra S., Qamhawi Z. (2014). Sex differences in Parkinson's disease. Front. Neuroendocrinol. 35, 370 384. 10.1016/j.yfrne.2014.02.002.

Chapter Four

1. Zablotsky B, Black LI, Maenner MJ, Schieve LA, Blumberg SJ. Estimated Prevalence of Autism and Other Developmental Disabilities Following Questionnaire Changes in the 2014 National Health Interview Survey. National Health Statistics Reports. Volume 87. http://www.cdc.gov/nchs/data/nhsr/nhsr087.pdf. Published 11/13/2015. Accessed 13/11/2015.

2. Boyle CA, Boulet S, Schieve LA, Cohen RA, Blumberg SJ, Yeargin-Allsopp M, et al (2011) Trends in the prevalence of developmental disabilities in US children, 1997–2008. Pediatrics 127: 1034–42.

3. Kern JK, et al. Developmental neurotoxicants and the vulnerable male brain: a systematic review of suspected neurotoxicants that disproportionally affect males. Acta Neurobiol Exp (Wars). 2017; 77(4):269-296.

4. Geier DA, Kern JK, Sykes LK, Geier MR (2016a) Examining genotypic variation in autism spectrum disorder and its relationship to parental age and phenotype. Appl Clin Genet 9: 121–9.

5. Stessman HA, Xiong B, Coe BP, et al (2017) Targeted sequencing identifies 91 neurodevelopmental-disorder risk genes with autism and developmental-

disability biases. Nat Genet 49: 515–26.

6. Shen Y, Dies KA, Holm IA, et al (2010) Autism Consortium Clinical Genetics/ DNA Diagnostics Collaboration. Clinical genetic testing for patients with autism spectrum disorders. Pediatrics 125: e727–35.

7. Hallmayer J, Cleveland S, Torres A, et al. "Genetic Heritability and Shared Environmental Factors Among Twin Pairs With Autism," Arch Gen Psychiatry. 2011; 68(11):1095-1102. doi:10.1001/archgenpsychiatry.2011.76.

8. https://www.nature.com/articles/s41559-016-0051.

9. https://www.scientificamerican.com/article/chemical-tainted-food/.

10. Gale RW, WL Cranor, DA Alvarez, JN Huckins, JD Petty and GL Robertson. Semivolatile organic compounds in residential air along the Arizona-Mexico border. Environmental Science and Technology doi: 10.1021/es803482u.

11. http://www.scientificamerican.com/article.cfm?id=newborn-babies-chemicals-exposure-bpa.

12. Woodruff TJ, et al. Environmental Chemicals in Pregnant Women in the US: NHANES 2003-2004. Environmental Health Perspectives, 2011; DOI: 10.1289/ehp.1002727.

13. https://www.nature.com/articles/d41586-018-02481-5.

14. https://www.chemicalsafetyfacts.org/chemistry-context/debunking-myth-chemicals-testing-safety/.

15. http://www.thelancet.com/journals/laneur/article/PIIS1474-4422%2813%2970278-3/abstract.

16. Bennett D, Bellinger DC, Birnaum LS et al (2016) Project TENDR: Targeting Environmental Neuro-Developmental Risks The TENDR Consensus Statement. Environ Health Perspect 124: A118–22.

17. Sealey LA, Hughes BW, Sriskanda AN, Guest JR, Gibson AD, Johnson-Williams L, Pace DG, Bagasra O (2016) Environmental factors in the development of autism spectrum disorders. Environ Int 88: 288–98.

LEAD

18. https://www.aap.org/en-us/about-the-aap/aap-press-.

19. https://www.unicef.org/reports/toxic-truth-childrens-exposure-to-lead-pollution-2020.

References

20. Bellinger, David C. Very low lead exposures and children's neurodevelopment. 2, April 2008, Current Opinion in Pediatrics, Vol. 20, pp. 172– 177.

21. http://www.ncbi.nlm.nih.gov/pmc/articles/PMC3230438/.

22. http://www.scientificamerican.com/article/lead-in-aviation-fuel/.

23. http://www.bbc.com/news/magazine-27067615.

24. Bellinger D. C. (2008). Very low lead exposures and children's neurodevelopment. Curr. Opin. Pediatr. 20 172–177. 10.1097/MOP.0b013e3282f4f97b; Wright J. P., Dietrich K. N., Ris M. D., Hornung R. W., Wessel S. D., Lanphear B. P., et al. (2008). Association of prenatal and childhood blood lead concentrations with criminal arrests in early adulthood. PLoS Med. 5:e101. 10.1371/journal.pmed.0050101.

25. https://undark.org/article/lead-ammunition-bullets-hunting-copper/.

26. https://www.npr.org/sections/health- shots/2017/05/10/527648768/lead-dust-from-firearms-can-pose-a-silent- health-risk.

27. Miranda ML, Kim D, Overstreet Galeano MA, Paul C, Hull A, Morgan SP. The relationship between early childhood blood lead levels and performance on end of grade tests. Environ Health Perspect. 2007; 115:1242–1247.

28. Johnston J, et al. Lead and Arsenic in Shed Deciduous Teeth of Children Living Near a Lead-Acid Battery Smelter. Environ. Sci. Technol. 2019, 53, 10, 6000–6006.

29. https://www.discovermagazine.com/health/the-pediatrician-who-woke-america-up-to-the-lead-crisis.

30. Pocock S. J., Ashby D., Smith M. A. (1987). Lead exposure and children's intellectual performance. Int. J. Epidemiol. 16 57–67. 10.1093/ije/16.1.57 [PubMed] [CrossRef] [Google Scholar].

31. Khanna MM (2015) Boys, not girls, are negatively affected on cognitive tasks by lead exposure: a pilot study. J Environ Health 77: 72–7.

32. Irgens A, Kruger K, Skorve AH, Irgens LM. Reproductive outcome in offspring of parents occupationally exposed to lead in Norway. Am J Ind Med 1998; 34:431–7; Torres-Sanchez LE, Berkowitz G, Lopez-Carrillo L, Torres-Arreola L, Rios C, Lopez-Cervantes M. Intrauterine lead exposure and preterm birth. Environ Res 1999; 81:297–301; Gonzalez-Cossio T, Peterson KE, Sanin LH, Fishbein E, Palazuelos E, Aro A, et al. Decrease in birth weight in relation to maternal bone-lead burden. Pediatrics 1997; 100:856–62; Hernandez-Avila M, Peterson KE, Gonzalez-Cossio T, Sanin LH, Aro A, Schnaas L, et al. Effect

of maternal bone lead on length and head circumference of newborns and 1-month-old infants. Arch Environ Health 2002; 57:482–8.

33. Jedrychowski W., Perera F., Jankowski J., Mrozek-Budzyn D., Mroz E., Flak E., et al. (2009). Gender specific differences in neurodevelopmental effects of prenatal exposure to very low-lead levels: the prospective cohort study in three-year olds. Early Hum. Dev. 85 503–510. 10.1016/j.earlhumdev.2009.04.006.

34. Ris M. D., Dietrich K. N., Succop P. A., Berger O. G., Bornschein R. L. (2004). Early exposure to lead and neuropsychological outcome in adolescence. J. Int. Neuropsychol. Soc. 10 261–270. 10.1017/S1355617704102154; Taylor C. M., Kordas K., Golding J., Emond A. M. (2017). Data relating to prenatal lead exposure and child IQ at 4 and 8 years old in the avon longitudinal study of parents and children. Neurotoxicology 62 224–230. 10.1016/j.neuro.2017.07.025.

35. Cecil K. M., Brubaker C. J., Adler C. M., Dietrich K. N., Altaye M., Egelhoff J. C., et al. (2008). Decreased brain volume in adults with childhood lead exposure. PLoS Med. 5:e112. 10.1371/journal.pmed.0050112 [PMC free article] [PubMed] [CrossRef] [Google Scholar].

36. Singh G, Singh V, Sobolewski M, Cory-Slechta DA, Schneider JS. Sex-Dependent Effects of Developmental Lead Exposure on the Brain. Front Genet. 2018; 9:89. Published 2018 Mar 16. doi:10.3389/fgene.2018.00089.

37. Yıldız S, Gözü Pirinççioğlu A, Arıca E. Evaluation of Heavy Metal (Lead, Mercury, Cadmium, and Manganese) Levels in Blood, Plasma, and Urine of Adolescents With Aggressive Behavior. Cureus. 2023 Jan 17;15(1):e33902. doi: 10.7759/cureus.33902. PMID: 36819371; PMCID: PMC9936102.

MERCURY, ARSENIC

1. Siblerud R, Mutter J, Moore E, Naumann J, Walach H. A Hypothesis and Evidence That Mercury May be an Etiological Factor in Alzheimer's Disease. Int J Environ Res Public Health. 2019;16(24):5152. Published 2019 Dec 17. doi:10.3390/ijerph16245152.

2. https://www.youtube.com/watch?v=ewNvcFJEHbA.

3. Centers for Disease Control, January 2003. Second National Report on Human Exposure to Environmetal Chemicals.

4. https://blogs.scientificamerican.com/observations/why-does-autism-impact-boys-more-often-than-girls/.

5. https://www.foodwhistleblower.org/fda-whistleblower-speaks-out-about-mercury-in-our-food/.

References

6. https://grist.org/article/sweetness-and-blight.

7. Woods JS, Heyer NJ, Russo JE, Martin MD, Farin FM (2014) Genetic polymorphisms affecting susceptibility to mercury neurotoxicity in children: summary findings from the Casa Pia Children's Amalgam clinical trial. Neurotoxicology 44: 288–302.

8. Clarkson TW, Vyas JB, Ballatori N (October 2007). "Mechanisms of mercury disposition in the body". American Journal of Industrial Medicine. 50 (10): 757–64.

9. Loren H, et a. Effects on and transfer across the blood-brain barrier in vitro—Comparison of organic and inorganic mercury species. BMC Pharmacol Toxicol. 2016; 17: 63.

10. Barrett J. Thimerosal and Animal Brains: New Data for Assessing Human Ethylmercury RiskEnviron Health Perspect. 2005 Aug; 113(8): A543–A544.

11. Sharpe M, et al. Thimerosal-Derived Ethylmercury Is a Mitochondrial Toxin in Human Astrocytes: Possible Role of Fenton Chemistry in the Oxidation and Breakage of mtDNA. Journal of Toxicology, Volume 2012 |Article ID 373678.

12. Dorea J, et al. Toxicity of ethylmercury (and Thimerosal): A comparison with methylmercury. Journal of Applied Toxicology 33(8) August 2013.

13. https://www.cdc.gov/vaccinesafety/pdf/cdcstudiesonvaccinesandautism.pdf.

14. Thompson WW, Price C, Goodson B, Shay DK, Benson P, Hinrichsen VL et al.; Vaccine Safety Datalink Team. Early thimerosal exposure and neuropsychological outcomes at 7 to 10 years. N Engl J Med 2007; 357: 1281-92.

15. Tozzi AE, Bisiacchi P, Tarantino V, De Mei B, D'Elia L, Chiarotti F, Salmaso S. Neuropsychological performance 10 years after immunization in infancy with thimerosal-containing vaccines. Pediatrics 2009; 123: 475-82.

16. https://www.nejm.org/doi/full/10.1056/nejmp078187.

17. Barile JP, Kuperminc GP, Weintraub ES, Mink JW, Thompson WW (2012) Thimerosal exposure in early life and neuropsychological outcomes 7-10 years later. J Pediatr Psychol 37; 106-18; Thompson WW, Price C, Goodson B, Shay DK, Benson P, Hinrichsen VL, Lewis E, Eriksen E, Ray P, Marcy SM, Dunn J, Jackson LA, Lieu TA, Black S, Stewart G, Weintraub ES, Davis RL, DeStefano F; Vaccine Safety Datalink Team (2007) Early thimerosal exposure and neuropsychological outcomes at 7 to 10 years. N Engl J Med 357: 1281–92.

18. Vahter M, et al. Gender differences in the deposition and toxicity of

metals. Environmental Research 104(1):85-95 ·June 2007.

19. Ruszkiewicz J., Bowman A., Farina M., Rocha J., Aschner M. (2016). Sex- and structure-specific differences in antioxidant responses to methylmercury during early development. Neurotoxicology 56 118–126. 10.1016/j.neuro.2016.07.009.

20. Cardenas A, Rifas-Shiman SL, Agha G, et al. Persistent DNA methylation changes associated with prenatal mercury exposure and cognitive performance during childhood. Sci Rep. 2017;7(1):288. Published 2017 Mar 21. doi:10.1038/s41598-017-00384-5.

21. Sager PR, Aschner M, Rodier PM (1984) Persistent, differential alterations in developing cerebellar cortex of male and female mice after methyl- mercury exposure. 2 Brain Res 314: 1–11.

22. Branch DR (2009) Gender-selective toxicity of thimerosal. Exp Toxicol Pathol 61: 133–6.

23. Edoff K., Raciti M., Moors M., Sundström E., Ceccatelli S. (2017). Gestational age and sex influence the susceptibility of human neural progenitor cells to low levels of MeHg. Neurotox. Res. 32 683–693. 10.1007/s12640-017-9786-x.

24. Woods J. S., Heyer N. J., Russo J. E., Martin M. D., Farin F. M. (2014). Genetic polymorphisms affecting susceptibility to mercury neurotoxicity in children: Summary findings from the Casa Pia Childrens Amalgam Clinical Trial. Neurotoxicology 44 288–302. 10.1016/j.neuro.2014.07.010.

25. Li X, Qu F, Xie W, Wang F, Liu H, Song S, Chen T, Zhang Y, Zhu S, Wang Y, Guo C, Tang TS (2014) Transcriptomic analyses of neurotoxic effects in mouse brain after intermittent neonatal administration of thimerosal. Toxicol Sci 139: 452–65.

26. Wasserman, G.A., Liu, X., LoIacono, N.J. et al. A cross-sectional study of well water arsenic and child IQ in Maine schoolchildren. Environ Health 13, 23 (2014). https://doi.org/10.1186/1476-069X-13-23.

27. Peng H, et al. Methylated Phenylarsenical Metabolites Discovered in Chicken Liver. Angewandte Chemie International Edition, 2017; DOI: 10.1002/anie.201700736.

.28. Hall AH. Chronic arsenic poisoning. Toxicol Lett 2002; 128(1):69–72.

29. Ahmed RG, El-Gareib AW. Gestational Arsenic Trioxide Exposure Acts as a Developing Neuroendocrine-Disruptor by Downregulating Nrf2/PPARγ and Upregulating Caspase-3/NF-κB/Cox2/BAX/iNOS/ROS. 2018 Sep 12:S0278-6915(18)30663-X. doi: 10.1016/j.fct.2018.09.019.

References

30. O'Bryant SE, Edwards M, Menon CV, Gong G, Barber R (2011) Long-term low-level arsenic exposure is associated with poorer neuropsychological functioning: a Project FRONTIER study. Int J Environ Res Public Health 8: 861–74; Tyler CR, Allan AM. The Effects of Arsenic Exposure on Neurological and Cognitive Dysfunction in Human and Rodent Studies: A Review. Curr Environ Health Rep. 2014; 1(2):132-147. Published 2014 Mar 21. doi:10.1007/s40572-014-0012-1.

31. Rosado JL, Ronquillo D, Kordas K, Rojas O, Alatorre J, Lopez P, Garcia-Vargas G, Del Carmen Caamaño M, Cebrián ME, Stoltzfus RJ (2007) Arsenic exposure and cognitive performance in Mexican schoolchildren. Environ Health Perspect 115: 1371–5.

32. Allan AM, Hafez AK, Labrecque MT, et al. Sex-Dependent effects of developmental arsenic exposure on methylation capacity and methylation regulation of the glucocorticoid receptor system in the embryonic mouse brain. Toxicol Rep. 2015;2 :1376-1390. doi:10.1016/j.toxrep.2015.10.003.

33. Mazumdar M, Ibne Hasan MO, Hamid R, Valeri L, Paul L, et al. Arsenic is associated with reduced effect of folic acid in myelomeningocele prevention: a case control study in Bangladesh. Environ Health 2015; 14:34.

34. Parvez F, Chen Y, Brandt-Rauf PW, et al. A prospective study of respiratory symptoms associated with chronic arsenic exposure in Bangladesh: findings from the Health Effects of Arsenic Longitudinal Study (HEALS). Thorax. 2010; 65:528–533.

35. Smith AH, Goycolea M, Haque R, Biggs ML. Marked increase in bladder and lung cancer mortality in a region of Northern Chile due to arsenic in drinking water. Am J Epidemiol. 1998; 147:660–669.

36. Khan M, et al. Prospective cohort study of respiratory effects at ages 14 to 26 following early life exposure to arsenic in drinking water. Environ Epidemiol. 2020 Apr; 4(2): e089. Published online 2020 Apr 9.

37. Yorifuji T, Kato T, Ohta H, Bellinger DC, Matsuoka K, Grandjean P. Neurological and neuropsychological functions in adults with a history of developmental arsenic poisoning from contaminated milk powder. Neurotoxicol Teratol. 2016; 53:75–80.

MANGANESE

38. https://www.worldoil.com/news/2020/2/3/us-crude-oil-and-natural-gas-production-increased-in-2018-with-10-fewer-wells.

39. Wright RO, Amarasiriwardena C, Woolf AD, Jim R, Bellinger DC. Neuropsychological correlates of hair arsenic, manganese, and cadmium levels

in school-age children residing near a hazardous waste site. Neurotoxicology 2006;27(2):210–6.

40. Rahman SM, Kippler M, Tofail F, Bölte S, Hamadani JD, et al. Manganese in drinking water and cognitive abilities and behavior at 10 years of age: a prospective cohort study. Environ Health Perspect 2017; 125(5):057003.

ALUMINUM

41. Çabuş N, Oğuz EO, Tufan AÇ, Adıgüzel E (2015) A histological study of toxic effects of aluminium sulfate on rat hippocampus. Biotech Histochem 90: 132–9; Crépeaux G, Eidi H, David MO, Tzavara E, Giros B, Exley C, Curmi PA, Shaw CA, Gherardi RK, Cadusseau J (2015) Highly delayed systemic translocation of aluminum-based adjuvant in CD1 mice following intramuscular injections. J Inorg Biochem 152: 199–205; Gherardi RK, Eidi H, Crépeaux G, Authier FJ, Cadusseau J (2015) Biopersistence and brain translocation of aluminum adjuvants of vaccines. Front Neurol 6: 4.

42. Exley, C., Clarkson, E. Aluminium in human brain tissue from donors without neurodegenerative disease: A comparison with Alzheimer's disease, multiple sclerosis and autism. Sci Rep 10, 7770 (2020).

43. Bondy SC. The neurotoxicity of environmental aluminum is still an issue. Neurotoxicology 2010;31(5):575-81.

44. Exley C. The coordination chemistry of aluminum in neurodegenerative disease. Coord Chem Rev 2012; 256(19-20):2142-6.

45. Howard JMH: Clinical import of small increases in serum aluminum. Clin Chem 30: 1722-1723, 1984.

46. Fernandez-Lorenzo JR, Cocho JA, Rey-Goldar ML, Couce M, Fraga JM: Aluminum contents of human milk, Cow's milk, and infant formulas. J Pediatr Gastroentero Nutr 28: 270-275, 1999.

47. Yumoto S, Nagai H, Kobayashi K, Tamate A, Kakimi S, Matsuzaki H: 26Al incorporation into the brain of suckling rats through maternal milk. J Inorg Biochem 97: 155-160, 2003.

48. Yasuda H, et al. High Accumulation of Aluminum in Hairs of Infants and Children. Biomed Res Trace Elements 19(1): 57-62, 2008.

49. Aluminum Toxicity in Infants and Children, Committee on Nutrition, American Academy of Pediatrics, Pediatrics Volume 97, Number 3 March, 1996, pp. 413-416.

50. (2008) Toxicological profile for aluminum. Agency for toxic substances and disease registry (ATSDR), USA, pp.1-357.

References

51. Petrovsky N. Comparative Safety of Vaccine Adjuvants: A Summary of Current Evidence and Future Needs. Drug Saf. 2015; 38(11): 1059–1074.

52. Warfving N, Laufs J, Weber K (2017) Short Review of Aluminum Hydroxide Related Lesions in Preclinical Studies and their Relevance. Int J Vaccines Vaccin 4(2): 00076. DOI: 10.15406/ijvv.2017.04.00076.

53. Yasuda H, Tsutsui T. Assessment of infantile mineral imbalances in autism spectrum disorders (ASDs) Int J Environ Res Public Health. 2013; 10(11):6027–6043; Mohamed Fel B, Zaky EA, El-Sayed AB, Elhossieny RM, Zahra SS, Salah Eldin W, Youssef WY, Khaled RA, Youssef AM. Assessment of Hair Aluminum, Lead, and Mercury in a Sample of Autistic Egyptian Children: Environmental Risk Factors of Heavy Metals in Autism. Behav Neurol. 2015; 2015:545674; Blaurock-Busch E, Amin OR, Dessoki HH, Rabah T. Toxic Metals and Essential Elements in Hair and Severity of Symptoms among Children with Autism. Maedica. 2012; 7(1):38–48.

54. Eisenkraft A, Falk A, Finkelstein A. The role of glutamate and the immune system in organophosphate-induced CNS damage. Neurotox Res. 2013; 24(2):265–279. doi: 10.1007/s12640-013-9388-1; Kern JK, Geier DA, Sykes LK, Haley BE, Geier MR. The relationship between mercury and autism: A comprehensive review and discussion. J Trace Elem Med Biol. 2016; 37:8–24. doi: 10.1016/j.jtemb.2016.06.002.

55. Warfving N, Laufs J, Weber K (2017) Short Review of Aluminum Hydroxide Related Lesions in Preclinical Studies and their Relevance. Int J Vaccines Vaccin 4(2): 00076. DOI: 10.15406/ijvv.2017.04.00076.

56. Inbar R, et al. Behavioral abnormalities in female mice following administration of aluminum adjuvants and the human papillomavirus (HPV) vaccine Gardasil, Immunol Res (2016). doi:10.1007/s12026-016-8826-6.

57. https://www.cdc.gov/vaccines/vpd/anthrax/public/index.html.

58. Shaw CA, Petrik MS (2009) Aluminum hydroxide injections lead to motor deficits and motor neuron degeneration. J Inorg Biochem 103(11): 1555-1562; Tomljenovic L, Shaw CA (2011) Aluminum Vaccine Adjuvants: Are they Safe? Curr Med Chem 18(17) 2630-2637.

59. Masson JD, et al. Calcium Phosphate: A Substitute for Aluminum Adjuvants? Expert Rev Vaccines. 2017 Mar;16(3):289-299; Ceo P, et al. Enhanced Oral Vaccine Efficacy of Polysaccharide-Coated Calcium Phosphate Nanoparticles. ACS Omega. 2020 Jul 17; 5(29):18185-18197. doi: 10.1021/acsomega.0c01792. eCollection 2020 Jul 28.

60. House E, Esiri M, Forster G, et al. Aluminium, iron and copper in human brain tissues donated to the medical research council's cognitive function and ageing study. Metallomics 2012; 4(1):56-65.

61. Wang Z, Wei X, Yang J, Suo J, Chen J, Liu X, Zhao X. Chronic exposure to aluminum and risk of Alzheimer's disease: A meta-analysis. Neurosci Lett. 2016; 610:200–206. doi: 10.1016/j.neulet.2015.11.014.

62. Kawahara M, Kato-Negishi M. Link between Aluminum and the Pathogenesis of Alzheimer's Disease The Integration of the Aluminum and Amyloid Cascade Hypotheses. Int J Alzheimers Dis. 2011; 276393.

63. Davenward S, Bentham P, Wright J, et al. Silicon-rich mineral water as a non-invasive test of the 'aluminium hypothesis' in Alzheimer's disease. J Alzheimers Dis 2013; 33(2):423-30.

CADMIUM

64. https://usludgefree.org/information/farm-risks.

65. https://www.washingtonpost.com/health/why-romaine-lettuce-keeps-getting-recalled-for-e-coli-contamination/2019/11/26/f20e7592-0fc4-11ea-b0fc-62cc38411ebb_story.html.

66. R. W. Thatcher, M. L. Lester, R. McAlaster, and R. Horst, "Effects of low levels of cadmium and lead on cognitive functioning in children," Archives of Environmental Health, vol. 37, no. 3, pp. 159–166, 1982; R. W. Thatcher, R. McAlaster, and M. L. Lester, "Evoked potentials related to hair cadmium and lead in children," Annals of the New York Academy of Sciences, vol. 425, pp. 384–390, 1984.

67. Ciesielski T, Weuve J, Bellinger DC, Schwartz J, Lanphear B, Wright RO. Cadmium exposure and neurodevelopmental outcomes in U.S. children. Environ Health Perspect. 2012 May; 120(5):758-63. doi: 10.1289/ehp.1104152.

68. Wang B, Du Y. Cadmium and its neurotoxic effects. Oxid Med Cell Longev. 2013; 2013:898034.

69. H. Ishitobi, K. Mori, K. Yoshida, and C. Watanabe, "Effects of perinatal exposure to low-dose cadmium on thyroid hormone-related and sex hormone receptor gene expressions in brain of offspring," NeuroToxicology, vol. 28, no. 4, pp. 790–797, 2007; H. Ishitobi and C. Watanabe, "Effects of low-dose perinatal cadmium exposure on tissue zinc and copper concentrations in neonatal mice and on the reproductive development of female offspring," Toxicology Letters, vol. 159, no. 1, pp. 38–46, 2005.

FLAME RETARDANTS, PCBS, FOREVER CHEMICALS, FLUORIDE

1. https://www.scientificamerican.com/article/chemical-tainted-food/.

2. http://bangordailynews.com/2012/11/28/health/toxic-flame- retardants-found-in-couches-in-maine-and-u-s/?ref=inline.

References

3. http://www.chicagotribune.com/news/watchdog/flames/ct-met- flames-regulators-20120510,0,6880244,full.story.

4. http://www.ewg.org/research/flame-retardants-2014.

5. http://greensciencepolicy.org/wp-content/uploads/2014/03/Sac-Bee- Op-Ed.pdf.

6. Daniels R, et al. Mortality and cancer incidence in a pooled cohort of US firefighters from San Francisco, Chicago and Philadelphia (1950–2009). Occup Environ Med oemed-2013-101662.

7. Kang D, Davis L, Hunt P, Kriebel. Cancer Incidence Among Male MassachusettsFirefighters, 1987–2003. AMERICAN JOURNAL OF INDUSTRIAL MEDICINE 51:329–335 (2008).

8. Costa L, et al. DEVELOPMENTAL NEUROTOXICITY OF POLYBROMINATED DIPHENYL ETHER (PBDE) FLAME RETARDANTS. Neurotoxicology. 2007 Nov; 28(6): 1047–1067. Published online 2007 Aug 24. doi: 10.1016/j.neuro.2007.08.007.

9. http://www.doomsteaddiner.net/forum/index.php?topic=559.1920.

10. Stapleton HM, et al. Novel and High Volume Use Flame Retardants in US Couches Reflective of the 2005 PentaBDE Phase Out. Environ. Sci. Technol., 2012, 46 (24), pp 13432–13439 DOI: 10.1021/es303471d.

11. https://www.durabilityanddesign.com/news/?fuseaction=view&id=115 63.

12. http://www.huffingtonpost.com/2014/06/24/flame-retardants-toxic-_n_5525973.html.

13. Harley K, et al. Association of prenatal and childhood PBDE exposure with timing of puberty in boys and girls. Environ Int. 2017 Mar; 100: 132–138.

14. Dingemans M, et al. Neurotoxicity of Brominated Flame Retardants: (In)direct Effects of Parent and Hydroxylated Polybrominated Diphenyl Ethers on the (Developing) Nervous System. Environ Health Perspect. 2011 Jul 1; 119(7): 900–907.

15. Czerska M, Zieliński M, Kamińska J, Ligocka D (2013) Effects of polybrominated diphenyl ethers on thyroid hormone, neurodevelopment and fertility in rodents and humans. Int J Occup Med Environ Health 26: 498–510.

16. Reverte I, Klein AB, Domingo JL, Colomina MT (2013) Long term effects of murine postnatal exposure to decabromodiphenyl ether (BDE-209) on learning and memory are dependent upon APOE polymorphism and age. Neurotoxicol Teratol 40: 17–27.

17. https://www.ewg.org/research/pcbs-farmed-salmon.

18. https://www.atsdr.cdc.gov/csem/csem.asp?csem=30&po=10: Winneke G (2011) Developmental aspects of environmental neurotoxicology: lessons from lead and polychlorinated biphenyls. J Neurol Sci 308: 9–15.

19. http://seafood.edf.org/pcbs-fish-and-shellfish.

20. Fonnum F, Mariussen E. Mechanisms Involved in the Neurotoxic Effects of Environmental Toxicants Such as Polychlorinated Biphenyls and Brominated Flame Retardants. Review J Neurochem. 2009 Dec; 111(6):1327-47. doi: 10.1111/j.1471-4159.2009.06427.x. Epub 2009 Oct 10; Fonnum F, Mariussen E, Reistad T. Molecular mechanisms involved in the toxic effects of polychlorinated biphenyls (PCBs) and brominated flame retardants (BFRs). J Toxicol Environ Health A. 2006 Jan 8; 69(1-2):21-35. doi: 10.1080/15287390500259020. PMID: 16291560.

21. University of California - Davis - Health System. (2009, April 14). How PCBs May Alter In Utero, Neonatal Brain Development. ScienceDaily. Retrieved May 12, 2020 from www.sciencedaily.com/releases/2009/04/090413204546.ht; Pessah I, et al. Minding the Calcium Store: Ryanodine Receptor Activation as a Convergent Mechanism of PCB Toxicity. Pharmacol Ther. 2010 Feb;125(2):260-85. doi: 10.1016/j.pharmthera.2009.10.009. Epub 2009 Nov 25: Wayman G, et al. PCB-95 Promotes Dendritic Growth via Ryanodine Receptor–Dependent Mechanisms. Environ Health Perspect. 2012 Jul; 120(7): 997–1002. Published online 2012 Apr 25. doi: 10.1289/ehp.1104832.

22. Gaum P, et al. Depressive Symptoms After PCB Exposure: Hypotheses for Underlying Pathomechanisms via the Thyroid and Dopamine SystemInt J Environ Res Public Health. 2019 Mar; 16(6): 950. Published online 2019 Mar 16. doi: 10.3390/ijerph16060950: Gaum P.M., Esser A., Schettgen T., Gube M., Kraus T., Lang J. Prevalence and incidence rates of mental syndromes after occupational exposure to polychlorinated biphenyls. Int. J. Hyg. Environ. Health. 2014; 217:765–774. doi: 10.1016/j.ijheh.2014.04.001.

23. Rude K, et al. The role of the gut microbiome in mediating neurotoxic outcomes to PCB exposure. NeuroToxicology Volume 75, December 2019, Pages 30-40.

24. https://www.ncbi.nlm.nih.gov/pmc/articles/PMC2072821/.

25. https://www.ewg.org/research/poisoned-legacy/lab-accident-global-pollutant#.WzEUGC2ZOA8.

26. https://www.nofluoride.com/3MSecrets.cfm.

27. https://theintercept.com/2018/07/31/3m-pfas-minnesota-pfoa-pfos/.

References

28. https://theintercept.com/2015/08/11/dupont-chemistry-deception/.

29. https://www.ewg.org/research/poisoned-legacy/lab-accident-global-pollutant#.WzEUGC2ZOA8.

30. https://www.treehugger.com/environmental-policy/what-you-need-know-about-pfoa-and-pfos-chemicals-behind-pruitts-recent-epa-scandal.html.

31. https://theintercept.com/2015/08/17/teflon-toxin-case-against-dupont/.

32. https://ehjournal.biomedcentral.com/articles/10.1186/s12940-018-0405-y.

33. https://www.politico.com/story/2018/05/14/emails-white-house-interfered-with-science-study-536950.

34. https://ehjournal.biomedcentral.com/articles/10.1186/s12940-018-0405-y.

35. https://theintercept.com/2016/03/03/new-teflon-toxin-causes-cancer-in-lab-animals/.

36. https://www.purdue.edu/newsroom/releases/2020/Q1/what-the-brain-really-thinks-about-forever-chemicals.html.

37. Liu Z, et al. Multiple crop bioaccumulation and human exposure of perfluoroalkyl substances around a mega fluorochemical industrial park, China: Implication for planting optimization and food safety. Environment International. Volume 127, June 2019, Pages 671-684.

38. LINDSTROM - HEASD-11-066 DECATUR WATER PAPER MARCH 23 2011.PDF.

39. Sammi S, et al. Perfluorooctane Sulfonate (PFOS) Produces Dopaminergic Neuropathology in Caenorhabditis elegans. Toxicological Sciences, Volume 172, Issue 2, December 2019, Pages 417–434.

40. Vuong AM, Yolton K, Webster GM, Sjödin A, Calafat AM, Braun JM, Dietrich KN, Lanphear BP, Chen A (2016) Prenatal polybrominated diphenyl ether and perfluoroalkyl substance exposures and executive function in school-age children. Environ Res 47: 556–64; Quaak I, de Cock M, de Boer M, Lamoree M, Leonards P, van de Bor M (2016) Prenatal exposure to perfluoroalkyl substances and behavioral development in children. Int J Environ Res Public Health 13.

41. https://fluoridealert.org/articles/wastenot414/.

42. https://www.projectcensored.org/18-manhattan-project-covered-up-effects-of-fluoride-toxicity/.

43. https://www.washingtonpost.com/news/wonk/wp/2013/05/21/a-brief-history-of-americas-fluoride-wars/.

44. https://www.sciencehistory.org/distillations/pipe-dreams-americas-fluoride-controversy.

45. Reilly G, "'This Poisoning of Our Drinking Water': The American Fluoridation Controversy in Historical Context, 1950–1990." PhD diss., George Washington University, 2001; C. Carstairs and R. Elder, "Expertise, Health and Popular Opinion: Debating Water Fluoridation," Canadian Historical Review 89, no. 3 (2008): 345–371.

46. https://fluoridealert.org/content/bfs-2012/.

47. Carlsson A. Current problems of the pharmacology and toxicology of fluorides. Lakartidningen. 1978; 75:1388–1392.

48. https://www.cdc.gov/mmwr/preview/mmwrhtml/mm4850bx.htm.

49. World Health Organization. In: Fawell J, Bailey K, Chilton E, Dahi E, Fewtrell L, Magara Y, editors. Fluoride in drinking-water. London: IWA Publishing; 2006.

50. Gori S, Inno A, Lunardi G, Gorgoni G, Malfatti V, Severi F, Alongi F, Carbognin G, Romano L, Pasetto S, et al. 18F-sodium fluoride PET-CT for the assessment of brain metastasis from lung adenocarcinoma. J Thorac Oncol. 2015; 10(8):e67–8.

51. Bhatnagar M, Rao P, Sushma J, Bhatnagar R. Neurotoxicity of fluoride: neurodegeneration in hippocampus of female mice. Indian J Exp Biol. 2002; 40(5):546–54; Pereira M, Dombrowski PA, Losso EM, Chioca LR, Da Cunha C, Andreatini R. Memory impairment induced by sodium fluoride is associated with changes in brain monoamine levels. Neurotox Res. 2011; 19(1):55–62.

52. Spittle B. Fluoride Fatigue: Fluoride Poisoning: Is Fluoride in your Drinking Water, and from Other Sources, Making you Sick? Paua Press Limited; Dunedin, New Zealand: 2008. p. 78.

53. Strunecka A, et al. Chronic Fluoride Exposure and the Risk of Autism Spectrum Disorder. Int J Environ Res Public Health. 2019 Sep; 16(18): 3431.

54. Gao Q, Liu YJ, Guan ZZ. Oxidative stress might be a mechanism connected with the decreased alpha 7 nicotinic receptor influenced by high-concentration of fluoride in SH-SY5Y neuroblastoma cells. Toxicol in Vitro. 2008; 22(4):837–43; Goschorska M, Baranowska-Bosiacka I, Gutowska I, Tarnowski M, Piotrowska K, Metryka E, Safranow K, Chlubek D. Effect of acetylcholinesterase inhibitors donepezil and rivastigmine on the activity and expression of cyclooxygenases in a model of the inflammatory action of fluoride

on macrophages obtained from THP-1 monocytes. Toxicology. 2018; 406-407:9–20.

55. National Research Council. Fluoride in Drinking Water: A Scientific Review of EPA's Standards. Washington, D.C.: National Academy Press; 2006.

56. Hill C, et al. Nonmonotonic Dose–Response Curves Occur in Dose Ranges That Are Relevant to Regulatory Decision-Making. Dose Response. 2018 Jul-Sep; 16(3): 1559325818798282. Published online 2018 Sep 13. doi: 10.1177/1559325818798282.

57. Choi A, et al. Developmental Fluoride Neurotoxicity: A Systematic Review and Meta-Analysis. Environmental Health Perspectives. October 2012 https://doi.org/10.1289/ehp.1104912.

58. Grandjean P. Developmental fluoride neurotoxicity: an updated review. Environmental Health volume 18, Article number: 110 (2019).

59. Bashash M, Thomas D, Hu H, Martinez-Mier EA, Sanchez BN, Basu N, Peterson KE, Ettinger AS, Wright R, Zhang Z, et al. Prenatal fluoride exposure and cognitive outcomes in children at 4 and 6-12 years of age in Mexico. Environ Health Perspect. 2017; 125(9):097017.

60. Tang Q.Q., Du J., Ma H.H., Jiang S.J., Zhou X.J. Fluoride and children's intelligence: A meta-analysis. Biol. Trace. Elem. Res. 2008; 126:115–120. doi: 10.1007/s12011-008-8204-x.

61. Green R, Lanphear B, Hornung R, Flora D, Martinez-Mier EA, Neufeld R, Ayotte P, Muckle G, Till C. Association between maternal fluoride exposure during pregnancy and IQ scores in offspring in Canada. JAMA Pediatr. in press; 2019, 173.

62. https://edhub.ama-assn.org/jn-learning/audio-player/17802991.

63. Till C, Green R, Flora D, Hornung R, Martinez-Mier EA, Blazer M, Farmus L, Ayotte P, Muckle G, Lanphear B. Fluoride exposure from infant formula and child IQ in a Canadian birth cohort. Environ Int. 2019; 134:105315.

64. Waugh D.T., Godfrey M., Limeback H., Potter W. Black tea source, production, and consumption: Assessment of health risks of fluoride intake in New Zealand. J. Environ. Public Health. 2017; 2017:5120504. doi: 10.1155/2017/5120504.

65. Bashash M, Marchand M, Hu H, Till C, Martinez-Mier EA, Sanchez BN, Basu N, Peterson KE, Green R, Schnaas L, et al. Prenatal fluoride exposure and attention deficit hyperactivity disorder (ADHD) symptoms in children at 6-12 years of age in Mexico City. Environ Int. 2018; 121(Pt 1):658–66.

66. He H, Cheng Z, Liu W. Effects of fluorine on the human fetus. Fluoride. 2008; 41(4):321–6; Du L. The effect of fluorine on the developing human brain. Chin. J. Pathol. 1992; 21:218–220.

67. Shao QL, Wang Y, Li L, Li J. Initial study of cognitive function impairment as caused by chronic fluorosis. Chinese Journal of Endemiology. 2003; 22(4):336–8.

68. ROWEN, R. Fluoridation Practices - A Missing Link in the Vaccine Autism Connection? Medical Research Archives, Vol. 5, Issue 2, February 2017.

69. https://www.nationalacademies.org/event/10-19-2020/review-of-the-revised-ntp-monograph-on-fluoride-exposure-and-neurodevelopmental-and-cognitive-health-effects-meeting-2.

70. https://www.epa.gov/sdwa/questions-and-answers-drinking-water-health-advisories-pfoa-pfos-genx-chemicals-and-pfbs

71. Jain R, Alan Ducatman A. Serum concentrations of selected perfluoroalkyl substances for US females compared to males as they age. Science of The Total Environment, Volume 842, 2022.

Chapter Five

ORGANOCHLORIDES

1. Bratsberg B, Rogeberg O. Psychological and Cognitive Sciences, Flynn effect and its reversal are both environmentally caused. Proc Natl Acad Sci U S A. 2018 Jun 26; 115(26): 6674–6678. Published online 2018 Jun 11. doi: 10.1073/pnas.1718793115.

2. Bradman A, Barr DB, Claus Henn BG, Drumheller T, Curry C, Eskenazi B. 2003. Measurement of pesticides and other toxicants in amniotic fluid as a potential biomarker of pre-natal exposure: a validation study. Environ Health Perspect 111:1779-178214594631.

3. Rauh V, Arunajadai S, Horton M, Perera F, Hoepner L, Barr DB, et al. 2011. Seven-Year Neurodevelopmental Scores and Prenatal Exposure to Chlorpyrifos, a Common Agricultural Pesticide. Environ Health Perspect 119:1196-1201. http://dx.doi.org/10.1289/ehp.1003160; Engel S, et al. Prenatal Exposure to Organophosphates, Paraoxonase 1, and Cognitive Development in Childhood. Environmental Health Perspectives, 2011; DOI: 10.1289/ehp.1003183; Horton M, et al. Impact of Prenatal Exposure to Piperonyl Butoxide and Permethrin on 36-Month Neurodevelopment. Pediatrics 2011; 127:3 e699-e706; doi:10.1542/peds.2010-0133; Horton M, Kahn L, Perera F, Barr D, Rauh V. Does the home environment and the sex of the child modify the adverse effects

References

of prenatal exposure to chlorpyrifos on child working memory? Neurotoxicology and Teratology, 2012; DOI: 10.1016/j.ntt.2012.07.004; Ross S, McManus IC, Harrison V, Mason O. Neurobehavioral problems following low-level exposure to organophosphate pesticides: a systematic and meta-analytic review. Critical Reviews in Toxicology, Ahead of Print: Pages 1-24 (doi: 10.3109/10408444.2012.738645).

4. Rauh V, et al. Brain anomalies in children exposed prenatally to a common organophosphate pesticide. PNAS 2012 109 (20) 7871-7876; published ahead of print April 30, 2012, doi:10.1073/pnas.1203396109.

5. Oulhote Y, Bouchard M, UrinaryMetabolitesofOrganophosphate and Pyrethroid Pesticides and Behavioral Problems in Canadian Children Environ Health Perspect; DOI:10.1289/ehp.1306667; Ostrea EM, et al. 2011. Fetal exposure to propoxur and abnormal child neurodevelopment at two years of age. Neurotoxicology http://dx.doi.org/10.1016/j.neuro.2011.11.006.

6. Greenop K, Peters S, Bailey H, et al. Exposure to pesticides and the risk of childhood brain tumors. Cancer Causes & Control. April 2013.

7. Greenop K, Peters S, Bailey H, et al. Exposure to pesticides and the risk of childhood brain tumors. Cancer Causes & Control. April 2013; Kimura-Kuroda J, Komuta Y, Kuroda Y, Hayashi M, Kawano H (2012) Nicotine-Like Effects of the Neonicotinoid Insecticides Acetamiprid and Imidacloprid on Cerebellar Neurons from Neonatal Rats. PLoS ONE 7(2): e32432. doi:10.1371/journal.pone.003243.

8. Pezzoli G, Cereda E. "Exposure to pesticides or solvents and risk of Parkinson disease" Neurology 2013; 80: 2035-2041; Ross S, McManus IC, Harrison V, Mason O. Neurobehavioral problems following low-level exposure to organophosphate pesticides: a systematic and meta-analytic review. Critical Reviews in Toxicology, Ahead of Print: Pages 1-24 (doi: 10.3109/10408444.2012.738645).

9. https://www.thedailybeast.com/how-rachel-carson-cost-millions-of-people-their-lives.

16. Wu H, Bertrand KA, Choi AL, Hu FB, Laden F, Grandjean P, Sun Q. Persistent Organic Pollutants and Type 2 Diabetes: A Prospective Analysis in the Nurses' Health Study and Meta-analysis. Environ Health Perspect (): .doi:10.1289/ehp.1205248.

17. Merrill M, Cirillo PM, Terry MB, Krigbaum NY, Flom JD, Cohn BA. Prenatal Exposure to the Pesticide DDT and Hypertension Diagnosed in Women Before Age 50: A Longitudinal Birth Cohort Study. Environ Health Perspect (): .doi:10.1289/ehp.1205921.

18. Cohn B, et al. DDT and Breast Cancer: Prospective Study of Induction

Time and Susceptibility Windows. JNCI: Journal of the National Cancer Institute, djy198, https://doi.org/10.1093/jnci/djy198 Published: 13 February 2019.

19. Richardson JR, et al. Elevated Serum Pesticide Levels and Risk for Alzheimer Disease. JAMA Neurol. Published online January 27, 2014. doi:10.1001/jamaneurol.2013.6030.

20. Eskenazi B, et al. In Utero Exposure to Dichlorodiphenyltrichloroethane (DDT) and Dichlorodiphenyldichloroethylene (DDE) and Neurodevelopment Among Young Mexican American Children. Pediatrics July 2006, 118 (1) 233-241; DOI: https://doi.org/10.1542/peds.2005-3117.

21. Brown AS, et al. Association of Maternal Insecticide Levels With Autism in Offspring From a National Birth Cohort. American Journal of Psychiatry, 2018 DOI: 10.1176/appi.ajp.2018.17101129.

22. Sioen I, Den Hond E, Nelen V, Van de Mieroop E, Croes K, Van Larebeke N, Nawrot TS, Schoeters G (2013) Prenatal exposure to environmental contaminants and behavioural problems at age 7–8 years. Environ Int 59: 225–31.

23. Manacaa MN, Grimaltb JO, Sunyerd J, Mandomandoa I, Gonzaleza R, Sacarlala J, Dobañoa C, Alonsoa PL, Menendez C. Concentration of DDT compounds in breast milk from African women (Manhiça, Mozambique) at the early stages of domestic indoor spraying with this insecticide. Chemosphere http://dx.doi.org/10.1016/j.chemosphere.2011.06.015.

24. Jason R. Richardson, PhD1,2; Ananya Roy, ScD2; Stuart L. Shalat, ScD1,2; Richard T. von Stein, PhD2; Muhammad M. Hossain, PhD1,2; Brian Buckley, PhD2; Marla Gearing, PhD4; Allan I. Levey, MD, PhD3; Dwight C. German, PhD5 Elevated Serum Pesticide Levels and Risk for Alzheimer Disease JAMA Neurol. Published online January 27, 2014. doi:10.1001/jamaneurol.2013.6030.

25. Kern J, et al. Developmental neurotoxicants and the vulnerable male brain: a systematic review of suspected neurotoxicants that disproportionally affect males. Acta Neurobiol Exp 2017, 77: 269–296.

26. Brehm E, Flaws JA. Transgenerational Effects of Endocrine-Disrupting Chemicals on Male and Female Reproduction. Endocrinology. 2019 Jun 1;160(6):1421-1435. doi: 10.1210/en.2019-00034. PMID: 30998239; PMCID: PMC6525581.

27. Van Cauwenbergh, O., Di Serafino, A., Tytgat, J. et al. Transgenerational epigenetic effects from male exposure to endocrine-disrupting compounds: a systematic review on research in mammals. Clin Epigenet 12, 65 (2020). https://doi.org/10.1186/s13148-020-00845-1

References

28. Edmund P. Russell, "Speaking of Annihilation": Mobilizing for War Against Human and Insect Enemies, 1914-1945. The Journal of American History, Vol. 82, No. 4 (Mar., 1996), pp. 1505-1529 (25 pages)

29. Li J, et al. Ecotoxicology and Environmental Safety Observation of organochlorine pesticides in the air of the Mt. Everest region. Ecotoxicology and Environmental Safety. Volume 63, Issue 1, January 2006, Pages 33-41

30. Jamieson, A., Malkocs, T., Piertney, S. et al. Bioaccumulation of persistent organic pollutants in the deepest ocean fauna. Nat Ecol Evol 1, 0051 (2017). https://doi.org/10.1038/s41559-016-0051

31. https://water.usgs.gov/nawqa/pnsp/pubs/fs152-95/atmos_4.html

32. Vandenberg L, et al. Hormones and Endocrine-Disrupting Chemicals: Low-Dose Effects and Nonmonotonic Dose Responses. Endocr Rev. 2012 Jun; 33(3): 378–455. Published online 2012 Mar 14. doi: 10.1210/er.2011-1050 PMCID: PMC3365860

33. https://www.ehn.org/when-safe-may-not-really-be-safe-2621578745/legal-doesnt-mean-safe

ORGANOPHOSPHATES

1. https://www.ehn.org/when-safe-may-not-really-be-safe-2621578745/legal-doesnt-mean-safe

2. Hertz-Picciotto I, Sass JB, Engel S, Bennett DH, Bradman A, Eskenazi B, Lanphear B, Whyatt R (2018) Organophosphate exposures during pregnancy and child neurodevelopment: Recommendations for essential policy reforms. PLoS Med 15: e1002671 Doi 10.1371/ journal.pmed.1002671

3. https://www.theguardian.com/environment/2018/oct/24/entire-pesticide-class-should-be-banned-for-effect-on-childrens-health

4. Gaylord A, et al. Trends in neurodevelopmental disability burden due to early life chemical exposure in the USA from 2001 to 2016: A population-based disease burden and cost analysis. Molecular and Cellular Endocrinology, 2020; 110666

5. Leiss, J. K., & Savitz, D. A. 1995. Home pesticide use and childhood cancer: a case-control study. American Journal of Public Health, 85(2), 249-252

6. Berteau, P.E. and W.A. Deen. 1978. A comparison of oral and inhalation toxicities of four insecticides to mice and rats. Bull. Environ. Contam. Toxicol. 19: 113-120.

7. Bellinger DC. A strategy for comparing the contributions of environmental

chemicals and other risk factors to neurodevelopment of children. Environ Health Perspect 2012;120:501-507.

8. Ishikawa S, and M. Miyata., "Development of myopia following chronic organophosphate pesticide intoxication: An epidemiological and experimental study," in Merigan, W.H. and B. Weiss (eds.) Neurotoxicity of the visual system, NY: Raven Press, 1980.

9. Lindsay A.E. " Memo to Douglas D. Campt, director, U.S. EPA Office of Pesticide Programs: Section 18-USDA quarantine exemptions for use of malathion and diazinon to eradicate exotic fruit fly species in Florida," 16 October 1991

10. Rauh V. Polluting Developing Brains — EPA Failure on Chlorpyrifos. N Engl J Med 2018; 378:1171-1174. March 29, 2018. DOI: 10.1056/NEJMp1716809.: Slotkin TA, Seidler FJ. Comparative developmental neurotoxicity of organophosphates in vivo: transcriptional responses of pathways for brain cell development, cell signaling, cytotoxicity and neurotransmitter systems. Brain Res Bull 2007; 72:232-274; Carr R, Alugubelly N and Mohammed A (2018) Possible Mechanisms of Developmental Neurotoxicity of Organophosphate Insecticides Linking Environmental Exposure to Neurodevelopmental Disorders, 10.1016/bs.ant. 2018.03.004, (145-188).

11. Eskenazi B, Marks AR, Bradman A, Harley K, Barr DB, Johnson C, et al. 2007. Organophosphate pesticide exposure and neurodevelopment in young Mexican- American children. Environ Health Perspect 115:792-798; doi:10.1289/ehp. 982817520070. Google Scholar; Jusko T, van den Dries M, Pronk A, Shaw P, Guxens M, Spaan S, Jaddoe V, Tiemeier H and Longnecker M (2019) Organophosphate Pesticide Metabolite Concentrations in Urine during Pregnancy and Offspring Nonverbal IQ at Age 6 Years, Environmental Health Perspectives, 127:1, Online publication date: 1- Jan-2019; Rauh VA, Garfinkel R, Perera FP, Andrews HF, Hoepner L, Barr DB, et al. 2006. Impact of prenatal chlorpyrifos exposure on neurodevelopment in the first 3 years of life among inner-city children. Pediatrics 118(6):1845-1859; Rauh V, Arunajadai S, Horton M, Perera F, Hoepner L, Barr DB, et al. 2011. Seven-Year Neurodevelopmental Scores and Prenatal Exposure to Chlorpyrifos, a Common Agricultural Pesticide. Environ Health Perspect 119:1196-1201. http://dx.doi.org/10.1289/ehp.1003160; Shelton JF, Geraghty EM, Tancredi DJ, Delwiche LD, Schmidt RJ, Ritz B, Hansen RL, Hertz-Picciotto I. 2014. Neurodevelopmental disorders and prenatal residential proximity to agricultural pesticides. the CHARGE study. Environ Health Perspect 122:1103–1109.

12. Shelton JF, Geraghty EM, Tancredi DJ, Delwiche LD, Schmidt RJ, Ritz B, Hansen RL, Hertz-Picciotto I. 2014. Neurodevelopmental disorders and prenatal residential proximity to agricultural pesticides: the CHARGE study. Environ Health Perspect 122:1103–1109.

References

13. Astiz M, Acaz-Fonseca E, Garcia-Segura LM. Sex Differences and Effects of Estrogenic Compounds on the Expression of Inflammatory Molecules by Astrocytes Exposed to the Insecticide Dimethoate. Neurotox Res. 2014; 25:271–85. This is the only in-vitro study to our knowledge that reports sex-specific effects of insecticide exposure.

14. Timofeeva OA, Roegge CS, Seidler F, Slotkin TA, Levin ED. 2008. Persistent cognitive alterations in rats after early postnatal exposure to low doses of the organophosphate pesticide, diazinon. Neurotoxicol Teratol 30(1):38–45, PMID: 18096363, 10.1016/j.ntt.2007.10.002; Comfort N, Re D. Sex-specific Neurotoxic Effects of Organophosphate Pesticides Across the Life Course Curr Environ Health Rep. 2017 Dec; 4(4): 392–404. doi: 10.1007/s40572-017-0171-y; Beard J, et al. Pesticide Exposure and Depression among Male Private Pesticide Applicators in the Agricultural Health Study. Environ Health Perspect; DOI:10.1289/ehp.1307450.

15. Starks SE, Gerr F, Kamel F, Lynch CF, Alavanja MC, Sandler DP, Hoppin JA. High pesticide exposure events and central nervous system function among pesticide applicators in the Agricultural Health Study. Int Arch Occup Environ Health; doi: 10.1007/s00420-011-0694-8 [Online 7 September 2011].

16. Roegge CS, Timofeeva OA, Seidler FJ, Slotkin TA, Levin ED. 2008. Developmental diazinon neurotoxicity in rats: later effects on emotional response. Brain Res Bull 75(1):166–172, PMID: 18158111, 10.1016/j.brainresbull.2007.08.008; Slotkin TA, Ryde IT, Levin ED, Seidler FJ. 2008. Developmental neurotoxicity of low dose diazinon exposure of neonatal rats: effects on serotonin systems in adolescence and adulthood. Brain Res Bull 75(5):640– 647, PMID: 18355640, 10.1016/j.brainresbull.2007.10.008.

PYRETHROIDS, ROUNDUP, NEONICOTINOIDS

1. Outhlote Y., Bouchard M. Urinary metabolites of organophosphate and pyrethroid pesticides and behavioral problems in Canadian children. Environ. Health Perspect. 2013; 121:1378–1384.

2. Stein E.A., Washburn M., Walczak C., Bloom A.S. Effects of pyrethroid insecticides on operant responding maintained by food. Neurotoxicol. Teratol. 1987; 9:27–31. doi: 10.1016/0892-0362(87)90066-3.

3. Bao W, et al. Association Between Exposure to Pyrethroid Insecticides and Risk of All-Cause and Cause-Specific Mortality in the General US Adult Population. JAMA Intern Med. December 30, 2019. doi:https://doi.org/10.1001/jamainternmed.2019.6019.

4. Costa L.G. The neurotoxicity of organochlorine and pyrethroid pesticides. Handb. Clin. Neurol. 2015; 131:135–148.

5. Glorennec P., Serrano T., Fravallo M., Warembourg C., Monfort C., Cordier S., Viel J., Le Gléau F., Le Bot B., Chevrier C. Determinants of children's exposure to pyrethroid insecticides in western France. Environ. Int. 2017; 104:76–82. doi: 10.1016/j.envint.2017.04.007; Corcellas C., Feo M.L., Torres J.P., Malm O., Ocampo-Duque W., Eljarrat E., Barceló D. Pyrethroids in human breast milk: Occurrence and nursing daily intake estimation. Environ. Int. 2014; 47:17–22. doi: 10.1016/j.envint.2012.05.007.

6. Lazarini C, Florio J, Lemonica I, Bernardi M. 2001. Effects of prenatal exposure to deltamethrin on forced swimming behavior, motor activity, and striatal dopamine levels in male and female rats. Neurotoxicol Teratol 23:665-67311792535; Laugeray A, Herzine A, Perche O, Richard O, Montecot-Dubourg C, Menuet A, et al. (2017) In utero and lactational exposure to low-doses of the pyrethroid insecticide cypermethrin leads to neurodevelopmental defects in male mice—An ethological and transcriptomic study. PLoS ONE 12(10): e0184475. https://doi.org/10.1371/journal.pone.0184475.

7. Horton M, et al. Impact of Prenatal Exposure to Piperonyl Butoxide and Permethrin on 36-Month Neurodevelopment. Pediatrics 2011; 127:3 e699-e706; doi:10.1542/peds.2010-0133.

8. Viel J-F, et al. Pyrethroid insecticide exposure and cognitive developmental disabilities in children: The PELAGIE mother–child cohort. Environment International, 2015; 82: 69 DOI: 10.1016/j.envint.2015.05.009: London L, Beseler C, Bouchard MF, Bellinger DC, Colosio C, Grandjean P, et al. Neurobehavioural and neurodevelopmental effects of pesticide exposures. Neurotoxicology. 2012; 33(4):887–96. pmid:22269431; Viel J-F, et al. Pyrethroid insecticide exposure and cognitive developmental disabilities in children: The PELAGIE mother–child cohort. Environment International, 2015; 82: 69 DOI: 10.1016/j.envint.2015.05.009; Oulhote Y, Bouchard MF. Urinary metabolites of organophosphate and pyrethroid pesticides and behavioral problems in Canadian children. Environ Health Perspect 121:1378–1384; http://dx.doi.org/10 1289/ehp.1306667.

9. Laugeray A, Herzine A, Perche O, Richard O, Montecot-Dubourg C, Menuet A, et al. (2017) In utero and lactational exposure to low-doses of the pyrethroid insecticide cypermethrin leads to neurodevelopmental defects in male mice—An ethological and transcriptomic study. PLoS ONE 12(10): e0184475. https://doi.org/10.1371/journal.pone.0184475.

10. Antoniou M, Habib MEM, Howard CV, Jennings RC, Leifert C, et al. (2012) Teratogenic Effects of Glyphosate Based Herbicides: Divergence of Regulatory Decisions from Scientific Evidence. J Environ Anal Toxicol S:4.

11. http://www.ksdk.com/story/news/health/2014/02/27/birth-defects- spike-yakima-valley/5861527/.

References

12. Rull R, et al. Neural tube defects and maternal residential proximity to agricultural pesticide applications. Epidemiology: July 2004 - Volume 15 - Issue 4 - p S188.

13. Vandenberg LN, Blumberg B, Antoniou MN, et al. Is it time to reassess current safety standards for glyphosate-based herbicides? J Epidemiol Community Health 2017; 71:613–618.

14. Majewski M, et al. Pesticides in Mississippi air and rain: A comparison between 1995 and 2007. Environ Toxicol Chem. 2014 Feb 19. Epub 2014 Feb 19. PMID: 24549493.

15. Vandenberg LN, Blumberg B, Antoniou MN, et al. Is it time to reassess current safety standards for glyphosate-based herbicides? J Epidemiol Community Health 2017; 71:613–618; Defarge N, et al. Toxicity of formulants and heavy metals in glyphosate-based herbicides and other pesticides. Toxicol Rep. 2018; 5: 156–163; https://www.ncbi.nlm.nih.gov/pmc/articles/PMC5756058/.

16. Mesnage R, Bernay B, Séralini GE. Ethoxylated adjuvants of glyphosate-based herbicides are active principles of human cell toxicity. Toxicology 2013; 313:122–8; Tsui MT, Chu LM. Aquatic toxicity of glyphosate-based formulations: comparison between different organisms and the effects of environmental factors. Chemosphere 2003; 52:1189–97; https://www.thehealthyhomeeconomist.com/cheerios-roundup-residue/.

17. https://pubmed.ncbi.nlm.nih.gov/29843257/.

18. Myers JP, vom Saal FS, Akingbemi BT, et al. Why public health agencies cannot depend on good laboratory practices as a criterion for selecting data: the case of bisphenol A. Environ Health Perspect 2009; 117:309–15.

19. Vandenberg LN, Blumberg B, Antoniou MN, et al. Is it time to reassess current safety standards for glyphosate-based herbicides? J Epidemiol Community Health 2017; 71:613–618.

20. https://detoxproject.org/glyphosate-in-food-water/

21. Bohn T, et al. (2014) Compositional differences in soybeans on the market: glyphosate accumulates in Roundup Ready GM soybeans. Food Chem 153: 207-215.

22. Independent Science News (2014) How "Extreme Levels" of Roundup in Food Became the Industry Norm. www.independentsciencenews.org/news/how-extreme-levels-of-roundup-in-food-became-the-industry-norm/

23. http://www.ithaka-journal.net/herbizide-im-urin?lang=en.

24. Cattani D, de Liz Oliveira Cavalli VL, Heinz Rieg CE, Domingues JT, Dal-Cim T, Tasca CI, Mena Barreto Silva FR, Zamoner A (2014) Mechanisms underlying the neurotoxicity induced by glyphosate-based herbicide in immature rat hippocampus: involvement of glutamate excitotoxicity. Toxicology 320: 34– Coullery RP, Ferrari ME, Rosso SB (2016) Neuronal development and axon growth are altered by glyphosate through a WNT non-canonical signal-ing pathway. Neurotoxicology 52: 150–61; Roy N, et al. Glyphosate Induces Neurotoxicity in Zebrafish. Environ Toxicol Pharmacol. 2016 Mar; 42:45-54. doi: 10.1016/j.etap.2016.01.003. Epub 2016 Jan 4; Bali Y, et al. Behavioral and Immunohistochemical Study of the Effects of Subchronic and Chronic Exposure to Glyphosate in Mice. Front. Behav. Neurosci., 08 August 2017.

25. Krüger M., Schledorn P., Schrödl W., Hoppe H. W., Lutz W., Shehata A. A. (2014). Detection of glyphosate residues in animals and humans. J. Environ. Anal. Toxicol. 4:210 10.4172/2161-0525.1000210.

26. Bali Y, et al. Behavioral and Immunohistochemical Study of the Effects of Subchronic and Chronic Exposure to Glyphosate in Mice. Front. Behav. Neurosci., 08 August 2017.

27. Kalender Y., Uzunhisarcikli M., Ogutcu A., Acikgoz F., Kalender S. (2006). Effects of diazinon on pseudocholinesterase activity and haematological indices in rats: the protective role of vitamin E. Environ. Toxicol. Pharmacol. 22, 46–51. 10.1016/j.etap.2005.11.007.

28. Hernández-Plata I., Giordano M., Díaz-Muñoz M., Rodríguez V. M. (2015). The herbicide glyphosate causes behavioral changes and alterations in dopaminergic markers in male Sprague-Dawley rat. Neurotoxicology 46, 79–91. 10.1016/j.neuro.2014.12.001.

29. Cattani D, et al. Mechanisms underlying the neurotoxicity induced by glyphosate-based herbicide in immature rat hippocampus: involvement of glutamate excitotoxicity. Toxicology. 2014 Mar 14. Epub 2014 Mar 14.

30. Shim Y, et al. Parental Exposure to Pesticides and Childhood Brain Cancer: U.S. Atlantic Coast Childhood Brain Cancer Study. Environ Health Perspect. 2009 Jun; 117(6): 1002–1006.

31. Anadón A., Del Pino J., Martínez M. A., Caballero V., Ares I., Nieto I., et al. (2008). "Neurotoxicological effects of the herbicide glyphosate," in Comunication 45th Congress of the European Societies of Toxicology (Eurotox 2008) Toxicol. Lett. (Rhodes, Greece), S164–S180.

32. Szepanowski F, et al. Glyphosate-based herbicide: a risk factor for demyelinating conditions of the peripheral nervous system? Year : 2019 | Volume : 14 | Issue : 12 | Page : 079-2080.

33. Rueda-Ruzafaa L, et al. Gut microbiota and neurological effects of

glyphosate. NeuroToxicology. Volume 75, December 2019, Pages 1-8.

34. Nakayama A, et al. The neonicotinoids acetamiprid and imidacloprid impair neurogenesis and alter the microglial profile in the hippocampal dentate gyrus of mouse neonates. Jan 2019 J Appl Toxicol; Kagawa N, Nagao T. Neurodevelopmental toxicity in the mouse neocortex following prenatal exposure to acetamiprid: Developmental Neonicotinoid Exposure-Induced Neurotoxicity. July 2018 Journal of Applied Toxicology 38(Suppl. 3) DOI: 10.1002/jat.3692.

THIS IS YOUR BRAIN ON RADIATION

1. Scherb H & Voigt K (2011). The human sex odds at birth after the atmospheric atomic bomb tests, after Chernobyl, and in the vicinity of nuclear facilities. Environmental Science and Pollution Research; DOI 10.1007/s11356-011-0462-z.

2. https://www.scientificamerican.com/article/sperm-count-dropping-in-western-world/.

3. https://www.bbc.com/news/health-53409521.

4. https://www.cdc.gov/reproductivehealth/infertility/.

5. https://www.ncbi.nlm.nih.gov/pmc/articles/PMC6396757/.

6. https://ratical.org/radiation/SecretFallout/SFchp16.html.

7. Almond D, et al. Prenatal Exposure to Radioactive Fallout and School Outcomes in Sweden" August 2007, NBER working paper 13347.

8. Sverdvik K, Mednick H, Sundet K, Rund B. Effect of low dose ionizing radiation exposure in utero on cognitive function in adolescence. Scandinavian Journal of Psychology. Volume 51, Issue 3, pages 210–215, June 2010.

9. McDiarmid M, et al. Health Effects of Depleted Uranium on Exposed Gulf War Veterans. Environ Res. 2000 Feb; 82(2):168-80. doi: 10.1006/enrs.1999.4012; McDiarmid M, et al. Health Effects and Biological Monitoring Results of Gulf War Veterans Exposed to Depleted Uranium Mil Med. 2002 Feb;167(2 Suppl):123-4.

10. Hinkle JJ, et al. Cranial irradiation mediated spine loss is sex-specific and complement receptor-3 dependent in male mice. Scientific Reports, 2019; 9 (1) DOI: 10.1038/s41598-019-55366-6.

11. Kovalchuk A, et al. Profound and Sexually Dimorphic Effects of Clinically-Relevant Low Dose Scatter Irradiation on the Brain and Behavior. Front. Behav. Neurosci., 03 June 2016 | https://doi.org/10.3389/fnbeh.2016.00084.

12. https://www.fda.gov/radiation-emitting-products/initiative-reduce-unnecessary-radiation-exposure-medical-imaging/appropriate-use.

13. https://www.nejm.org/doi/full/10.1056/NEJMra072149; de González AB, et al. Projected Cancer Risks From Computed Tomographic Scans Performed in the United States in 2007. Arch Intern Med. 2009; 169(22):2071-2077. doi: 10.1001/archinternmed.2009.440.

CELL PHONE RADIATION

15. https://www.greenamerica.org/do-cell-phones-cause-cancer/our-interview-dr-devra-davis-0.

16. Henz D, et al. Mobile Phone Chips Reduce Increases in EEG Brain Activity Induced by Mobile Phone-Emitted Electromagnetic Fields. Front Neurosci. 2018; 12: 190. Published online 2018 Apr 4. doi: 10.3389/fnins.2018.00190: Nanou E, Catterall WA. Calcium channels, synaptic plasticity, and neuropsychiatric disease. Neuron. 2018; 98:466–481. doi: 10.1016/j.neuron.2018.03.017.

17. Wyde ME, Horn TL, Capstick MH, Ladbury JM, Koepke G, Wilson PF, Kissling GE, Stout MD, Kuster N, Melnick RL, Gauger J, Bucher JR, Mccormick DL. Effect of cell phone radiofrequency radiation on body temperature in rodents: Pilot studies of the National Toxicology Program's reverberation chamber exposure system. Bioelectromagnetics. 2018; 39:190–199. doi: 10.1002/bem.22116.

18. https://www.youtube.com/watch?v=E_WJ_aJPWIA: https://www.the-scientist.com/news-opinion/opinion-cell-phone-health-risk-40449; Tang, J, et al. Exposure to 900 MHz electromagnetic fields activates the mkp-1/ERK pathway and causes blood-brain barrier damage and cognitive impairment in rats. Brain Research. Volume 1601, 19 March 2015, Pages 92-101; https://ehtrust.org/science/key-scientific-lectures/national-press-club-expert-lecture-2012/.

19. Akdag M, Dasdag S, Canturk F, Akdag MZ. Exposure to non-ionizing electromagnetic fields emitted from mobile phones induced DNA damage in human ear canal hair follicle cells. Electromagn Biol Med. (2018) 37:66–75. 10.1080/15368378.2018.1463246; Xu S, Zhou Z, Zhang L, Yu Z, Zhang W, Wang Y, Wang X, Li M, Chen Y, Chen C, He M, Zhang G, Zhong M. Exposure to 1800 MHz radiofrequency radiation induces oxidative damage to mitochondrial DNA in primary cultured neurons. Brain Res. 2010; 1311:189–196. doi: 10.1016/j.brainres.2009.10.062.

20. Volkow N, et al. Effects of Cell Phone Radiofrequency Signal Exposure on Brain Glucose Metabolism. JAMA. 2011 Feb 23; 305(8): 808–813. doi: 10.1001/jama.2011.186.

References

21. Kim JH, Yu DH, Kim HJ, Huh YH, Cho SW, Lee JK, Kim HG, Kim HR. Exposure to 835 MHz radiofrequency electromagnetic field induces autophagy in hippocampus but not in brain stem of mice. Toxicol. Ind. Health. 2018b; 34:23–35. doi: 10.1177/0748233717740066; Jiang D-P, Li J-H, Zhang J, Xu S-L, Kuang F, Lang H-Y, Wang Y-F, An G-Z, Li J, Guo G-Z. Long-term electromagnetic pulse exposure induces Abeta deposition and cognitive dysfunction through oxidative stress and overexpression of APP and BACE1. Brain Res. 2016; 1642:10–19. doi: 10.1016/j.brainres.2016.02.053.

22. Redmayne M, Johansson O. Could myelin damage from radiofrequency electromagnetic field exposure help explain the functional impairment electrohypersensitivity? A review of the evidence. J Toxicol Environ Health B Crit Rev. 2014; 17:247–258. doi: 10.1080/10937404.2014.923356.

23. Aldad, T., Gan, G., Gao, X. et al. Fetal Radiofrequency Radiation Exposure From 800-1900 MHz-Rated Cellular Telephones Affects Neurodevelopment and Behavior in Mice. Sci Rep 2, 312 (2012). https://doi.org/10.1038/srep00312.

24. Odaci E, et al. Effects of Prenatal Exposure to a 900 MHz Electromagnetic Field on the Dentate Gyrus of Rats: A Stereological and Histopathological Study. Brain Res. 2008 Oct 31; 1238:224-9; Orhan Bas O, et al. 900 MHz Electromagnetic Field Exposure Affects Qualitative and Quantitative Features of Hippocampal Pyramidal Cells in the Adult Female Rat. Brain Res. 2009 Apr 10; 1265:178-85.

25. Foerster M., Thielens A., Joseph W., Eeftens M., Röösli M. A prospective cohort study of adolescents' memory performance and individual brain dose of microwave radiation from wireless communication. Environmental Health Perspectives, 2018 DOI: 10.1289/EHP2427; Anna Schoeni, Katharina Roser, Martin Röösli. Memory performance, wireless communication and exposure to radiofrequency electromagnetic fields: A prospective cohort study in adolescents. Environment International, 2015; 85: 343 DOI: 10.1016/j.envint.2015.09.025.

26. Deniz O, et al. Effects of short and long term electromagnetic fields exposure on the human hippocampus. Journal of Microscopy and Ultrastructure. Volume 5, Issue 4, December 2017, Pages 191-197.

27. Pall ML. Microwave frequency electromagnetic fields (EMFs) produce widespread neuropsychiatric effects including depression. J Chem Neuroanat. (2016) 75:43–51. 10.1016/j.jchemneu.2015.08.001.

28. Byun Y-H, Ha M, Kwon H-J, Hong Y-C, Leem J-H, Sakong J, et al. (2013) Mobile Phone Use, Blood Lead Levels, and Attention Deficit Hyperactivity Symptoms in Children: A Longitudinal Study. PLoS ONE 8(3): e59742. https://doi.org/10.1371/journal.pone.0059742; Choi KH, Ha M, Ha EH, Park H, Kim Y, Hong YC, et al. Neurodevelopment for the first three years following

prenatal mobile phone use, radio frequency radiation and lead exposure. Environ Res. (2017) 156:810–17. 10.1016/j.envres.2017.04.029.

29. https://blogs.scientificamerican.com/observations/we-have-no-reason-to-believe-5g-is-safe/.

30. https://ntp.niehs.nih.gov/whatwestudy/topics/cellphones/index.html?utm_source=direct&utm_medium=prod&utm_campaign=ntpgolinks&utm_term=cellphone.

31. Hardell L, et al. Long-term use of cellular phones and brain tumours: increased risk associated with use for ⩾10 years. Occup Environ Med. 2007 Sep; 64(9): 626–632. Published online 2007 Apr 4. doi: 10.1136/oem.2006.029751.

32. Benson VS, Pirie K, Schüz J, Reeves GK, Beral V, Green J; for the Million Women Study Collaborators. Mobile phone use and risk of brain neoplasms and other cancers: prospective study. Int J Epidemiol. 2013 May 8. [Epub ahead of print].

33. Miller AB, Morgan LL, Udasin I, Davis DL. Cancer epidemiology update, following the 2011 IARC evaluation of radiofrequency electromagnetic fields (Monograph 102). Environ Res. (2018) 167:673–83. 10.1016/j.envres.2018.06.043 [PubMed] [CrossRef] [Google Scholar]; Hardell L, Carlberg M. Mobile phone and cordless phone use and the risk for glioma - analysis of pooled case-control studies in Sweden, 1997-2003 and 2007-2009. Pathophysiology. (2015) 22:1–13. 10.1016/j.pathophys.2014.10.001 [PubMed] [CrossRef] [Google Scholar]; Hardell L, Carlberg M, Söderqvist F, Kjell HM. Pooled analysis of case-control studies on acoustic neuroma diagnosed 1997-2003 and 2007-2009 and use of mobile and cordless phones. Int J Oncol. (2013) 43:1036–44. 10.3892/ijo.2013.2025.

34. Adams JA, Galloway TS, Mondal D, Esteves SC, Mathews F. Effect of mobile telephones on sperm 421 quality: a systematic review and meta-analysis. Environ Int. (2014) 70:106–12. 10.1016/j.envint.2014.04.015; Houston BJ, Nixon B, King BV, De Iuliis GN, Aitken RJ. The effects of radiofrequency electromagnetic radiation on sperm function. Reproduction. (2016) 152:R263–76. 10.1530/REP-16-0126; Kesari KK, Agarwal A, Henkel R. Radiations and male fertility. Reprod Biol Endocrinol. (2018) 16:118. 10.1186/s12958-018-0431-1; Rago R, Salacone P, Caponecchia L, Sebastianelli A, Marcucci I, Calogero AE, et al. The semen quality of the mobile phone users. J Endocrinol Invest. (2013) 36:970–4. 10.3275/8996; Zhang G, Yan H, Chen Q, Liu K, Ling X, Sun L, et al. Effects of cell phone use on semen parameters: results from the MARHCS cohort study in Chongqing, China. Environ Int. (2016) 91:116–21. 10.1016/j.envint.2016.02.028; Gautam R, Singh KV, Nirala J, Murmu NN, Meena R, Rajamani P. Oxidative stress-mediated alterations on sperm parameters in male Wistar rats exposed to 3G mobile phone radiation.

Andrologia. (2019) 51:e13201. 10.1111/and.13201.

35. Divan HA, Kheifets L, Obel C, Olsen J. Prenatal and postnatal exposure to cell phone use and behavioral problems in children. Epidemiology. (2008) 19:523–9. 10.1097/EDE.0b013e318175dd47; Sudan M, Olsen J, Arah OA, Obel C, Kheifets L. Prospective cohort analysis of cellphone use and emotional and behavioural difficulties in children. J Epidemiol Community Health. (2016) 70:1207–13. 10.1136/jech-2016-207419.

36. https://blogs.scientificamerican.com/observations/we-have-no-reason-to-believe-5g-is-safe/.

37. http://www.5gappeal.eu.

38. https://emfscientist.org/EMF_Scientist_Press_Release_22_July_2019.pdf.

39. https://thehill.com/opinion/technology/4437988-why-did-nih-abruptly-halt-research-on-the-harms-of-cell-phone-radiation/

BPA (AND OTHER ENDOCRINE DISRUPTORS)

1. Barboza, LG, et al. Microplastics in wild fish from North East Atlantic Ocean and its potential for causing neurotoxic effects, lipid oxidative damage, and human health risks associated with ingestion exposure. Science of The Total Environment Volume 717, 15 May 2020, 134625.

2. Cox K, et al. Human Consumption of Microplastics. Environmental Science & Technology 2019 53 (12), 7068-7074 DOI: 10.1021/acs.est.9b01517.

3. https://www.scientificamerican.com/article/microplastics-have-been-found-in-peoples-poop-mdash-what-does-it-mean/.

4. https://www.acs.org/content/acs/en/pressroom/newsreleases/2020/august/micro-and-nanoplastics-detectable-in-human-tissues.html.

5. Asimakopoulos AG, Thomaidis NS, Koupparis MA. Recent trends in biomonitoring of bisphenol A, 4-t-octylphenol, and 4-nonylphenol. Toxicol Lett. 2012; 210:141–154. [PubMed] [Google Scholar].

6. Grohs, M.N., Reynolds, J.E., Liu, J. et al. Prenatal maternal and childhood bisphenol a exposure and brain structure and behavior of young children. Environ Health 18, 85 (2019). https://doi.org/10.1186/s12940-019-0528-9.

7. https://www.sciencemag.org/news/2018/09/bpa-substitutes-may-be-just-bad-popular-consumer-plastic.

8. Yeo M, et al. Bisphenol A delays the perinatal chloride shift in cortical neurons by epigenetic effects on the Kcc2 promoter. PNAS, February 25, 2013

DOI: 10.1073/pnas.1300959110.

9. Corbel T, Perdu E, Gayrard V, Puel S, Lacroix MZ, Viguie C, et al. Conjugation and deconjugation reactions within the feto-placental compartment in a sheep model: a key factor determining bisphenol a fetal exposure. Drug Metab Dispos. 2015; 43(4):467–76.

10. Masuo Y., Ishido M. (2011). Neurotoxicity of endocrine disruptors: possible involvement in brain development and neurodegeneration. J. Toxicol. Environ. Health B Crit. Rev. 14 346–369. 10.1080/10937404.2011.578557.

11. Kundakovic M., Gudsnuk K., Herbstman J., Tang D., Perera F., Champagne F. (2015). DNA methylation of BDNF as a biomarker of early-life adversity. Proc. Natl. Acad. Sci. U.S.A. 112 6807–6813. 10.1073/pnas.1408355111.

12. Bao W, et al. Association Between Bisphenol A Exposure and Risk of All-Cause and Cause-Specific Mortality in US Adults. JAMA Netw Open. 2020;3(8):e2011620. doi:10.1001/jamanetworkopen.2020.11620.

13. Roen EL, Wang Y, Calafat AM, Wang S, Margolis A, Herbstman J, Hoepner LA, Rauh V, Perera FP (2015) Bisphenol A exposure and behavioral problems among inner city children at 7–9 years of age. Environ Res 142: 739–45; Lande MB, Adams H, Falkner B, Waldstein SR, Schwartz GJ, Szilagyi PG, Wang H, Palumbo D (2009) Parental assessments of internalizing and externalizing behavior and executive function in children with primary hypertension. J Pediatr 154: 207–12; Casas M, Forns J, Martínez D, Avella-García C, Valvi D, Ballesteros-Gómez A, Luque N, Rubio S, Julvez J, Sunyer J, Vrijheid M (2015) Exposure to bi- sphenol A during pregnancy and child neuropsychological development in the INMA-Sabadell cohort. Environ Res 142: 671–9; Sobolewski M, Conrad K, Allen JL, Weston H, Martin K, Lawrence BP, Cory-Slechta DA (2014) Sex-specific enhanced behavioral toxicity induced by maternal exposure to a mixture of low dose endocrine-disrupting chemicals. Neurotoxicology 45: 121–30; Evans SF, Kobrosly RW, Barrett ES, Thurston SW, Calafat AM, Weiss B, Stahlhut R, Yolton K, Swan SH (2014) Prenatal bisphenol A exposure and maternally reported behavior in boys and girls. Neurotoxicology 45: 91–9; Perera F, Vishnevetsky J, Herbstman JB, Calafat AM, Xiong W, Rauh V, Wang S (2012) Prenatal bisphenol a exposure and child behavior in an inner-city cohort. Environ Health Perspect 120: 1190–4.

14. https://www.abstractsonline.com/pp8/#!/4482/presentation/8696.

15. Grohs, M.N., Reynolds, J.E., Liu, J. et al. Prenatal maternal and childhood bisphenol exposure and brain structure and behavior of young children. Environ Health 18, 85 (2019). https://doi.org/10.1186/s12940-019-0528-9.

16. https://www.scientificamerican.com/article/lowered-thyroid-hormones-found-in-baby-boys-exposed-to-bispenol-a/.

17. Chevrier J, Gunier RB, Bradman A, Holland NT, Calafat AM, Eskenazi B, Harley KG. Maternal Urinary Bisphenol A during Pregnancy and Maternal and Neonatal Thyroid Function in the CHAMACOS Study. Environ Health Perspect, 2012 DOI: 10.1289/ehp.1205092.

18. https://www.scientificamerican.com/article/bpa-free-plastic-containers-may-be-just-as-hazardous/.

19. Marfella R, Prattichizzo F, Sardu C, Fulgenzi G, Graciotti L, Spadoni T, D'Onofrio N, Scisciola L, La Grotta R, Frigé C, Pellegrini V, Municinò M, Siniscalchi M, Spinetti F, Vigliotti G, Vecchione C, Carrizzo A, Accarino G, Squillante A, Spaziano G, Mirra D, Esposito R, Altieri S, Falco G, Fenti A, Galoppo S, Canzano S, Sasso FC, Matacchione G, Olivieri F, Ferraraccio F, Panarese I, Paolisso P, Barbato E, Lubritto C, Balestrieri ML, Mauro C, Caballero AE, Rajagopalan S, Ceriello A, D'Agostino B, Iovino P, Paolisso G. Microplastics and Nanoplastics in Atheromas and Cardiovascular Events. N Engl J Med. 2024 Mar 7;390(10):900-910. doi: 10.1056/NEJMoa2309822. PMID: 38446676.

PERCHLORATE, PHTHALATES

1. https://www.regulations.gov/document?D=EPA-HQ-OW-2016-0438-0002.

2. https://www.ncbi.nlm.nih.gov/books/NBK279032/.

3. Sahay RK, Nagesh VS. Hypothyroidism in pregnancy. Indian J Endocrinol Metab. 2012;16(3):364-370. doi:10.4103/2230-8210.95667.

4. Knight B, et al. OC3.1. Presented at: Society for Endocrinology BES; Nov. 6-8, 2017; Harrogate, UK.

5. Haddow J, Palomaki G, Allan W, et al. Maternal thyroid deficiency during pregnancy and subsequent neuropsychological development of the child. New Engl J Med. 1999;341(8):549-555.

6. https://www.courthousenews.com/wp-content/uploads/2020/05/aap-letter.pdf.

7. https://www.nrdc.org/experts/erik-d-olson/epa-refuses-protect-children-perchlorate-contaminated-tap-water.

8. https://www.nrdc.org/sites/default/files/fairfresheners.pdf.

9. Heudorf U, Mersch-Sundermann V, Angerer J (2007) Phthalates: toxicology and exposure. Int J Hyg Environ Health 210:623–634. doi:10.1016/j.ijheh.2007.07.011 pmid:17889607.

10. Factor-Litvak P, et al. Persistent Associations between Maternal Prenatal Exposure to Phthalates on Child IQ at Age 7 Years. Plos One Published: December 10, 2014. https://doi.org/10.1371/journal.pone.0114003.

11. https://www.cdc.gov/exposurereport/.

12. Kobrosly RW, Evans S, Miodovnik A, Barrett ES, Thurston SW, Calafat AM, Swan SH (2014) Prenatal phthalate exposures and neurobehavioral development scores in boys and girls at 6-10 years of age. Environ Health Perspect 122: 521–8.

13. Huang HB, Chen HY, Su PH, et al. Fetal and Childhood Exposure to Phthalate Diesters and Cognitive Function in Children Up to 12 Years of Age: Taiwanese Maternal and Infant Cohort Study. PLoS One. 2015;10(6):e0131910. Published 2015 Jun 29. doi:10.1371/journal.pone.0131910.

14. Kougias D, et al. Perinatal Exposure to an Environmentally Relevant Mixture of Phthalates Results in a Lower Number of Neurons and Synapses in the Medial Prefrontal Cortex and Decreased Cognitive Flexibility in Adult Male and Female Rats. Journal of Neuroscience 1 August 2018, 38 (31) 6864-6872; DOI: https://doi.org/10.1523/JNEUROSCI.0607-18.2018.

15. Oulhote Y, et al. Gestational Exposures to Phthalates and Folic Acid, and Autistic Traits in Canadian Children. Environmental Health Perspectives. Published:19 February 2020.

16. Balalian AA, et al. Prenatal and childhood exposure to phthalates and motor skills at age 11 years. Environmental Research. Volume 171, April 2019, Pages 416-427.

AIR POLLUTION

1. Calderón-Garcidueñas L, Reed W, Maronpot RR, Henríquez-Roldán C, Delgado- Chavez R, Calderón-Garcidueñas A, Dragustinovis I, Franco Lira M, Aragón-Flores M, Solt AC, Altenburg M, Torres-Jardón R, Swenberg JA. Brain inflammation and Alzheimer's-like pathology in individuals exposed to severe air pollution. Toxicol Pathol. 2004 Nov- Dec; 32(6):650-8; Calderon-Garciduenas, L. et al. (2003) DNA damage in nasal and brain tissues of canines exposed to air pollutants is associated with evidence of chronic brain inflammation and neurodegeneration. Toxicol. Pathol. 31, 524–538; Gackière F, Saliba L, Baude A, Bosler O, Strube C. Ozone inhalation activates stress-responsive regions of the central nervous system. J Neurochem. 2011 Apr 6. doi: 10.1111/j.1471-4159.2011.07267.x. [Epub ahead of print]; Levesque S, Surace MJ, McDonald J, Block ML. Air pollution and the brain: Subchronic diesel exhaust exposure causes neuroinflammation and elevates early markers of neurodegenerative disease. J Neuroinflammation. 2011 Aug 24;8(1):105. [Epub ahead of print]5; Calderón-Garcidueñas L, et al. Air pollution, a rising

References

environmental risk factor for cognition, neuroinflammation and neurodegeneration: The clinical impact on children and beyond. Rev Neurol (Paris). 2015 Dec 21. pii: S0035-3787(15)00923-6. doi: 10.1016/j.neurol.2015.10.008. [Epub ahead of print; Brockmeyer S, D'Angiulli A. How air pollution alters brain development: the role of neuroinflammation. Transl Neurosci. 2016 Mar 21;7(1):24-30. doi: 10.1515/tnsci-2016-0005. eCollection 2016.

2. Hartz A, Bauer B, Block M, Diesel exhaust particles induce oxidative stress, proinflammatory signaling, and P-glycoprotein, up-regulation at the blood-brain barrier. The FASEB Journal 2008; 22:2723-2733; Calderon-Garciduenas L, Solt AC, et al. Long-term air pollution exposure is associated with neuroinflammation, an altered innate immune response, disruption of the blood-brain barrier, ultrafine particulate deposition, and accumulation of amyloid beta-42 and alpha-synuclein in children and young adults. Toxicol Pathol. 2008;36(2): 289-310. Epub 2008 Mar 18; Calderón-Garcidueñas L, et al. Air Pollution and Children: Neural and Tight Junction Antibodies and Combustion Metals, the Role of Barrier Breakdown and Brain Immunity in Neurodegeneration. Journal of Alzheimer's Disease, August 2014 DOI: 10.3233/JAD-141365.

3. Wardlaw J, et al. What are White Matter Hyperintensities Made of? J Am Heart Assoc. 2015 Jun; 4(6): e001140. Published online 2015 Jun 23. doi: 10.1161/JAHA.114.0011404; Calderón-Garcidueñas L, Mora-Tiscareño A, Styner M, Gómez-Garza G, Zhu H,Torres-Jardón R. et al. White matter hyperintensities, systemic inflammation, brain growth, and cognitive functions in children exposed to air pollution. J. Alzheimers Dis. 2012; 31:183–191; Koppenborg RP, Nederkoorn PJ, Geerlings MI, van den Berg E. Presence and progression of white matter hyperintensities and cognition: a meta-analysis. Neurology. 2014; 82:2127–2138

4. Calderon-Garciduenas L, Mora-Tiscareno A, Ontiveros E, et al. Air pollution, cognitive deficits and brain abnormalities: a pilot study with children and dogs. Brain Cogn. 2008 Nov;68(2):117-27. Epub 2008 Jun 11.

5. G. Oberdörster, Z. Sharp, V. Atudorei, A. Elder, R. Gelein, W. Kreyling and C. Cox. Translocation of Inhaled Ultrafine Particles to the Brain. Inhalation Toxicology 2004, Vol. 16, No. 6-7, Pages 437-445; Lewis J, Bench G, Myers O, Tinner B, Staines W, Barr E, Divine KK, Barrington W, Karlsson J (2005) Trigeminal uptake and clearance of inhaled manganese chloride in rats and mice. Neurotoxicology 26:113–23.

6. Maher, B, et al. Magnetite pollution nanoparticles in the human brain. PNAS 2016; published ahead of print September 6, 2016, doi:10.1073/pnas.1605941113.

7. González-Maciel A, Reynoso-Robles R, Torres-Jardón R, Mukherjee PS,

Calderón-Garcidueñas L. Combustion-Derived Nanoparticles in Key Brain Target Cells and Organelles in Young Urbanites: Culprit Hidden in Plain Sight in Alzheimer's Disease Development. J Alzheimers Dis. 2017 Jun 3. doi: 10.3233/JAD-170012. [Epub ahead of print].

8. Bolton JL, Huff NC, Smith SH, Mason SN, Foster WM, Auten RL, et al. 2013. Maternal stress and effects of prenatal air pollution on offspring mental health outcomes in mice. Environ Health Perspect 121:1075-1082.

9. Peterson B, et al. Effects of Prenatal Exposure to Air Pollutants (Polycyclic Aromatic Hydrocarbons) on the Development of Brain White Matter, Cognition, and Behavior in Later Childhood. JAMA Psychiatry. Published online March 25, 2015. doi: 10.1001/jamapsychiatry.2015.57.

10. Perera FP, Tang D, Wang S, Vishnevetsky J, Zhang B, Diaz D, Camann D, Rauh V. Prenatal Polycyclic Aromatic Hydrocarbon (PAH) Exposure and Child Behavior at age 6-7. Environ Health Perspect. 2012 Mar 22. [Epub ahead of print; Calderón-Garcidueñas L, Engle R, Mora-Tiscareño A, Styner M, Gómez-Garza G, Zhu H, Jewells V, Torres-Jardón R, Romero L, Monroy- Acosta ME, Bryant C, González- González LO, Medina-Cortina H, D'Angiulli A. Exposure to severe urban air pollution influences cognitive outcomes, brain volume and systemic inflammation in clinically healthy children. Brain Cogn. 2011 Oct 25. [Epub ahead of print]; Perera, FP, L Zhigang, R Whyatt, L Hoepner, S Wang, D Camann and V Rauh. 2009. Prenatal airborne polycyclic aromatic hydrocarbon exposure and child IQ at age 5 years. Pediatrics doi: 10.1542/peds.2008-3506; Edwards SC, Jedrychowski W, Butscher M, Camann D, Kieltyka A, Mroz E, et al. 2010. Prenatal Exposure to Airborne Polycyclic Aromatic Hydrocarbons and Children's Intelligence at Age 5 in a Prospective Cohort Study in Poland. Environ Health Perspect:-. doi:10.1289/ehp.0901070.

11. Beckwith T, et al. Reduced gray matter volume and cortical thickness associated with traffic-related air pollution in a longitudinally studied pediatric cohort. PLOS ONE, 2020; 15 (1): e0228092 DOI: 10.1371/journal.pone.0228092.

12. Perera, FP, L Zhigang, R Whyatt, L Hoepner, S Wang, D Camann and V Rauh. 2009. 2009. Prenatal airborne polycyclic aromatic hydrocarbon exposure and child IQ at age 5 years. Pediatrics doi: 10.1542/peds.2008- 3506; Edwards SC, Jedrychowski W, Butscher M, Camann D, Kieltyka A, Mroz E, et al. 2010. Prenatal Exposure to Airborne Polycyclic Aromatic Hydrocarbons and Children's Intelligence at Age 5 in a Prospective Cohort Study in Poland. Environ Health Perspect:-. doi:10.1289/ehp.090107; Zhou Z, Yuan T, Chen Y, Qu L, Rauh V, Zhang Y, Tang D, Perera F, Li T. Benefits of Reducing Prenatal Exposure to Coal-Burning Pollutants to Children's Neurodevelopment in China Research Article, published 14 Jul 2008 | doi:10.1289/ ehp.11480; Perera FP, Tang D, Wang S, Vishnevetsky J, Zhang B, Diaz D, Camann D, Rauh V. Prenatal Polycyclic Aromatic Hydrocarbon (PAH) Exposure and Child Behavior

References

at age 6-7. Environ Health Perspect. 2012 259; Perera F, Weiland K, Neidell M, Wang S. Prenatal exposure to airborne polycyclic aromatic hydrocarbons and IQ: Estimated benefit of pollution reduction. J Public Health Policy. 2014 May 8. doi: 10.1057/jphp.2014.14. [Epub ahead of print]; Prenatal exposure to PM10 and NO2 and children's neurdevelopment from birth to 24 months of age: mothers and Children's Environmental Health (MOCEH) study. Sci Total Environ. 2014 May 15; 481:439-45. doi: 10.1016/j.scitotenv. 2014.01.107. Epub 2014 Mar 12; Jedrychowski WA, Perera FP, Camann D, Spengler J, Butscher M, Mroz E, Majewska R, Flak E, Jacek R, Sowa A. Prenatal exposure to polycyclic aromatic hydrocarbons and cognitive dysfunction in children. Environ Sci Pollut Res Int. 2014 Sep 26. [Epub ahead of print]; Perera FP, Chang H-w, Tang D, Roen EL, Herbstman J, et al. (2014) Early-Life Exposure to Polycyclic Aromatic Hydrocarbons and ADHD Behavior Problems. PLoS ONE 9(11): e111670. doi:10.1371/journal.pone.0111670; Lertxundi A, et al. Exposure to fine particle matter, nitrogen dioxide and benzene during pregnancy and cognitive and psychomotor developments in children at 15months of age. Environ Int. 2015 Apr10; 80:33-40. doi: 10.1016/j.envint.2015.03.007. [Epub ahead of print]; Vishnevetskya J, et al. Combined effects of prenatal polycyclic aromatic hydrocarbons and material hardship on child IQ. Neurotoxicology and Teratology. doi: 10.1016/j.ntt.2015.04.002. Available online 23 April 2015; Yorifuji T, Kashima S, Higa Diez M, Kado Y, Sanada S, Doi H. Prenatal Exposure to Traffic-related Air Pollution and Child Behavioral Development Milestone Delays in Japan. Epidemiology. 2015 Aug 5. [Epub ahead of print]; Cooper L, Eskenazi B, Romero C, Balmes J, Smith KR. Neurodevelopmental performance among school age children in rural Guatemala is associated with prenatal and postnatal exposure to carbon monoxide, a marker for exposure to woodsmoke. Neurotoxicology. 2012 Mar; 33(2):246-54. doi: 10.1016/j.neuro.2011.09.004. Epub 2011 Sep 24.

13. Allen JL, Liu X, Pelkowski S, Palmer B, Conrad K, Oberdörster G, Weston D, Mayer-Pröschel M, Cory-Slechta DA (2014a) Early postnatal exposure to ultrafine particulate matter air pollution: persistent ventriculomegaly, neurochemical disruption, and glial activation preferentially in male mice. Environ Health Perspect 122: 939–45.

14. Allen J, et al. Early Postnatal Exposure to Ultrafine Particulate Matter Air Pollution: Persistent Ventriculomegaly, Neurochemical Disruption, and Glial Activation Preferentially in Male Mice. Environ Health Perspect; DOI:10.1289/ehp.1307984.

15. Chen JC, et al. Ambient Air Pollution and Neurotoxicity on Brain Structure: Evidence From Women's Health Initiative Memory Study. Ann Neurol 2015; 78:466–476.

16. https://www.theguardian.com/science/2013/sep/15/zebrafish-human-genes-project.

17. Bronstein J, et al. Diesel exhaust extract exposure induces neuronal toxicity by disrupting autophagy. Toxicological Sciences, 2020; DOI: 10.1093/toxsci/kfaa055.

18. Levesque S, Taetzsch T, Lull ME, Kodavanti U, Stadler K, Wagner A. et al. Diesel exhaust activates and primes microglia: air pollution, neuroinflammation and regulation of dopaminergic neurotoxicity. Environ. Health Perspect. 2011; 119:1149–1155. [PMC free article] [PubMed]; Levesque S, Taetzsch T, Lull ME, Johnson JA, McGraw C, Block ML. The role of MAC1 in diesel exhaust particle-induced microglial activation and loss of dopaminergic neuron function. J. Neurochem. 2013; 125:756– 765. [PMC free article] [PubMed]; Cacciottolo M, et al. Particulate air pollutants, APOE alleles and their contributions to cognitive impairment in older women and to amyloidogenesis in experimental models. Translational Psychiatry (2017) 7, e1022; doi:10.1038/tp.2016.280 Published online 31 January; Calderón-Garcidueñas L, Reed W, Maronpot RR, Henríquez-Roldán C, Delgado- Chavez R, Calderón-Garcidueñas A, Dragustinovis I, Franco- Lira M, Aragón-Flores M, Solt AC, Altenburg M, Torres-Jardón R, Swenberg JA. Brain inflammation and Alzheimer's-like pathology in individuals exposed to severe air pollution. Toxicol Pathol. 2004 Nov- Dec;32(6):650-8; Calderón-Garcidueñas L, Kavanaugh M, Block M, D'Angiulli A, Delgado-Chávez R, Torres-Jardón R. et al. Neuroinflammation, Alzheimer's disease-associated pathology and down regulation of the prion-related protein in air pollution exposed children and young adults. J. Alzheimers Dis. 2012; 28:93–107 [PubMed.]: Fonken LK, Xu X, Weil ZM, Chen G, Sun Q, Rajagopalan S. et al. Air pollution impairs cognition, provokes depressive-like behaviors and alters hippocampal cytokine expression and morphology. Mol. Psychiatry. 2011; 16:987–995. [PMC free article] [PubMed]; Rivas-Arancibia S, Guevara-Guzmán R, López-Vidal Y, Rodríguez- Martínez E, Zanardo-Gomes M, Angoa-Pérez M. et al. Oxidative stress caused by ozone exposure induces loss of brain repair in the hippocampus of adult rats. Toxicol.Sci. 2010;113:187–197. [PubMed].

19. Jung CR, Lin YT, Hwang BF. Ozone, particulate matter, and newly diagnosed Alzheimer's disease: a population-based cohort study in Taiwan. J Alzheimers Dis. 2015; 44(2):573-84. doi: 10.3233/JAD-140855.

20. Calderón-Garcidueñas L, et al. Hallmarks of Alzheimer disease are evolving relentlessly in Metropolitan Mexico City infants, children and young adults. APOE4 carriers have higher suicide risk and higher odds of reaching NFT stage V at ≤ 40 years of age. Environmental Research, 2018; 164: 475 DOI: 10.1016/j.envres.2018.03.023.

21. Cheng H, et al. Nanoscale Particulate Matter from Urban Traffic Rapidly Induces Oxidative Stress and Inflammation in Olfactory Epithelium with Concomitant Effects on Brain. Environ Health Perspect; DOI:10.1289/EHP13; Colicino E, et al. Telomere Length, Long-Term Black Carbon Exposure, and Cognitive Function in a Cohort of Older Men: The VA Normative Aging Study.

References

Environ Health Perspect. 2016 Jun 3. [Epub ahead of print]; Kim KN, et al. Long-Term Fine Particulate Matter Exposure and Major Depressive Disorder in a Community-Based Urban Cohort. Environ Health Perspect. 2016 Apr 29. [Epub ahead of print]; Oudin, A, et al. Traffic-Related Air Pollution and Dementia Incidence in Northern Sweden: A Longitudinal Study. Environ Health Perspect; DOI:10.1289/ehp.1408322; Best EA, Juarez-Colunga E, James K, LeBlanc WG, Serdar B. Biomarkers of Exposure to Polycyclic Aromatic Hydrocarbons and Cognitive Function among Elderly in the United States (National Health and Nutrition Examination Survey: 2001-2002). PLoS One. 2016 Feb 5; 11(2):e0147632. doi: 10.1371/journal.pone.0147632; Laura A,, et al. Effects of particulate matter exposure on multiple sclerosis hospital admission in Lombardy region, Italy. Environ Res. 2015. Nov 25; 145:68-73. doi: 10.1016/j.envres.2015.11.017. [Epub ahead of print]; Power MC, et al. The relation between past exposure to fine particulate air pollution and prevalent anxiety: observational cohort study. BMJ, 2015; 350 (mar23 11): h1111 DOI: 10.1136/bmj.h1111; Ailshire JA, Crimmins EM. Fine Particulate Matter Air Pollution and Cognitive Function Among Older US Adults. Am J Epidemiol. 2014 Jun 24. pii: kwu155. [Epub ahead of print]; Pun VC, et al. Association of Ambient Air Pollution with Depressive and Anxiety Symptoms in Older Adults: Results from the NSHAP Study. Environ Health Perspect; DOI:10.1289/EHP494; Lee H, Myung W, Kim DK, Kim SE, Kim CT, Kim H. Short-term air pollution exposure aggravates Parkinson's disease in a population-based cohort. Sci Rep. 2017 Mar 16; 7:44741. doi: 10.1038/srep44741; Porta D, Narduzzi S, Badaloni C, Bucci S, Cesaroni G, Colelli V, Davoli M, Sunyer J, Zirro E, Schwartz J, Forastiere F. Air pollution and cognitive development at age seven in a prospective Italian birth cohort. Epidemiology. 2015 Sep 30. [Epub ahead of print].

22. Ho HC, et al. Spatiotemporal influence of temperature, air quality, and urban environment on cause-specific mortality during hazy days. Environment International, Volume 112, March 2018, Pages 10-22; Jia Z, et al. Exposure to Ambient Air Particles Increases the Risk of Mental Disorder: Findings from a Natural Experiment in Beijing. Int J Environ Res Public Health. 2018 Jan 19; 15(1). pii: E160. doi: 10.3390/ijerph15010160; Oudin A, et al. The association between daily concentrations of air pollution and visits to a psychiatric emergency unit: a case-crossover study. Environ Health. 2018 Jan 10; 17(1):4. doi: 10.1186/s12940-017-0348- 8; Casas L, et al. Does air pollution trigger suicide? A case-crossover analysisofsuicidedeathsoverthelifespan. EuropeanJournalof Epidemiology. November 2017, Volume 32, Issue 11, pp 973–981.

23. Mez J, et al. Clinicopathological Evaluation of Chronic Traumatic Encephalopathy in Players of American Football. JAMA. 2017; 318(4):360-370. doi:10.1001/jama.2017.8334.

24. Yang Y, Glenn AL, Raine A. Brain abnormalities in antisocial individuals: implications for the law. Behav Sci Law. 2008; 26(1):65-83. doi:

10.1002/bsl.788.

25. Lu J, et al. Polluted Morality: Air Pollution Predicts Criminal Activity and Unethical Behavior. Psychological Science, 2018; 095679761773580 DOI: 10.1177/0956797617735807.

26. Huang F, et al. Particulate Matter and Hospital Admissions for Stroke in Beijing, China: Modification Effects by Ambient Temperature. J Am Heart Assoc. 2016 Jul 13; 5(7). pii: e003437. doi: 10.1161/JAHA.116.003437; Shah A, et al. Short term exposure to air pollution and stroke: systematic review and meta-analysis. BMJ 2015; 350:h1295; Wellenius G, et al. Ambient Air Pollution and the Risk of Acute Ischemic Stroke. Arch Intern Med. 2012; 172(3):229-234; Han M, et al. Association between hemorrhagic stroke occurrence and meteorological factors and pollutants. BMC Neurol. 2016 May 4;16(1):59. doi: 10.1186/s12883-016-0579-2; Chiu HF, Yang CY. Short-term effects of fine particulate air pollution on ischemic stroke occurrence: a case-crossover study. J Toxicol Environ Health A. 2013; 76(21): 1188-97. doi:10.1080/15287394.2013.842463; Chen R, Zhang Y, Yang C, Zhao Z, Xu X, Kan H. Acute Effect of 296. Mateen F, Brook R. Air Pollution as an Emerging Global Risk Factor for Stroke JAMA 2011; 305(12):1240-1241.doi:10.1001/jama.2011.352; Kettunen, J. et al. (2007) Associations of fine and ultrafine particulate air pollution with stroke mortality in an area of low air pollution levels. Stroke 38, 918–922.

27. https://www.who.int/news-room/detail/29-10-2018-more-than-90-of-the-worlds-children-breathe-toxic-air-every-day.

28. Sharma A, et al. Quantification of air pollution exposure to in-pram babies and mitigation strategies. Environment International, 2020; 139: 105671 DOI: 10.1016/j.envint.2020.105671.

29. Sunyer J, et al. Traffic-related Air Pollution and Attention in Primary School Children: Short-term Association. Epidemiology: March 2017 – Volume 28 – Issue 2 – p 181–189. doi: 10.1097/EDE.0000000000000603.

30. Giordano G., Tait L., Furlong C. E., Cole T. B., Kavanagh T. J., Costa L. G. (2013). Gender differences in brain susceptibility to oxidative stress are mediated by levels of paraoxonase-2 expression. Free Radic. Biol. Med. 58 98–108. 10.1016/j.freeradbiomed.2013.01.019.

31. Cole T., Coburn J., Dao K., Roqué P., Chang Y.-C., Kalia V., et al. (2016). Sex and genetic differences in the effects of acute diesel exhaust exposure on inflammation and oxidative stress in mouse brain. Toxicology 374 1–9. 10.1016/j.tox.2016.11.010.

32. Chen X. Smog, Cognition and Real-World Decision-Making. Int J Health Policy Manag. 2019 Feb 1;8(2):76-80. doi: 10.15171/ijhpm.2018.105. PMID:

References

30980620; PMCID: PMC6462201.

NEWBORN ICU

1. Aylward, G. P. Neurodevelopmental outcomes of infants born prematurely. J. Dev. Behav. Pediatr. 35, 394–407 (2014).

2. Benavides, A. & Metzger, A. et al (2018). Sex Specific Alterations in Preterm Brain, Pediatric Research. 85, pages55–62(2019).

3. Skiold, B. et al. Sex differences in outcome and associations with neonatal brain morphology in extremely preterm children. J. Pediatr. 164, 1012–1018 (2014); Reiss, A. L. et al. Sex differences in cerebral volumes of 8-year-olds born preterm. J. Pediatr. 145, 242–249 (2004).

4. Benavides, A. & Metzger, A. et al (2018). Sex Specific Alterations in Preterm Brain, Pediatric Research. 85, pages 55–62(2019).

5. Domellof, M. et al. Sex differences in iron status during infancy. Pediatrics 110, 545–552 (2002).

6. Iribarne-Durán, L.M., et al. (2019) Presence of bisphenol A and parabens in a neonatal intensive care unit: An exploratory study of potential sources of exposure. Environmental Health Perspectives. doi.org/10.1289/EHP5564.

7. Calafat AM, Needham LL, Silva MJ, Lambert G. Exposure to di-(2-ethylhexyl) phthalate among premature neonates in a neonatal intensive care unit. Pediatrics. 2004;113(5):e429–34.

8. Green R, Hauser R, Calafat AM, et al. Use of di(2-ethylhexyl) phthalate-containing medical products and urinary levels of mono(2-ethylhexyl) phthalate in neonatal intensive care unit infants. Environmental Health Perspectives. 2005; 113(9):1222–5; Calafat AM, Weuve J, Ye X, et al. Exposure to bisphenol A and other phenols in neonatal intensive care unit premature infants. Environmental health perspectives. 2009;117(4):639–44.

9. Metcalf MEM, Borgens RB. Weak Applied Voltages Interfere with Amphibian Morphogenesis and Pattern. J Exp Zool. 1994; 268:323–338; Hotary KB, Robinson KR. Endogenous Electrical Currents and Voltage Gradients in Xenopus embryos and the Consequences of their Disruption. Dev Biol. 1994; 166(2):789–800.

10. Peacock, J., Marston, L., Marlow, N. et al. Neonatal and infant outcome in boys and girls born very prematurely. Pediatr Res 71, 305–310 (2012). https://doi.org/10.1038/pr.2011.50.

Chapter Six

The Great Brain Robbery – Brian Moench

1. Wang L, et al. Sexual dimorphism in glutathione metabolism and glutathione-dependent responses. Redox Biology, Volume 31, April 2020, 101410.

2. Betteridge DJ. What is oxidative stress? Metabolism. 2000 Feb; 49(2 Suppl 1):3-8. doi: 10.1016/s0026-0495(00)80077-3.

3. Lavoie JC. Chessex P (1997) Gender and maturation affect glutathione status in human neonatal tissues. Free Radical Biol Med 23: 648–57; Rush JW, Sandiford SD (2003) Plasma glutathione peroxidase in healthy young adults: Influence of gender and physical activity. Clinical Bio-chemistry 36: 345–51; Wang, H, et al. Gender Difference in Glutathione Metabolism During Aging in Mice. Exp Gerontol. 2003 May; 38(5):507-17; Hamon I, et al. [Gender-dependent Differences in Glutathione (GSH) Metabolism in Very Preterm Infants]. Arch Pediatr. 2011 Mar; 18(3):247-52.

4. P.K. Mandal, M. Tripathi, S. Sugunan, Brain oxidative stress: detection and map-ping of anti-oxidant marker 'Glutathione' in different brain regions of healthy male/female, MCI and Alzheimer patients using non-invasive magnetic resonance spectroscopy, Biochem. Biophys. Res. Commun. 417 (1) (2012) 43–48.

5. Al-Yafee YA, et al. Novel metabolic biomarkers related to sulfur-dependent detoxification pathways in autistic patients of Saudi Arabia. BMC Neurol. 2011; 11: 139. Published online 2011 Nov 4. doi: 10.1186/1471-2377-11-139.

6. K. Aoyama, T. Nakaki, Impaired glutathione synthesis in neurodegeneration, Int.J. Mol. Sci. 14 (10) (2013) 21021–21044; K. Schuessel, S. Leutner, N. Cairns, et al., Impact of gender on upregulation of antioxidant defence mechanisms in Alzheimer's disease brain, 111 (9) (2004)1167–1182.

7. Kern JK, Haley BE, Geier DA, Sykes LK, King PG, Geier, MR (2013) Thimerosal exposure and the role of sulfation chemistry and thiol availability in autism. Int J Environ Res Public Health 10: 3771–800.

8. Zarate S, et al. Role of Estrogen and Other Sex Hormones in Brain Aging. Neuroprotection and DNA Repair. Front. Aging Neurosci., 22 December 2017.

9. Simpson ER. Sources of estrogen and their importance. J Steroid Biochem Mol Biol. 2003 Sep; 86(3-5):225-30.

10. Kenealy BP, et al. Neuroestradiol in the Hypothalamus Contributes to the Regulation of Gonadotropin Releasing Hormone Release. Journal of Neuroscience, 2013; 33 (49): 19051 DOI: 10.1523/JNEUROSCI.3878-13.2013.

11. Miller DB, Ali SF, O'Callaghan JP, Laws SC (1998) The impact of gender and estrogen on striatal dopaminergic neurotoxicity. Ann N Y Acad Sci 844: 153–65; Schaeffer V, Patte-Mensah C, Eckert A, Mensah-Nyagan AG (2008)

References

Selective regulation of neurosteroid biosynthesis in human neuroblastoma cells under hydrogen peroxide-induced oxidative stress condition. Neuroscience 151: 758–70; Simpkins J. et al. The Potential for Estrogens in Preventing Alzheimer's Disease and Vascular Dementia. Ther Adv Neurol Disord. 2009 Jan; 2(1): 31–49. doi: 10.1177/1756285608100427.

12. Emerson C.S., Headrick J.P., Vink R. Estrogen improves biochemical and neurologic outcome following traumatic brain injury in male rats, but not in females. Brain Res. 1993; 608(1):95–100.

13. Zlotnik A., Leibowitz A., Gurevich B., Ohayon S., Boyko M., Klein M., Knyazer B., Shapira Y., Teichberg V.I. Effect of estrogens on blood glutamate levels in relation to neurological outcome after TBI in male rats. Intensive Care Med. 2012; 38(1):137–144. [http://dx.doi.org/10.1007/s00134-011-2401-3].

14. Soustiel J.F., Palzur E., Nevo O., Thaler I., Vlodavsky E. Neuroprotective anti-apoptosis effect of estrogens in traumatic brain injury. J. Neurotrauma. 2005; 22(3):345–352; Naderi V., Khaksari M., Abbasi R., Maghool F. Estrogen provides neuroprotection against brain edema and blood brain barrier disruption through both estrogen receptors α and β following traumatic brain injury. Iran. J. Basic Med. Sci. 2015; 18(2):138–144; Day N.L., Floyd C.L., D'Alessandro T.L., Hubbard W.J., Chaudry I.H. 17β-estradiol confers protection after traumatic brain injury in the rat and involves activation of G protein-coupled estrogen receptor 1. J. Neurotrauma. 2013; 30(17):1531–1541.

15. Berry C., Ley E.J., Tillou A., Cryer G., Margulies D.R., Salim A. The effect of gender on patients with moderate to severe head injuries. J. Trauma.

16. Brann D.W., Dhandapani K., Wakade C., Mahesh V.B., Khan M.M. Neurotrophic and neuroprotective actions of estrogen: basic mechanisms and clinical implications. Steroids. 2007; 72(5):381–405; Bruce-Keller A.J., Keeling J.L., Keller J.N., Huang F.F., Camondola S., Mattson M.P. Antiinflammatory effects of estrogen on microglial activation. Endocrinology. 2000; 141(10):3646–3656.

17. Hu R., Sun H., Zhang Q., Chen J., Wu N., Meng H., Cui G., Hu S., Li F., Lin J., Wan Q., Feng H. G-protein coupled estrogen receptor 1 mediated estrogenic neuroprotection against spinal cord injury. Crit. Care Med. 2012; 40(12):3230–3237; Samantaray S., Smith J.A., Das A., Matzelle D.D., Varma A.K., Ray S.K., Banik N.L. Low dose estrogen prevents neuronal degeneration and microglial reactivity in an acute model of spinal cord injury: effect of dosing, route of administration, and therapy delay. Neurochem. Res. 2011; 36(10):1809–1816.

18. Korosia A. E. F. G., Nanincka C. A., Oomenb M., Schoutena H., Krugersa C., Fitzsimonsa P. J. Lucassena. Early-life stress mediated modulation of adult neurogenesis and behavior. Behav. Brain Res. 2012; 227:400–409; Bredy T.W.,

The Great Brain Robbery – Brian Moench

Grant R.J., Champagne D.L., Meaney M.J. Maternal care influences neuronal survival in the hippocampus of the rat. Eur. J. Neurosci. 2003; 18(10):2903–2909; Pawluski J.L., Brummelte S., Barha C.K., Tamara M. Crozier; Galea, L. A. M. Effects of steroid hormones on neuro- genesis in the hippocampus of the Frontiers. Neuroendocrinology. 2009; 30:343–357; Saravia F., Beauquis J., Pietranera L., De Nicola A.F. Neuroprotective effects of estradiol in hippocampal neurons and glia of middle age mice. Psychoneuroendocrinology. 2007; 32(5):480–492; Christie D., Yan L. F., Zuoxin W. Estrogen and adult neurogenesis in the amygdala and hypothalamus. Brain Res. Rev. 2008; 57:342–351.

19. Singh M., Su C. Progesterone and neuroprotection. Horm. Behav. 2013; 63(2):284–290; Teichberg V.I., Cohen-Kashi-Malina K., Cooper I., Zlotnik A. Homeostasis of glutamate in brain fluids: an accelerated brain-to-blood efflux of excess glutamate is produced by blood glutamate scavenging and offers protection from neuropathologies. Neuroscience. 2009; 158(1):301–308.

20. Zárate S, et al. Role of Estrogen and Other Sex Hormones in Brain Aging. Neuroprotection and DNA Repair. Front Aging Neurosci. 2017; 9: 430.

21. https://www.ahajournals.org/doi/full/10.1161/01.str.0000054051.88378.25.

22. Johann S., Beyer C. Neuroprotection by gonadal steroid hormones in acute brain damage requires cooperation with astroglia and microglia. J. Steroid Biochem. Mol. Biol. 2013; 137:71–81

23. Fox M, Berzuini C, Knapp L, Glynn LM. Women's Pregnancy Life History and Alzheimer's Risk: Can Immunoregulation Explain the Link? Am J Alzheimers Dis Other Demen. 2018 Dec; 33(8):516-526. doi: 10.1177/1533317518786447. Epub 2018 Jul 30.

24. https://www.healthline.com/health-news/can-estrogen-protect-women-against-dementia#4.

25. https://www.alz.org/aaic/releases_2018/AAIC18-Mon-women-dementia-risk.asp; https://www.npr.org/sections/health-shots/2018/07/23/630688342/might-sex-hormones-help-protect-women-from-alzheimer-s-after-all-maybe.

26. Green P.S., Yang S.H., Simpkins J.W. Neuroprotective effects of phenolic A ring oestrogens. Novartis Found. Symp. 2000; 230:202–213; Behl C. Oestrogen as a neuroprotective hormone. Nat. Rev. Neurosci. 2002; 3(6):433–442; Singh M., Su C. Progesterone and neuroprotection. Horm. Behav. 2013;63(2):284–290.

27. https://www.funpic.hu/en/image/57092_that-tiny-spare-tire-on-the-back-d.

28. McEwen B. S., Milner T. A. (2017). Understanding the broad influence of

References

sex hormones and sex differences in the brain. J. Neurosci. Res. 95, 24–39. 10.1002/jnr.23809 [PMC free article].

29. Scott E., Zhang Q. G., Wang R., Vadlamudi R., Brann D. (2012). Estrogen neuroprotection and the critical period hypothesis. Front. Neuroendocrinol. 33, 85–104. 10.1016/j.yfrne.2011.10.001; Miller V. M., Harman S. M. (2017). An update on hormone therapy in postmenopausal women: mini-review for the basic scientist. Am. J. Physiol. Heart Circ. Physiol. 313, H1013–H1021. 10.1152/ajpheart.00383.2017 [PMC free article] [PubMed] [CrossRef] [Google Scholar].

30. https://www.alz.org/aaic/releases_2018/AAIC18-Mon-women-dementia-risk.asp.

31. Woolley C. S., McEwen B. S. (1992). Estradiol mediates fluctuation in hippocampal synapse density during the estrous cycle in the adult rat. J. Neurosci. 12, 2549–2554.

32. Suzuki S., Brown C. M., Wise P. M. (2009). Neuroprotective effects of estrogens following ischemic stroke. Front. Neuroendocrinol. 30, 201–211. 10.1016/j.yfrne.2009.04.007.

33. https://www.ahajournals.org/doi/full/10.1161/01.str.0000054051.88378.25.

34. Maddox SA, et al. Estrogen-dependent association of HDAC4 with fear in female mice and women with PTSD. Molecular Psychiatry (2018) 23, 658–665.

35. Goyal MS, et al. Loss of brain aerobic glycolysis in normal human aging. Cell Metab. 2017 Aug 1; 26(2): 353–360.e3.

36. Goyal MS, Blazey TM, Su Y, Couture LE, Durbin TJ, Bateman RJ, Benzinger TLS, Morris JC, Raichle ME, Vlassenko AG. Persistent metabolic youth in the aging female brain. Proceedings of the National Academy of Sciences, Feb. 4, 2019 DOI: 10.1073/pnas.1815917116.

37. Satterthwaite TD, et al. Impact of puberty on the evolution of cerebral perfusion during adolescence. Proc Natl Acad Sci USA. 2014; 111:8643–8648; Aanerud J, Borghammer P, Rodell A, Jonsdottir KY, Gjedde A. Sex differences of human cortical blood flow and energy metabolism. J Cereb Blood Flow Metab. 2016; 37:2433–2440.

38. Berchtold NC, et al. Gene expression changes in the course of normal brain aging are sexually dimorphic. Proc Natl Acad Sci USA. 2008; 105:15605–15610.

39. Jack CR, Jr, et al. Age, sex, and APOE ε4 effects on memory, brain structure, and β-amyloid across the adult life span. JAMA Neurol. 2015; 72:511–519.

40. Risher JF, Tucker P (2017) Alkyl Mercury-induced toxicity: multiple mechanisms of action. Rev Environ Contam Toxicol 240: 105–149.

41. Borrás C, Sastre J, García-Sala D, Lloret A, Pallardó FV, Viña J (2003) Mito-chondria from females exhibit higher antioxidant gene expression and lower oxidative damage than males. Free Radic Biol Med 34: 546-52.

42. Miller DB, Ali SF, O'Callaghan JP, Laws SC (1998) The impact of gender and estrogen on striatal dopaminergic neurotoxicity. Ann N Y Acad Sci 844: 153–65; Yang, S, et al. Testosterone increases neurotoxicity of glutamate in vitro and ischemia-reperfusion injury in an animal model. Journal of Applied Physiology 92(1):195-201 February 2002.

43. Haley BE (2005) Mercury toxicity: genetic susceptibility and synergistic effects. Med Veritas 2: 535–42.

44. Djavadian R.L. Serotonin and neurogenesis in the hippocampal dentate gyrus of adult mammals. Acta Neurobiol. Exp. (Warsz.) 2004; 64(2):189–200.

45. Barkan A.L., Dimaraki E.V., Jessup S.K., Symons K.V., Ermolenko M., Jaffe C.A. Ghrelin secretion in humans is sexually dimorphic, suppressed by somatostatin, and not affected by the ambient growth hormone levels. J. Clin. Endocrinol. Metab. 2003; 88(5):2180–2184.

46. Roof RL, Hall ED (2000) Gender differences in acute CNS trauma and stroke: neuroprotective effects of estrogen and progesterone. J Neurotrauma 17: 367–88; Meffre D, Labombarda F, Delespierre B, Chastre A, De Nicola AF, Stein DG, Schumacher M, Guennoun R (2013) Distribution of membrane progesterone receptor alpha in the male mouse and rat brain and its regulation after traumatic brain injury. Neuroscience 231: 111–24.

47. https://www.lifeextension.com/magazine/2009/11/progesterone-may-improve-outcomes-from-brain-injury; Stein DG, Hurn PD. Effects of Sex Steroids on Damaged Neural Systems. In: Pfaff DW, Arnold AP, Etgen AM, eds. Hormones, Brains, and Behavior. 2nd ed. Oxford: Elsevier; 2009.

48. Singh M. Progesterone-induced neuroprotection. Endocrine. 2006; 29(2):271–274; Singh M., Su C. Progesterone and neuroprotection. Horm. Behav. 2013; 63(2):284–290.

49. Neurosci Lett. 2007 Sep 25; 425(2):94-8.

50. Ann Emerg Med. 2007 Apr; 49(4):391-402. Brain Res Rev. 2008 Mar; 57(2):386-97.

51. Behl C., Manthey D. Neuroprotective activities of estrogen: an update. J. Neurocytol. 2000; 29(5-6):351–358.

References

52. Roof R.L., Duvdevani R., Heyburn J.W., Stein D.G. Progesterone rapidly decreases brain edema: treatment delayed up to 24 hours is still effective. Exp. Neurol. 1996; 138(2):246–251; Wright D.W., Bauer M.E., Hoffman S.W., Stein D.G. Serum progesterone levels correlate with decreased cerebral edema after traumatic brain injury in male rats. J. Neurotrauma. 2001; 18(9):901–909; Guo Q, Sayeed I, Baronne LM, Hoffman SW, Guennoun R, Stein DG, et al. Progesterone administration modulates AQP4 expression and edema after traumatic brain injury in male rats. Exp Neurol. 2006; 198:469–78.

53. Roof R.L., Duvdevani R., Heyburn J.W., Stein D.G. Progesterone rapidly decreases brain edema: treatment delayed up to 24 hours is still effective. Exp. Neurol. 1996;138(2):246–251.

54. Wright D.W., Kellermann A.L., Hertzberg V.S., Clark P.L., Frankel M., Goldstein F.C., Salomone J.P., Dent L.L., Harris O.A., Ander D.S., Lowery D.W., Patel M.M., Denson D.D., Gordon A.B., Wald M.M., Gupta S., Hoffman S.W., Stein D.G. ProTECT: a randomized clinical trial of progesterone for acute traumatic brain injury. Ann. Emerg. Med. 2007; 49(4):391–402.

55. Wright D.W., Kellermann A.L., Hertzberg V.S., Clark P.L., Frankel M., Goldstein F.C., Salomone J.P., Dent L.L., Harris O.A., Ander D.S., Lowery D.W., Patel M.M., Denson D.D., Gordon A.B., Wald M.M., Gupta S., Hoffman S.W., Stein D.G. ProTECT: a randomized clinical trial of progesterone for acute traumatic brain injury. Ann. Emerg. Med. 2007; 49(4):391–402; Aminmansour B., Nikbakht H., Ghorbani A., Rezvani M., Rahmani P., Torkashvand M., Nourian M., Moradi M. Comparison of the administration of progesterone versus progesterone and vitamin D in improvement of outcomes in patients with traumatic brain injury: A randomized clinical trial with placebo group. Adv. Biomed. Res. 2012; 1:58; Xiao G., Wei J., Yan W., Wang W., Lu Z. Improved outcomes from the administration of progesterone for patients with acute severe traumatic brain injury: a randomized controlled trial. Crit. Care. 2008; 12(2):R61.

56. Lin C., He H., Li Z., Liu Y., Chao H., Ji J., Liu N. Efficacy of progesterone for moderate to severe traumatic brain injury: a meta-analysis of randomized clinical trials. Sci. Rep. 2015; 5:13442.

57. Zhi-Yong P, et al. Effect of progesterone administration on the prognosis of patients with severe traumatic brain injury: a meta-analysis of randomized clinical trials. Drug Des Devel Ther. 2019; 13: 265–273. Published online 2019 Jan 11.

58. Brotfain E, et al. Neuroprotection by Estrogen and Progesterone in Traumatic Brain Injury and Spinal Cord Injury. Curr Neuropharmacol. 2016 Aug; 14(6): 641–653. Published online 2016 Aug.; Groswasser Z., Cohen M., Keren O. Female TBI patients recover better than males. Brain Inj. 1998; 12(9):805–808.

59. Roof RL, Duvdevani R, Stein DG, et al. Gender influences outcome of brain injury: progesterone plays a protective role. Brain Res. 1993a;607:333–6.

60. Guo Q, Sayeed I, Baronne LM, Hoffman SW, Guennoun R, Stein DG, et al. Progesterone administration modulates AQP4 expression and edema after traumatic brain injury in male rats. Exp Neurol. 2006; 198:469–78; Leonelli E, Bianchi R, Cavaletti G, Caruso D, Crippa D, Garcia-Segura LM, Lauria G, Magnaghi V, Roglio I, Melcangi RC, et al. Progesterone and its derivatives are neuroprotective agents in experimental diabetic neuropathy: A multimodal analysis. Neuroscience. 2007; 144:1293–304; O'Connor CA, Cernak I, Vink R, et al. Both estrogen and progesterone attenuate edema formation following diffuse traumatic brain injury in rats. Brain Res. 2005; 1062:171–4; Wright DW, Bauer ME, Hoffman SW, Stein DG, et al. Serum progesterone levels correlate with decreased cerebral edema after traumatic brain injury in male rats. J Neurotrauma. 2001; 18:901–9.

61. Thomas A.J., Nockels R.P., Pan H.Q., Shaffrey C.I., Chopp M. Progesterone is neuroprotective after acute experimental spinal cord trauma in rats. Spine. 1999; 24(20):2134–2138. De Nicola A.F., Labombarda F., Gonzalez D.M., Gonzalez S.L., Garay L., Meyer M., Gargiulo G., Guennoun R., Schumacher M. Progesterone neuroprotection in traumatic CNS injury and motoneuron degeneration. Front. Neuroendocrinol. 2009; 30(2):173–187; Guennoun R., Meffre D., Labombarda F., Gonzalez S.L., Gonzalez Deniselle M.C., Stein D.G., De Nicola A.F., Schumacher M. The membrane-associated progesterone-binding protein 25-Dx: expression, cellular localization and up-regulation after brain and spinal cord injuries. Brain Res. Brain Res. Rev. 2008; 57(2):493–505.

62. Wise P.M., Smith M.J., Dubal D.B., Wilson M.E., Rau S.W., Cashion A.B., Böttner M., Rosewell K.L. Neuroendocrine modulation and repercussions of female reproductive aging. Recent Prog. Horm. Res. 2002; 57:235–256. [http://dx.doi.org/10.1210/ rp.57.1.235]. [PMID: 12017546].

63. Behl C., Manthey D. Neuroprotective activities of estrogen: an update. J. Neurocytol. 2000; 29(5-6):351–358; Woolley C.S., McEwen B.S. Roles of estradiol and progesterone in regulation of hippocampal dendritic spine density during the estrous cycle in the rat. J. Comp. Neurol. 1993; 336(2):293–306.

64. Dubal D.B., Shughrue P.J., Wilson M.E., Merchenthaler I., Wise P.M. Estradiol modulates bcl-2 in cerebral ischemia: a potential role for estrogen receptors. J. Neurosci. 1999; 19(15):6385–6393; Zhang Q.G., Wang R., Khan M., Mahesh V., Brann D.W. Role of Dickkopf-1, an antagonist of the Wnt/beta-catenin signaling pathway, in estrogen-induced neuroprotection and attenuation of tau phosphorylation. J. Neurosci. 2008; 28(34):8430–8441; Yang L.C., Zhang Q.G., Zhou C.F., Yang F., Zhang Y.D., Wang R.M., Brann D.W. Extranuclear estrogen receptors mediate the neuroprotective effects of estrogen in the rat hippocampus. PLoS One. 2010; 5(5):e9851.

References

65. Buchanan FF, Myles PS, Cicuttini F. Effect of patient sex on general anaesthesia and recovery. BJA: British Journal of Anaesthesia, Volume 106, Issue 6, June 2011, Pages 832–839; Goto T, Nakata Y, Morita S. The minimum alveolar concentration of xenon in the elderly is sex-dependent, Anesthesiology, 2002, vol. 97 (pg. 1129-32).

66. Domino KB, Posner KL, Caplan RA, Cheney FW. Awareness during anaesthesia—a closed claims analysis, Anesthesiology, 1999, vol. 90 (pg. 1053-61; Ghoneim MM, Block RI, Haffarnan M, Mathews MJ. Awareness during anaesthesia: risk factors, causes and sequelae. A review of reported cases in the literature, Anesth Analg, 2009, vol. 108 (pg. 529-35).

67. Taenzer AH, Clark C, Curry CS. Gender affects report of pain and function after arthroscopic anterior cruciate ligament reconstruction, Anesthesiology, 2000, vol. 93 (pg. 670-5); Harmon D, O'Connor P, Gleasa O, Gardiner J. Menstrual cycle irregularity and the incidence of nausea and vomiting after laparoscopy, Anaesthesia, 2000, vol. 55 (pg. 1164-7).

68. Tsesis S., Gruenbaum B.F., Ohayon S., Boyko M., Gruenbaum S.E., Shapira Y., Weintraub A., Zlotnik A. The effects of estrogen and progesterone on blood glutamate levels during normal pregnancy in women. Gynecol. Endocrinol. 2013; 29(10):912–916.

69. Al-Suwailem E., Abdi S., El-Ansary A. (2017). Sex differences in the glutamate signaling pathway in juvenile rats. J. Neurosci. Res. 96 459–466. 10.1002/jnr.24144.

70. Zlotnik A., Gurevich B., Tkachov S., Maoz I., Shapira Y., Teichberg V.I. Brain neuroprotection by scavenging blood glutamate. Exp. Neurol. 2007; 203(1):213–220.

71. Stover J.F., Kempski O.S. Anesthesia increases circulating glutamate in neurosurgical patients. Acta Neurochir. (Wien) 2005;147(8):847–853.

72. https://www.psychologytoday.com/us/blog/balanced/202001/the-link-between-bdnf-and-neuroplasticity.

73. Park H, Poo MM. Neurotrophin regulation of neural circuit development and function. Nat Rev Neurosci. 2013; 14(1):7–23.

74. Zuccato C, Cattaneo E. Brain-derived neurotrophic factor in neurodegenerative diseases. Nat Rev Neurol. 2009; 5(6):311–322; Howells DW, et al. Reduced BDNF mRNA expression in the Parkinson's disease substantia nigra. Exp Neurol. 2000; 166:127–135.

75. Dias BG, et al. Differential regulation of brain derived neurotrophic factor transcripts by antidepressant treatments in the adult rat brain. Neuropharmacology. 2003; 45:553–563; Tsai SJ. Is mania caused by

overactivity of central brain-derived neurotrophic factor? Med Hypotheses. 2004; 62:19–22.

76. Mattson M. Energy intake, meal frequency, and health: a neurobiological perspective. Annu Rev Nutr. 2005; 25:237-60.

77. Russo-Neustadt A, Beard RC, Cotman CW. Exercise, antidepressant medications, and enhanced brain derived neurotrophic factor expression. Neuropsychopharmacology. 1999; 21:679–682; Griffin E, et al. Aerobic exercise improves hippocampal function and increases BDNF in the serum of young adult males. Physiol Behav. 2011 Oct 24; 104(5):934-41.

78. Snigdha S, Neill JC, McLean SL, Shemar GK, Cruise L, Shahid M, Henry B. Phencyclidine (PCP)-induced disruption in cognitive performance is gender-specific and associated with a reduction in brain-derived neurotrophic factor (BDNF) in specific regions of the female rat brain. J Mol Neurosci. 2011; 43(3):337–345.

79. Hayley S, Du L, Litteljohn D, Palkovits M, Faludi G, Merali Z, Poulter MO, Anisman H. Gender and brain regions specific differences in brain derived neurotrophic factor protein levels of depressed individuals who died through suicide. Neurosci Lett. 2015; 600:12–16.

80. Gibbs RB. 1998. Levels of TrkA and BDNF mRNA but not NGF mRNA fluctuate across the estrous cycle and increase in response to acute hormone replacement. Brain Res 787:259–268.

81. Singh M, Meyer EM, Simpkins JW. 1995. The effect of ovariectomy and estradiol replacement on brain-derived neurotrophic factor messenger ribonucleic acid expression in cortical and hippocampal brain regions of female Sprague-Dawley rats. Endocrinology 136:2320–2324.

82. Bakos J, Hlavacova N, Rajman M, Ondicova K, Koros C, Kitraki E, Steinbusch HW, Jezova D. Enriched environment influences hormonal status and hippocampal brain derived neurotrophic factor in a sex dependent manner. Neuroscience. 2009; 164(2):788–797.

83. Ohlsson C, Engdahl C, Borjesson AE, Windahl SH, Studer E, Westberg L, Eriksson E, Koskela A, Tuukkanen J, Krust A, Chambon P, Carlsten H, Lagerquist MK. Estrogen receptor-alpha expression in neuronal cells affects bone mass. Proc Natl Acad Sci U S A. 2012; 109(3):983–988.

84. Komulainen P., Pedersen M., Hänninen T., Bruunsgaard H., Lakka T.A., Kivipelto M., Hassinen M., Rauramaa T.H., Pedersen B.K., Rauramaa R. BDNF is a novel marker of cognitive function in ageing women: the DR's EXTRA Study. Neurobiol. Learn. Mem.

85. Castre'n E., Rantamaki T. The Role of BDNF and Its Receptors in

References

Depression and Antidepressant Drug Action: Reactivation of Developmental Plasticity. Dev. Neurobiol. 2010; 22:289–297.

86. Allen A.L., McCarson K.E. Estrogen increases nociception-evoked brain-derived neurotrophic factor gene expression in the female rat. Neuroendocrinology. 2005; 81(3):193–199. doi: 10.1159/000087002.

87. Fusani L, Metzdorf R, Hutchison JB, Gahr M. 2003. Aromatase inhibition affects testosterone-induced masculinization of song and the neural song system in female canaries. J Neurobiol 54:370–379.

88. Yang F, Je H-S, Ji Y, Nagappan G, Hempstead B, Lu B. 2009. Pro-BDNF-induced synaptic depression and retraction at developing neuromuscular synapses. J Cell Biol 185:727–741; Verhovshek T, Cai Y, Osborne MC, Sengelaub DR. 2010. Androgen regulates brain-derived neurotrophic factor in spinal motoneurons and their target musculature. Endocrinology 151:253–261; Ottem EN, Poort JE, Wang H, Jordan CL, Breedlove SM. 2010. Differential expression and regulation of brain-derived neurotrophic factor (BDNF) mRNA isoforms in androgen-sensitive motoneurons of the rat lumbar spinal cord. Mol Cell Endocrinol 328:40–46.

89. Chan CB, Ye K. Sex Differences in Brain-Derived Neurotrophic Factor Signaling and Functions. J Neurosci Res. 2017 Jan 2; 95(1-2): 328–335; Brenowitz E. Testosterone and BDNF interactions in the avian song control system. Neuroscience. 2013 Jun 3; 239: 115–123; Wei, Y-C, et al. Sex differences in brain-derived neurotrophic factor signaling: Functions and implications. JNR. 07 November 2016 https://doi.org/10.1002/jnr.23897.

90. Pakkenberg B, et al. (2003) Aging and the human neocortex. Exp Gerontol 38:95–99.

91. Coffey CE, et al. (1998) Sex differences in brain aging: A quantitative magnetic resonance imaging study. Arch Neurol 55:169–179; Gur RC, et al. (1999) Sex differences in brain gray and white matter in healthy young adults: Correlations with cognitive performance. J Neurosci 19:4065–4072; Gur RC, Gunning-Dixon FM, Turetsky BI, Bilker WB, Gur RE (2002) Brain region and sex differences in age association with brain volume: A quantitative MRI study of healthy young adults. Am J Geriatr Psychiatry 10:72–80; Murphy DG, et al. (1996) Sex differences in human brain morphometry and metabolism: An in vivo quantitative magnetic resonance imaging and positron emission tomography study on the effect of aging. Arch Gen Psychiatry 53:585–594.

92. Berchtold NC, et al. Gene expression changes in the course of normal brain aging are sexually dimorphic. Proc Natl Acad Sci USA. 2008; 105:15605–15610.

93. Seghaye, M. C., M. Qing, and G. von Bernuth. 2001. Systemic

inflammatory response to cardiac surgery: does female sex really protect? Crit. Care (London) 5:280-282.

94. Casimir, G. J., S. Mulier, L. Hanssens, K. Zylberberg, and J. Duchateau. 2010. Gender differences in inflammatory markers in children. Shock 33:258-262; Casimir, G. J., et al. 2010. Chronic inflammatory diseases in children are more severe in girls. Shock 34:23-26; Casimir, G. J., et al. 2010. Gender differences and inflammation: an in vitro model of blood cells stimulation in prepubescent children. J. Inflamm. (London) 7:28-34.

95. Fleiss B, Nilsson MK, Blomgren K, Mallard C (2012) Neuroprotection by the histone deacetylase inhibitor trichostatin A in a model of lipopolysaccharide-sensitised neonatal hypoxic-ischaemic brain injury. J Neuroinflammation 9: 70; Kentner AC, McLeod SA, Field EF, Pittman QJ (2010) Sex-dependent effects of neonatal inflammation on adult inflammatory markers and behavior. Endocrinology 151: 2689–99. Smith JA, Das A, Butler JT, Ray SK, Banik NL (2011) Estrogen or estrogen receptor agonist inhibits lipopolysaccharide induced microglial activation and death. Neurochem Res 36: 1587–93; Villa A, Vegeto E, Poletti A, Maggi A (2016) Estrogens, neuroinflammation and neurodegeneration. Endocr Rev 37: 372–402; Doran S, et al. Sex Differences in Acute Neuroinflammation after Experimental Traumatic Brain Injury Are Mediated by Infiltrating Myeloid Cells. Journal of NeurotraumaVol. 36, No. 7.

96. Weatherhead, JE, et al. Long-Term Neurological Outcomes in West Nile Virus–Infected Patients: An Observational Study. Am J Trop Med Hyg. 2015 May 6; 92(5): 1006–1012. doi: 10.4269/ajtmh.14-0616

97. Lindsey N, et al. Eastern Equine Encephalitis Virus in the United States, 2003-2016. Am J Trop Med Hyg. 2018 May; 98(5): 1472–1477. Published online 2018 Mar 19. doi: 10.4269/ajtmh.17-0927

98. Persky, R. W., Turtzo, L. C., & McCullough, L. D. (2010). Stroke in women: disparities and outcomes. Current Cardiology Reports, 12(1), 6–13.

99. Bushnell, C. A., McCullough, L. D., Awad, I. A., Chireau, M. V., Fedder, W. N., Furie, K. L., Walters, M. R. (2014). Guidelines for the Prevention of Stroke in Women. (link is external) Stroke, 47(9).

100. Petrea RE, Beiser AS, Seshadri S, Kelly-Hayes M, Kase CS, Wolf PA. Gender differences in stroke incidence and poststroke disability in the Framingham heart study. Stroke. 2009; 40(4):1032–7. doi:10.1161/STROKEAHA.108.542894; Benjamin, E. J., Virani, S. S., Callaway, C. W., Chamberlain, A. M., Chang, A. R., Cheng, S, Muntner, P. (2018). Heart Disease and Stroke Statistics—2018 Update: A Report From the American Heart Association (link is external). Circulation, 137, e67–e492; Ahnstedt, H., McCullough, L. D., & Cipolla, M. J. (2016). The Importance of Considering Sex Differences in Translational Stroke Research. Translational

References

Stroke Research, 7(4), 261–273.

101. Liu F, Yuan R, Benashski SE, McCullough LD. Changes in experimental stroke outcome across the life span. J Cereb Blood Flow Metab. 2009;29(4):792–802; https://www.sciencedaily.com/releases/2009/11/091103171715.htm.

102. McCullough LD, Hurn PD. Estrogen and ischemic neuroprotection: an integrated view. Trends Endocrinol Metab. 2003; 14(5):228–35.

103. Hall ED, Pazara KE, Linseman KL. Sex differences in postischemic neuronal necrosis in gerbils. J Cereb Blood Flow Metab. 1991; 11:292–8; Alkayed NJ, Harukuni I, Kimes AS, London ED, Traystman RJ, Hurn PD. Gender-linked brain injury in experimental stroke. Stroke. 1998; 29:159–65. [PubMed] [Google Scholar] 29; Zhang YQ, Shi J, Rajakumar G, Day AL, Simpkins JW. Effects of gender and estradiol treatment on focal brain ischemia. Brain Res. 1998; 784:321–4. [PubMed] [Google Scholar]30; Carswell HV, Anderson NH, Clark JS, Graham D, Jeffs B, Dominiczak AF, Macrae IM. Genetic and gender influences on sensitivity to focal cerebral ischemia in the stroke-prone spontaneously hypertensive rat. Hypertension. 1999; 33:681–5. [PubMed] [Google Scholar]31; McCullough LD, Zeng Z, Blizzard KK, Debchoudhury I, Hurn PD. Ischemic nitric oxide and poly (ADP-ribose) polymerase-1 in cerebral ischemia: male toxicity, female protection. J Cereb Blood Flow Metab. 2005; 25:502–12.

104. Carcel C, et al. Sex differences in treatment and outcome after stroke. Neurology, 2019; 10.1212/WNL.0000000000008615 DOI: 10.1212/WNL.0000000000008615; Reeves MJ, Bushnell CD, Howard G, Gargano JW, Duncan PW, Lynch G, Khatiwoda A, Lisabeth L. Sex differences in stroke: epidemiology, clinical presentation, medical care, and outcomes. Lancet Neurol. 2008; 7:915–926.

105. Appelros P, et al. Sex Differences in Stroke Epidemiology A Systematic Review (Stroke. 2009; 40:1082-1090.)

106. Mahowald MK, Alqahtani F, Alkhouli M. Comparison of outcomes of coronary revascularization for acute myocardial infarction in men versus women. Am J Cardiol. 2020; Epub ahead of print.

107. Lang JT, McCullough LD. Pathways to ischemic neuronal cell death: are sex differences relevant? J Transl Med. 2008; 6:33. doi:10.1186/1479-5876-6-33; Golomb MR, Fullerton HJ, Nowak-Gottl U, Deveber G. Male predominance in childhood ischemic stroke: findings from the international pediatric stroke study. Stroke. 2009; 40(1):52–7. doi:10.1161/STROKEAHA.108.521203.

Chapter Seven

The Great Brain Robbery –Brian Moench

1. https://www.cdc.gov/aging/publications/aag/alzheimers.html.

2. Nebel R, et al. Understanding the impact of sex and gender in Alzheimer's disease: A call to action. Alzheimers Dement. 2018 Sep; 14(9): 1171–1183. Published online 2018 Jun 12.

3. Association As. 2017 Alzheimer's Disease Facts and Figures. 2017.

4. https://www.alzheimers.net/8-12-15-why-is-alzheimers-more-likely-in-women.

5. https://www.livescience.com/51616-alzheimers-risk-women-decline-faster.html.

6. Pankratz VS, Roberts RO, Mielke MM, Knopman DS, Jack CR Jr., Geda YE, et al. Predicting the risk of mild cognitive impairment in the Mayo Clinic Study of Aging. Neurology. 2015; 84:1433–42; Azad NA, Al Bugami M, Loy-English I. Gender differences in dementia risk factors. Gend Med. 2007; 4:120–9.

7. Ownby RL, Crocco E, Acevedo A, John V, Loewenstein D. Depression and risk for Alzheimer disease: systematic review, meta-analysis, and metaregression analysis. Arch Gen Psychiatry. 2006; 63:530–8.

8. Kessler RC, McGonagle KA, Swartz M, Blazer DG, Nelson CB. Sex and depression in the National Comorbidity Survey. I: Lifetime prevalence, chronicity and recurrence. J Affect Disord. 1993; 29:85–96.

9. Bromberger JT, Kravitz HM, Chang YF, Cyranowski JM, Brown C, Matthews KA. Major depression during and after the menopausal transition: Study of Women's Health Across the Nation (SWAN). Psychol Med. 2011; 41:1879–88.

10. Goveas JS, Espeland MA, Woods NF, Wassertheil-Smoller S, Kotchen JM. Depressive symptoms and incidence of mild cognitive impairment and probable dementia in elderly women: the Women's Health Initiative Memory Study. J Am Geriatr Soc. 2011; 59:57–66.

11. Elbejjani M, Fuhrer R, Abrahamowicz M, Mazoyer B, Crivello F, Tzourio C, et al. Hippocampal atrophy and subsequent depressive symptoms in older men and women: results from a 10-year prospective cohort. Am J Epidemiol. 2014; 180:385–93; Goveas JS, Espeland MA, Hogan P, Dotson V, Tarima S, Coker LII, et al. Depressive symptoms, brain volumes and subclinical cerebrovascular disease in postmenopausal women: the Women's Health Initiative MRI Study. J Affect Disord. 2011; 132:275–84.

12. Mielke MM, Vemuri P, Rocca WA. Clinical epidemiology of Alzheimer's disease: assessing sex and gender differences. Clin Epidemiol. 2014; 6:37–48.

References

13. Langa KM, Larson EB, Crimmins EM, Faul JD, Levine DA, Kabeto MU, et al. A Comparison of the Prevalence of Dementia in the United States in 2000 and 2012. JAMA Intern Med. 2017;177:51–8; Matthews FE, Arthur A, Barnes LE, Bond J, Jagger C, Robinson L, et al. A two-decade comparison of prevalence of dementia in individuals aged 65 years and older from three geographical areas of England: results of the Cognitive Function and Ageing Study I and II. Lancet. 2013; 382:1405–12.

14. Rovio S, Kareholt I, Helkala EL, Viitanen M, Winblad B, Tuomilehto J, et al. Leisure-time physical activity at midlife and the risk of dementia and Alzheimer's disease. Lancet Neurol. 2005; 4:705–11.

15. Nomaguchi Kei M., Bianchi SM. Exercise Time: Gender Differences in the Effects of Marriage, Parenthood, and Employment. Journal of Family and Marriage. 2004; 66:413–30.

16. Pankratz VS, Roberts RO, Mielke MM, Knopman DS, Jack CR Jr., Geda YE, et al. Predicting the risk of mild cognitive impairment in the Mayo Clinic Study of Aging. Neurology. 2015; 84:1433–42; Miech RA, Breitner JC, Zandi PP, Khachaturian AS, Anthony JC, Mayer L. Incidence of AD may decline in the early 90s for men, later for women: The Cache County study. Neurology. 2002; 58:209–18.

17. Lim AS, Kowgier M, Yu L, Buchman AS, Bennett DA. Sleep Fragmentation and the Risk of Incident Alzheimer's Disease and Cognitive Decline in Older Persons. Sleep. 2013; 36:1027–32; Spira AP, Gamaldo AA, An Y, Wu MN, Simonsick EM, Bilgel M, et al. Self-reported sleep and beta-amyloid deposition in community-dwelling older adults. JAMA Neurol. 2013; 70:1537–43.

18. Mielke MM, Milic NM, Weissgerber TL, White WM, Kantarci K, Mosley TH, et al. Impaired Cognition and Brain Atrophy Decades After Hypertensive Pregnancy Disorders. Circ Cardiovasc Qual Outcomes. 2016; 9:S70–6.

19. Klosinski LP, Yao J, Yin F, Fonteh AN, Harrington MG, Christensen TA, Trushina E, Brinton RD. White Matter Lipids as a Ketogenic Fuel Supply in Aging Female Brain: Implications for Alzheimer's Disease. EBioMedicine. 2015 Dec; 2(12):1888-904. Epub 2015 Nov 3 PubMed.

20. Mosconi L, Berti V, Guyara-Quinn C, McHugh P, Petrongolo G, Osorio RS, Connaughty C, Pupi A, Vallabhajosula S, Isaacson RS, de Leon MJ, Swerdlow RH, Brinton RD. Perimenopause and emergence of an Alzheimer's bioenergetic phenotype in brain and periphery. PLoS One. 2017; 12(10):e0185926. Epub 2017 Oct 10 PubMed.

21. Schulte PJ, et al. Association between exposure to anaesthesia and surgery and long-term cognitive trajectories in older adults: report from the Mayo Clinic

Study of Aging. British Journal of Anaesthesia, 2018; DOI: 10.1016/j.bja.2018.05.060.

22. https://www.alz.org/aaic/_downloads/tues-8am-women-risk.pdf.

23. Lejri I, Grimm A, Eckert A. Mitochondria, estrogen and female brain aging. Front. Aging Neurosci. 10 (2018.

24. Rocca WA, Grossardt BR, Shuster LT, Stewart EA. Hysterectomy, oophorectomy, estrogen, and the risk of dementia. Neurodegener Dis. 2012; 10(1-4):175-178. doi:10.1159/000334764.

25. https://www.alzheimers.net/8-12-15-why-is-alzheimers-more-likely-in-women.

26. Lagunas N., Calmarza-Font I., Diz-Chaves Y., Garcia-Segura L.M. Long-term ovariectomy enhances anxiety and depressive-like behaviors in mice submitted to chronic unpredictable stress. Horm. Behav. 2010; 58(5):786–791; Cizza G., Gold P.W., Chrousos G.P. High-dose transdermal estrogen, corticotropin-releasing hormone, and postnatal depression. J. Clin. Endocrinol. Metab. 1997; 82(2):704. doi: 10.1210/jc.82.2.703; Studd J., Nappi R. E. Reproductive depression. Gynecol. Endocrinol. 2012; 28:42–45. doi: 10.3109/09513590.2012.651932; Worsley R., Davis S.R., Gavrilidis E., Gibbs Z., Lee S., Burger H., Kulkarni J. Hormonal therapies for new onset and relapsed depression during perimenopause. Maturitas. 2012; 73(2):127–133.

27. Vermeulen A, et al. Estradiol in elderly men. Aging Male. 2002 Jun; 5(2):98-102.

28. Davis E, et al. A second X chromosome contributes to resilience in a mouse model of Alzheimer's disease. Science Translational Medicine, 2020; 12 (558): eaaz5677 DOI: 10.1126/scitranslmed.aaz5677.

Chapter Eight

1. https://www.aappublications.org/news/2018/11/26/autism112618.

2. https://blogs.scientificamerican.com/observations/why-does-autism-impact-boys-more-often-than-girls/.

3. https://www.cdc.gov/mmwr/volumes/65/ss/ss6513a1.htm?s_cid=ss6513a1_w.

4. Baio J., Wiggins L., Christensen D.L., Maenner M.J., Daniels J., Warren Z., Kurzius-Spencer M., Zahorodny W., Robinson Rosenberg C., White T., et al. Prevalence of autism spectrum disorder among children aged 8 years—Autism and developmental disabilities monitoring network, 11 Sites, United States, 2014. MMWR Surveill. Summ. 2018.;67:1–23. doi: 10.15585/mmwr.ss6706a1.

References

5. Adak B., Halder S. Systematic review on prevalence for autism spectrum disorder with respect to gender and socio-economic status. J. Ment. Dis. Treat. 2017; 3 doi: 10.4172/2471-271X.1000133.

6. Kites DM, Gullifer J, Tyson GA. Views on the diagnostic labels of autism and Asperger's disorder and the proposed changes in the DSM. Journal of Autism and Developmental Disorders. 2013; 43(7):1692–1700.

7. Leonard H, Dixon G, Whitehouse AJO, et al. Unpacking the complex nature of the autism epidemic. Research in Autism Spectrum Disorders. 2010; 4(4):548–554.

8. Limperopoulos C. Autism spectrum disorders in survivors of extreme prematurity. Clinics in Perinatology. 2009; 36(4):791–805.

9. https://www.spectrumnews.org/news/autism-rates-united-states-explained/.

10. Brett D, et al. Factors Affecting Age at ASD Diagnosis in UK: No Evidence that Diagnosis Age has Decreased Between 2004 and 2014. Journal of Autism and Developmental Disorders, 2016.

11. https://www.autism-society.org/what-is/facts-and-statistics/.

12. Parner ET, Baron-Cohen S, Luritsen MB, et al. Parental age and autism spectrum disorder. Annals of Epidemiology. 2012; 22(3):143–150.

13. Wan H, et al. Association of maternal diabetes with autism spectrum disorders in offspring: A systemic review and meta-analysis. Medicine (Baltimore). 2018 Jan; 97(2): e9438.

14. https://www.scientificamerican.com/article/maternal-obesity-diabetes-tied-to-increased-autism-risk-in-kids/.

15. Hallmayer J, Cleveland S, Torres A, et al. "Genetic Heritability and Shared Environmental Factors Among Twin Pairs With Autism," Arch Gen Psychiatry. 2011; 68(11):1095-1102. doi:10.1001/archgenpsychiatry.2011.76; Almandil N.B., Alkuroud D.N., Abdul Azeez S., Al Sulaiman A., Elaissari A., Borgio J.F. Environmental and genetic factors in autism spectrum disorders: Special emphasis on data from arabian studies. Int. J. Environ. Res. Public Health. 2019; 16:658. doi: 10.3390/ijerph16040658; Sealey LA, Hughes BW, Sriskanda AN, Guest JR, Gibson AD, Johnson-Williams L, Pace DG, Bagasra O (2016) Environmental factors in the development of autism spectrum disorders. Environ Int 88: 288–98.

16. James SJ, Slikker W, Melnyk S, New E, Pogribna M, Jernigan S. "Thimerosol Neurotoxicity is Associated with Glutathione Depletion: Protection with Glutathione Precursors," NeuroToxicology 26.(2005) 1-8.

17. Croen L, Grether J, Yoshida C, Odouli R, Hendrick V, "Antidepressant Use During Pregnancy and Childhood Autism Spectrum Disorders," Arch Gen Psychiatry. 2011; 68(11):1104-1112. doi:10.1001/archgenpsychiatry.2011.73; Volk H, Hertz-Picciotto I, Delwiche L, Lurmann F, McConnell R. "Residential Proximity to Freeways and Autism in the CHARGE study," Environ Health Perspect. 2010 December 13. (Epub ahead of print.) PMID: 21156395; Whyatt RM, Liu X, Rauh VA, Calafat AM, Just AC, Hoepner L, et al. 2011. "Maternal Prenatal Urinary Phthalate Metabolite Concentrations and Child Mental, Psychomotor and Behavioral Development at 3 Years of Age," Environ Health Perspect 120:290-295; Kern J, Geier D, Adams J, Mehta J, Grannemann B, Geier M. "Toxicity biomarkers in autism spectrum disorder: A blinded study of urinary porphyrins," Pediatrics International. (2011) 53, 147–153 doi: 10.1111/j.1442-200X.2010.03196.x; Miodovnik, A, SM Engel, C Zhu, X Ye, LV Soorya, MJ Silva, AM Calafat and MS Wolff. 2011. "Endocrine disruptors and childhood social impairment," Neurotoxicology; Roberts, EM et al. "Maternal residence near agricultural pesticide applications and autism spectrum disorders among children in the California Central Valley," Environmental Health Perspectives. 115(10):1482-1489; Henrik Viberg anders Fredriksson, Sonja Buratovic, Per Eriksson. "Dose-dependent behavioral disturbances after a single neonatal Bisphenol A dose," Toxicology, 2011; DOI: 10.1016/j.tox.2011.09.006; Whyatt RM, Liu X, Rauh VA, Calafat AM, Just AC, Hoepner L, et al. 2011. "Maternal Prenatal Urinary Phthalate Metabolite Concentrations and Child Mental, Psychomotor and Behavioral Development at Age Three Years," Environ Health Perspect; Holmes AS, Blaxill MF, Haley BE; "Reduced levels of mercury in first baby haircuts of autistic children," Int J Toxicol. 2003 Jul-Aug; 22(4):277-85; Allen J, Shanker G, Tan K, Aschner M. "The Consequences of Methylmercury Exposure on Interactive Functions between Astrocytes and Neurons," Neurotoxicology 23.(2002) 755-759; Schmidt RJ, et al. Combined Prenatal Pesticide Exposure and Folic Acid Intake in Relation to Autism Spectrum Disorder. Environ Health Perspect. 2017 Sep 8; 125(9):097007. doi: 10.1289/EHP604; Shelton J, Geraghty E, Tancredi D, et al. Neurodevelopmental Disorders and Prenatal Residential Proximity to Agricultural Pesticides: The CHARGE Study. Environ Health Perspect; DOI:10.1289/ehp.1307044; von Ehrenstein O, et al. Prenatal and infant exposure to ambient pesticides and autism spectrum disorder in children: population based case-control study. BMJ 2019; 364:l962.

18. Mohamed F, et al. Assessment of Hair Aluminum, Lead, and Mercury in a Sample of Autistic Egyptian Children: Environmental Risk Factors of Heavy Metals in Autism. Volume 2015 |Article ID 545674.

19. Adams J, Baral M, Geis E, et al. "The Severity of Autism Is Associated with Toxic Metal Body Burden and Red Blood Cell Glutathione Levels," Journal of Toxicology Volume 2009. (2009), Article ID 532640, 7 pages. doi:10.1155/2009/532640.

20. Kim D, et al. The joint effect of air pollution exposure and copy number

References

variation on risk for autism. Autism Res. 2017 Apr 27. doi: 10.1002/aur.1799. [Epub ahead of print]; Lam J, Sutton P, Kalkbrenner A, Windham G, Halladay A, Koustas E, Lawler C, Davidson L, Daniels N, Newschaffer C, Woodruff T. A Systematic Review and Meta-Analysis of Multiple Airborne Pollutants and Autism Spectrum Disorder. PLoS One. 2016 Sep 21; 11(9):e0161851. doi: 10.1371/journal.pone.0161851; Flores-Pajot MC, Ofner M, Do MT, Lavigne E, Villeneuve PJ. Childhood autism spectrum disorders and exposure to nitrogen dioxide, and particulate matter air pollution: A review and meta-analysis. Environ Res. 2016 Aug 25. pii: S0013-9351(16)30317-6. doi: 10.1016/j.envres.2016.07.030. [Epub ahead of print]; Allen JL, et al. Developmental Neurotoxicity of Inhaled Ambient Ultrafine Particle Air Pollution: Parallels with Neuropathological and Behavioral Features of Autism and Other Neurodevelopmental Disorders. Neurotoxicology. 2015 Dec 22. pii: S0161-813X(15)30048-6. doi: 10.1016/j.neuro.2015.12.014. [Epub ahead of print; Dickerson AS, et al. Autism spectrum disorder prevalence and proximity to industrial facilities releasing arsenic, lead or mercury. Sci Total Environ. 2015 Jul 25; 536:245-251. doi: 10.1016/j.scitotenv.2015.07.024. [Epub ahead of print]; Talbott E, et al. Fine particulate matter and the risk of autism spectrum disorder. Environmental Research. Volume 140, July 2015, Pages 414–420; Kalkbrenner AE, Windham GC, Serre ML, Akita Y, Wang X, Hoffman K, Thayer BP, Daniels JL. Particulate Matter Exposure, Prenatal and Postnatal Windows of Susceptibility, and Autism Spectrum Disorders. Epidemiology. 2014 Oct 3. [Epub ahead of print]; von Ehrenstein OS, Aralis H, Cockburn M, Ritz B. In Utero Exposure to Toxic Air Pollutants and Risk of Childhood Autism. Epidemiology. 2014 Jul 21. [Epub ahead of print]; Volk HE, Kerin T, Lurmann F, Hertz-Picciotto I, McConnell R, Campbell DB. Autism spectrum disorder: interaction of air pollution with the MET receptor tyrosine kinase gene. Epidemiology. 2014 Jan; 25(1):44-7. doi: 10.1097/EDE.0000000000000030; Volk HE, Hertz-Picciotto I, Delwiche L, Lurmann F, McConnell R. Residential proximity to freeways and autism in the CHARGE study. Environmental Health Perspectives. 2011; 119(6):873–877; Rzhetsky A, Bagley SC, Wang K, Lyttle CS, Cook EH Jr, et al. (2014) Environmental and State-Level Regulatory Factors Affect the Incidence of Autism and Intellectual Disability. PLoS Comput Biol 10(3): e1003518. doi:10.1371/journal.pcbi. 1003518; Becerra T, Wilhelm M, Olsen J, Cockburn M, Ritz B. Ambient Air Pollution and Autism in Los Angeles County, California. Environ Health Perspect 121:380–386 (2013). http://dx.doi.org/10.1289/ehp.1205827 [Online 18 December 2012]; Jung CR, Lin YT, Hwang BF. Air Pollution and Newly Diagnostic Autism Spectrum Disorders: A Population-Based Cohort Study in Taiwan. PLoS One. 2013 Sep 25; 8(9):e75510; Windham GC, Zhang L, Gunier R, Croen LA, Grether JK. Autism spectrum disorders in relation to distribution of hazardous air pollutants in the San Francisco Bay area. Environmental Health Perspectives. 2006; 114(9):1438–1444; Rossignol D A, Genuis S J, Frye R E. Environmental toxicants and autism spectrum disorders: a systematic review. Trans. Psychiatry. 2014; 4(2):e360. [PMC free article] [PubMed]; Lyall K, Schmidt R J, Hertz-Picciotto I. Maternal lifestyle and environmental risk factors for autism spectrum disorders. Int. J. Epi. 2014; 43:443–464. [PMC free article] [PubMed]; Raz R, Roberts AL, Lyall K, Hart JE, Just AC, Laden F. et al. Autism spectrum disorder and particulate matter air pollution before, during, and after pregnancy: a nested case-control analysis within the Nurses' Health Study II Cohort. Env. Health Perspect. 2015; 123(3):264–270. [PMC free article] [PubMed].

21. http://archive.sltrib.com/article.php?id=53816934&itype=CMSID.

22. Jo H, et al. Sex-specific associations of autism spectrum disorder with residential air pollution exposure in a large Southern California pregnancy cohort. Environmental Pollution, Volume 254, Part A, November 2019, 113010.

23. Goodrich AJ, et al. Joint effects of prenatal air pollutant exposure and maternal folic acid supplementation on risk of autism spectrum disorder. Autism Res. 2017 Nov 9. doi: 10.1002/aur.1885. [Epub ahead of print].

24. Sender R, et al. Revised Estimates for the Number of Human and Bacteria Cells in the Body. PLoS Biol. 2016 Aug; 14(8): e1002533.

25. https://www.ebi.ac.uk/about/news/press-releases/2000-unknown-gut-bacteria-discovered.

26. https://ehp.niehs.nih.gov/ehp3127/.

27. https://www.sciencedirect.com/journal/neurotoxicology/special-issue/106W6B3HLNX.

28. https://www.sciencedirect.com/journal/neurotoxicology/special-issue/106W6B3HLNX.

29. Murch S, et al. Autism, inflammatory bowel disease, and MMR vaccine. The Lancet, Volume 351, Issue 9106, Page 908, 21 March 1998.: Walker S, et al. Identification of Unique Gene Expression Profile in Children with Regressive Autism Spectrum Disorder (ASD) and Ileocolitis. March 08, 2013 DOI: 10.1371/journal.pone.0058058; Chen B. et al. Abnormal gastrointestinal histopathology in children with autism spectrum disorders. J Pediatr Gastroenterol Nutr. February 2011.

30. Hosie S, et al. Gastrointestinal dysfunction in patients and mice expressing the autism-associated R451C mutation in neuroligin-3. Autism Research, 2019; DOI: 10.1002/AUR.2127.

31. Sudo N, Chida Y, Aiba Y, Sonoda J, Oyama N, Yu X-N, et al. 2004. Postnatal microbial colonization programs the hypothalamic-pituitary- adrenal system for stress response in mice. J Physiol (Lond) 558(Pt 1):263– 275, PMID: 15133062, 10.1113/jphysiol.2004.063388.

References

32. Clarke G, Grenham S, Scully P, Fitzgerald P, Moloney RD, Shanahan F, et al. 2013. The microbiome-gut-brain axis during early life regulates the hippocampal serotogenic system in a sex-dependent manner. Mol Psychiatry 18(6):666–673, PMID: 22688187, 10.1038/mp.2012.77.

33. Hsiao EY. 2014. Gastrointestinal issues in autism spectrum disorder. Harv Rev Psychiatry 22(2):104–111, PMID: 24614765, 10.1097/HRP .0000000000000029; Kang DW, Adams JB, Gregory AC, Borody T, Chittick L, Fasano A, et al. 2017. Microbiota Transfer Therapy alters gut ecosystem and improves gastrointestinal autism symptoms: an open label study. Microbiome 5(1):10, PMID: 28122648, 10.1186/s40168-016-0225-7.

34. Pardo C, et al. Immunity, neuroglia and neuroinflammation in autism. International Review of Psychiatry, December 2005; 17(6): 485–495.

35. Herath M, et al. The Role of the Gastrointestinal Mucus System in Intestinal Homeostasis: Implications for Neurological Disorders. Frontiers in Cellular and Infection Microbiology, 2020; 10 DOI: 10.3389/fcimb.2020.00248.

36. Hamad A, et al. Prenatal antibiotics exposure and the risk of autism spectrum disorders: A population-based cohort study. PLoS One. 2019; 14(8): e0221921.

37. Lee E, Cho J, Kim K. The Association between Autism Spectrum Disorder and Pre- and Postnatal Antibiotic Exposure in Childhood—A Systematic Review with Meta-Analysis. Int. J. Environ. Res. Public Health 2019, 16, 4042; doi:10.3390/ijerph16204042.

38. https://www.gastrojournal.org/article/S0016-5085(19)40573-8/pdf.

39. Lee M, et al. Association of Autism Spectrum Disorders and Inflammatory Bowel Disease. Vol.:(0123456789)1 3Journal of Autism and Developmental Disorders; Doshi-Velez F, et al. Prevalence of Inflammatory Bowel Disease Among Patients with Autism Spectrum Disorders. Inflamm Bowel Dis. 2015 Oct; 21(10):2281-8.

40. Kempermann G, Song H, Gage FH. Neurogenesis in the adult hippocampus. Cold Spring Harb. Perspect. Biol. 2015; 7:a018812.

41. M. Henry et al. "A common pesticide decreases foraging success and survival in honey bees," Science. doi: 10.1126/science.1215039; P.R. Whitehorn et al. "Neonicotinoid pesticide reduces bumble bee colony growth and queen production," Science. doi: 10.1126/science.1215025; C. Lu, K.M. Warchol and R.A. Callahan. "In situ replication of honey bee colony collapse disorder," Bulletin of Insectology, Vol. 65, June 2012.

42. http://www.theguardian.com/environment/2014/may/09/honeybees dying-insecticide-harvard-study.

43. http://onlinelibrary.wiley.com/doi/10.1111/1365-2435.12292/full.

44. http://www.ithaka-journal.net/herbizide-im-urin?lang=en.

45. http://www.nejm.org/doi/full/10.1056/NEJMoa1307491.

46. http://www.pnas.org/content/114/36/9653; http://www.sciencemag.org/news/2017/07/antisocial-bees-share- genetic-profile-people-autism.

47. Elsabbagh M., Divan G., Koh Y.-J., Kim Y.S., Kauchali S., Marcín C., Montiel-Nava C., Patel V., Paula C.S., Wang C., et al. Global prevalence of autism and other pervasive developmental disorders. Autism Res. 2012; 5:160–179. doi: 10.1002/aur.239; European Commission Health & Consumer Protection Directorate-General. Some Elements About the Prevalence of Autism Spectrum Disorders (ASD) in the European Union. European Commission; Luxembourg: 2005. 16p.

48. Strunecká A., Strunecký O., Guan Z. The resemblance of fluorosis pathology to that of autism spectrum disorder: A mini-review. Fluoride. 2019; 52:105–115.

49. Strunecka A., Blaylock R.L., Patocka J., Strunecky O. Immunoexcitotoxicity as the central mechanism of etiopathology and treatment of autism spectrum disorders: A possible role of fluoride and aluminum. Surg. Neurol. Int. 2018; 9:74. doi: 10.4103/sni.sni_407_17; Hassan M.H., Desoky T., Sakhr H.M., Gabra R.H., Bakri A.H. Possible metabolic alterations among autistic male children: Clinical and biochemical approaches. J. Mol. Neurosci. 2019; 67:204–216. doi: 10.1007/s12031-018-1225-9; Rossignol D.A., Frye R.E. Evidence linking oxidative stress, mitochondrial dysfunction, and inflammation in the brain of individuals with autism. Front. Physiol. 2014; 5:150. doi: 10.3389/fphys.2014.00150; Rose S., Melnyk S., Pavliv O., Bai S., Nick T.G., Frye R.E., James S.J. Evidence of oxidative damage and inflammation associated with low glutathione redox status in the autism brain. Transl. Psychiatry. 2012; 2:e134. doi: 10.1038/tp.2012.61; Frye R.E., James S.J. Metabolic pathology of autism in relation to redox metabolism. Biomark. Med. 2014; 8:321–330. doi: 10.2217/bmm.13.158; Strunecka A., editor. Cellular and Molecular Biology of Autism Spectrum Disorders. Bentham e Books Bentham Science; Sharjah, UEA: 2010. Biochemical Changes in ASD; pp. 100–120.

50. Vargas D.L., Nascimbene C., Krishnan C., Zimmerman A.W., Pardo C.A. Neuroglial activation and neuroinflammation in the brain of patients with autism. Ann. Neurol. 2005;5 7:67–81. doi: 10.1002/ana.20315.

51. Pagan C., Delorme R., Callebert J., Goubran-Botros H., Amsellem F., Drouot X., Boudebesse C., Le Dudal K., Ngo-Nguyen N., Laouamri H., et al. The serotonin-N-acetylserotonin-melatonin pathway as a biomarker for autism

References

spectrum disorders. Transl. Psychiatry. 2014; 4:e479. doi: 10.1038/tp.2014.120.

52. Veatch O.J., Goldman S.E., Adkins K.W., Malow B.A. Melatonin in children with autism spectrum disorders: How does the evidence fit together? J. Nat. Sci. 2015; 1:e125; Tordjman S., Anderson G.M., Bellissant E., Botbol M., Charbuy H., Camus F., Graignic R., Kermarrec S., Fougerou C., Cohen D., et al. Day and nighttime excretion of 6-sulphatoxymelatonin in adolescents and young adults with autistic disorder. Psychoneuroendocrinology. 2012; 37:1990–1997. doi: 10.1016/j.psyneuen.2012.04.013.

53. Bernaerts, S., Boets, B., Bosmans, G. et al. Behavioral effects of multiple-dose oxytocin treatment in autism: a randomized, placebo-controlled trial with long-term follow-up. Molecular Autism 11, 6 (2020). https://doi.org/10.1186/s13229-020-0313-1.

Chapter Nine

1. http://www.insideradio.com/free/prevagen-ads-are-memorable-and-fraudulent-says-ftc/article_11d8ba46-d7d2-11e6-bb1c-bfacae58b40e.html.

2. https://www.nbcnews.com/health/health-news/jellyfish-memory-supplement-prevagen-hoax-ftc-says-n704886.

3. https://www.health.harvard.edu/mind-and-mood/dont-buy-into-brainhealth-supplements.

4. https://www.nytimes.com/2011/06/21/us/politics/21hatch.html.

5. https://www.health.harvard.edu/blog/fda-curbs-unfounded-memory-supplement-claims-2019053116772.

6. https://www.gao.gov/new.items/d10662t.pdf.

7. http://maristpoll.marist.edu/1114-alzheimers-most-feared-disease/#sthash.W3prb6y6.WzMr0da3.dpbs.

8. https://www.cnn.com/2019/03/21/health/alzheimers-drug-trial-failure-aducanumab-bn/index.html.

9. https://www.linkedin.com/pulse/advice-article-david-sinclair/.

10. https://khn.org/news/a-fountain-of-youth-pill-sure-if-youre-a-mouse/.

11. https://www.technologyreview.com/2017/01/06/154714/critics-blast-star-studded-advisory-board-of-anti-aging-company/.

12. https://www.newshub.co.nz/home/world/2018/09/when-the-apocalypse-is-due-according-to-isaac-newton.html.

13. https://www.syfy.com/syfywire/8_incredibly_dumb_theorie.

14. https://www.wired.com/2014/08/fantastically-wrong-life-on-the-sun/.

15. https://teslaresearch.jimdofree.com/death-ray/.

16. https://techcrunch.com/2017/01/16/a-new-lawsuit-alleges-anti-aging-startup-elysium-health-hasnt-paid-its-supplier-and-is-in-breach-of-agreement/.

17. https://khn.org/news/a-fountain-of-youth-pill-sure-if-youre-a-mouse/.

18. https://www.ftc.gov/news-events/press-releases/2019/04/geniux-dietary-supplement-sellers-barred-unsupported-cognitive.

19. Jenkins D, et al. Supplemental Vitamins and Minerals for CVD Prevention and Treatment. Volume 71, Issue 22, 5 June 2018, Pages 2570-2584.

20. https://www.hopkinsmedicine.org/health/wellness-and-prevention/is-there-really-any-benefit-to-multivitamins.

21. https://www.health.harvard.edu/staying-healthy/do-omega-3s-protect-your-thinking-skills.

22. https://www.hsph.harvard.edu/nutritionsource/fish/.

23. Kable J, et al. No Effect of Commercial Cognitive Training on Neural Activity During Decision-Making. The Journal of Neuroscience. DOI: 10.1523/JNEUROSCI.2832-16.2017.

24. https://onlinelibrary.wiley.com/doi/epdf/10.1002/ana.24689.

25. https://www.medscape.com/viewarticle/866172?src=ppc_google_rlsa-lapsed-traf_news-perspectives_md_us.

26. Rosario E, et al. The Effect of Hyperbaric Oxygen Therapy on Functional Impairments Caused by Ischemic Stroke. Neurology Research International. Volume 2018 |Article ID 3172679.

27. Amir H, et al. Cognitive enhancement of healthy older adults using hyperbaric oxygen: a randomized controlled trial. Aging, 2020; DOI: 10.18632/aging.103571.

28. Morris MC, et al. MIND diet slows cognitive decline with aging. 2015 Sep;11(9):1015-22. doi: 10.1016/j.jalz.2015.04.011. Epub 2015 Jun 15.

29. Holland TM, Agarwal P, Wang Y, et al. Dietary flavonols and risk of Alzheimer dementia. Neurology. 2020; 94:1-8. doi:10.1212/WNL.

30. https://www.health.harvard.edu/mind-and-mood/foods-linked-to-better-

References

brainpower.

31. Amen D, et al. Quantitative Erythrocyte Omega-3 EPA Plus DHA Levels are Related to Higher Regional Cerebral Blood Flow on Brain SPECT. Alzheimers Dis. 2017; 58(4):1189-1199.

32. O'brien J, et al. Long-term intake of nuts in relation to cognitive function in older women. J Nutr Health Aging. 2014 May; 18(5): 496–502; https://ods.od.nih.gov/factsheets/VitaminE-HealthProfessional/; La Fata G, et al. Effects of Vitamin E on Cognitive Performance during Ageing and in Alzheimer's Disease. Nutrients. 2014 Dec; 6(12): 5453–5472.

33. Andrade S, et al. Resveratrol Brain Delivery for Neurological Disorders Prevention and Treatment. Front. Pharmacol., 20 November 2018 https://doi.org/10.3389/fphar.2018.01261.

34. Nehlig A, et al. The neuroprotective effects of cocoa flavanol and its influence on cognitive performance. Br J Clin Pharmacol. 2013 Mar; 75(3): 716–727; Berk L, et al. Dark chocolate (70% organic cacao) increases acute and chronic EEG power spectral density (μV2) response of gamma frequency (25–40 Hz) for brain health: enhancement of neuroplasticity, neural synchrony, cognitive processing, learning, memory, recall, and mindfulness meditation. 01 April 2018. https://doi.org/10.1096/fasebj.2018.32.1_supplement.878.10.

35. Subash S, et al. Neuroprotective effects of berry fruits on neurodegenerative diseases. Neural Regen Res. 2014 Aug 15; 9(16): 1557–1566.

36. https://ods.od.nih.gov/factsheets/VitaminE-HealthProfessional/.

37. Chang D, et al. Caffeine Caused a Widespread Increase of Resting Brain Entropy. Sci Rep. 2018; 8: 2700.

38. Smith, AD, et al. Homocysteine-Lowering by B Vitamins Slows the Rate of Accelerated Brain Atrophy in Mild Cognitive Impairment: A Randomized Controlled Trial. Published: September 8, 2010 https://doi.org/10.1371/journal.pone.0012244.

39. Giacoppo S, et al. An overview on neuroprotective effects of isothiocyanates for the treatment of neurodegenerative diseases. Fitoterapia. 2015 Oct; 106:12-21.

40. Meeusen R, et al. Exercise, Nutrition and the Brain. Sports Med. 2014; 44(Suppl 1): 47–56.

41. Alisi L, et al. The Relationships Between Vitamin K and Cognition: A Review of Current Evidence. Front Neurol. 2019; 10: 239.

42. Yuan T, et al. Pomegranate's Neuroprotective Effects against Alzheimer's

Disease Are Mediated by Urolithins, Its Ellagitannin-Gut Microbial Derived Metabolites. ACS Chem. Neurosci. 2016, 7, 1, 26–33.

43. Erickson, K. I. et al. Exercise training increases size of hippocampus and improves memory. Proc. Natl. Acad. Sci. U. S. A. 108, 3017–3022; doi:10.1073/pnas.1015950108 (2011); Chaddock, L. et al. A neuroimaging investigation of the association between aerobic fitness, hippocampal volume, and memory performance in preadolescent children. Brain Res. 1358, 172–183; doi:10.1016/j.brainres.2010.08.049 (2010).

44. Baker LD, Frank LL, Foster-Schubert K, Green PS, Wilkinson CW, McTiernan A, et al. Effects of aerobic exercise on mild cognitive impairment: a controlled trial. Arch Neurol. 2010; 67(1):71–79. [PMC free article] [PubMed] [Google Scholar]; Baker LD, Frank LL, Foster-Schubert K, Green PS, Wilkinson CW, Tiernan AM, et al. Aerobic Exercise Improves Cognition for Older Adults with Glucose Intolerance, A Risk for Alzheimer's Disease. J Alzheimers Dis. 2010; 22(2):569–579. [PMC free article] [PubMed].

45. Justice N. The relationship between stress and Alzheimer's disease. Neurobiol Stress. 2018 Feb; 8: 127–133.

46. Du X., Pang T.Y. Is dysregulation of the HPA-Axis a core pathophysiology mediating Co-Morbid depression in neurodegenerative diseases? Front. Psychiatr. 2015; 6:32.

47. Mitchell R, Kumari V. Hans Eysenck's interface between the brain and personality: Modern evidence on the cognitive neuroscience of personality. Personality and Individual Differences 103 (2016) 74–81.

48. Arsenis N, et al. Physical activity and telomere length: Impact of aging and potential mechanisms of action. Oncotarget. 2017 Jul 4; 8(27): 45008–45019. Published online 2017 Mar 30. doi: 10.18632/oncotarget.16726.

49. Werner C, et al. Differential effects of endurance, interval, and resistance training on telomerase activity and telomere length in a randomized, controlled study. European Heart Journal, Volume 40, Issue 1, 01 January 2019, Pages 34–46.

50. Tucker L. Physical activity and telomere length in U.S. men and women: An NHANES investigation. Preventive Medicine, 2017; 100: 145. DOI: 10.1016/j.ypmed.2017.04.027.

51. Lourenco M, et al. Exercise-linked FNDC5/irisin rescues synaptic plasticity and memory defects in Alzheimer's models. Nature Medicine, 2019; 25 (1): 165 DOI: 10.1038/s41591-018-0275-4.

52. Huh JY, Panagiotou G, et al. FNDC5 and irisin in humans: I. Predictors of circulating concentrations in serum and plasma and II. mRNA expression and

References

circulating concentrations in response to weight loss and exercise. Metabolism. 2012;61(12):1725–1738. doi: 10.1016/j.metabol.2012.09.002.

53. Zügel M, et al. The role of sex, adiposity, and gonadectomy in the regulation of irisin secretion. Endocrine. 2016; 54(1): 101–110.

54. Killgore, W, et al. Physical Exercise Habits Correlate with Gray Matter Volume of the Hippocampus in Healthy Adult Humans. Scientific Reports. 3: 3457 | DOI: 10.1038/srep03457; Erickson, K. I., et al. Exercise training increases size of hippocampus and improves memory. Proc. Natl. Acad. Sci. U. S. A. 108, 3017–3022; doi:10.1073/ pnas.1015950108 (2011); Chaddock,, L. et al. A neuroimaging investigation of the association between aerobic fitness, hippocampal volume, and memory performance in preadolescent children. Brain Res. 1358, 172–183; doi:10.1016/j.brainres.2010.08.049 (2010).

55. Erickson K, et al. Physical activity, fitness, and gray matter volume. Neurobiol Aging. 2014 Sep; 35 Suppl 2: S20–S28.

56. Bherer L, et al. A Review of the Effects of Physical Activity and Exercise on Cognitive and Brain Functions in Older Adults. J Aging Res. 2013; 2013: 657508; Dimech C, et al. Sex differences in the relationship between cardiorespiratory fitness and brain function in older adulthood. Journal of Applied Physiology, 2019; DOI: 10.1152/japplphysiol.01046.2018.

57. Hölzel B, et al. Mindfulness practice leads to increases in regional brain gray matter density. Psychiatry Res. 2011 Jan 30; 191(1): 36–43; Kang D, et al. The effect of meditation on brain structure: cortical thickness mapping and diffusion tensor imaging. Soc Cogn Affect Neurosci. 2013 Jan; 8(1): 27–33.

58. Hölzel B, et al. Stress reduction correlates with structural changes in the amygdala. Soc Cogn Affect Neurosci. 2010 Mar; 5 (1): 11–17.

59. Greenberg J, Reiner K, Meiran N. "Mind the Trap": Mindfulness Practice Reduces Cognitive Rigidity. Plos One. Published: May 15, 2012 https://doi.org/10.1371/journal.pone.0036206

60. Tang Y, et al. Short-term meditation training improves attention and self-regulation. Proc Natl Acad Sci U S A. 2007 Oct 23; 104(43): 17152–17156.

61. Greenberg J, et al. Reduced interference in working memory following mindfulness training is associated with increases in hippocampal volume. Brain Imaging Behav. 2019 Apr; 13(2):366-376. doi: 10.1007/s11682-018-9858-4.

62. https://www.healthybabyfood.org/sites/healthybabyfoods.org/files/2019-10/BabyFoodReport_FULLREPORT_ENGLISH_R5b.pdf.

63. https://www.bbc.com/news/world-asia-50805822.

64. Soutschek, A., Burke, C.J., Raja Beharelle, A. et al. The dopaminergic reward system underpins gender differences in social preferences. Nat Hum Behav 1, 819–827 (2017). https://doi.org/10.1038/s41562-017-0226-y.

65. https://www.independent.co.uk/life-style/women-kinder-more-generous-men-study-behavioral-experiments-university-zurich-a7991961.html.

66. Schwartz S, Rubel-Lifschitz T. Cross-National Variation in the Size of Sex Differences in Values: Effects of Gender Equality. Journal of Personality and Social Psychology © 2009 American Psychological Association 2009, Vol. 97, No. 1, 171–185; Schwartz, S. H., & Rubel, T. (2005). Sex differences in value priorities: cross-cultural and multimethod studies. Journal of Personality and Social Psychology, 89, 1010-1028.

67. https://www.researchgate.net/publication237511237_Altruism_in_Contemporary_America_A_Report_from_the_National_Altruism_Study

68. Sisco, M.R., Weber, E.U. Examining charitable giving in real-world online donations. Nat Commun 10, 3968 (2019). https://doi.org/10.1038/s41467-019-11852-z.

69. Piper, G., & Schnepf, S. V. (2008). Gender differences in charitable giving in Great Britain. Voluntas, 19, 103-124.

70. Hampson, E., van Anders, S. M., & Mullin, L. I. (2006). A female advantage in the recognition of emotional facial expressions: Test of an evolutionary hypothesis. Evolution and Human Behavior, 27, 401-416.

71. Baron-Cohen, S., & Wheelwright, S. (2004). The empathy quotient: An investigation of adults with Asperger syndrome or high functioning autism, and normal sex differences. Journal of Autism and Developmental Disorders, 34, 163–175.

72. Heintz, S., Kramm, C., & Ruch, W. (2017). A meta-analysis of gender differences in character strengths and age, nation, and measure as moderators. The Journal of Positive Psychology, 1-10.

73. Jaffee, S., & Hyde, J. S. (2000). Gender differences in moral orientation: a meta-analysis. Psychological Bulletin, 126, 703-726.

74. Su et al. (2009). Men and things, women and people: A meta-analysis of sex differences in interests. Psychological Bulletin, 135, 859-884.

75. Schmitt, D.P., et al. Personality and gender differences in global perspective. International Journal of Psychology, 2017 Vol. 52, No. S1, 45–56, DOI: 10.1002/ijop.12265; Schmitt, D. P., Realo, A., Voracek, M., & Allik, J. (2008). Why can't a man be more like a woman? Sex differences in Big Five personality traits across 55 cultures. Journal of Personality and Social

References

Psychology, 94, 168-192.

76. Rand, D. G., Brescoll, V., Everett, J. A., Capraro, V., & Barcelo, H. (2016). Social heuristics and social roles: Intuition favors altruism for women but not for men. Forthcoming in Journal of Experimental Psychology: General.

77. Grosch, K., & Rau, H. (2017). Gender differences in honesty: The role of social value orientation. Journal of Economic Psychology. https://doi.org/10.1016/j.joep.2017.07.008.

78. Carlo, G. (2006). Care-based and altruistically-based morality. In M. Killen & J. G. Smetana (Eds.), Handbook of moral development (pp. 551–579). Mahwah, NJ: Erlbaum.

79. Tsugawa Y, et al. Comparison of Hospital Mortality and Readmission Rates for Medicare Patients Treated by Male vs Female Physicians. JAMA Intern Med. 2017; 177(2):206-213. doi:10.1001/jamainternmed.2016.7875.

80. https://www.nbcnews.com/health/health-news/female-doctors-outperform-male-doctors-according-study-n697876.

81. Greenwood B, et al. Patient–physician gender concordance and increased mortality among female heart attack patients. PNAS August 21, 2018 115 (34) 8569-8574; first published August 6, 2018.

82. https://www.nytimes.com/2018/08/14/well/doctors-male-female-women-men-heart.html.

83. https://www.acpjournals.org/doi 10.7326/0003-4819-140-2-200401200-00017.

84. https://www.cnn.com/2019/10/16/success/women-ceos-and-cfos-outperform/index.html.

85. Bart C, et al. Why women make better directors. International Journal of Business Governance and Ethics, 2013; 8 (1): 93 DOI: 10.1504/IJBGE.2013.052743.

86. https://www.catalyst.org/wp-content/uploads/2019/01/The_Bottom_Line_Corporate_Performance_and_Womens_Representation_on_Boards.pdf.

87. https://www.researchgate.net/publication/228299596_Director_Characteristics_Gender_Balance_and_Insolvency_Risk_An_Empirical_Study.

88. https://www.forbes.com/sites/kathycaprino/2016/05/12/how-decision-making-is-different-between-men-and-women-and-why-it-matters-in-business/#7b326ab24dcd.

89. https://papers.ssrn.com/sol3/papers.cfm?abstract_id=3617953.

90. Volden C, Wiseman A, and Wittmer D. Women's Issues and Their Fates in the US Congress. Volume 6, Issue 4 October 2018, pp. 679-696.

91. https://www.nytimes.com/2016/11/10/upshot/women-actually-do-govern-differently.html.

92. https://journals.sagepub.com/doi/abs/10.1177/0160323x12463945.

93. http://people.tamu.edu/~mtkoch/Koch%20Fulton%20JoP.pdf.

94. https://www.nytimes.com/2016/11/10/upshot/women-actually-do-govern-differently.html.

95. https://ir.law.fsu.edu/cgi/viewcontent.cgi?article=1301&context=lr.

96. Schultz, T. Paul. "Returns to Women's Schooling," in Elizabeth King and M. Anne Hill, eds., Women's Education in Developing Countries: Barriers, Benefits and Policy, Baltimore: Johns Hopkins University Press, 2003.

97. https://www.rainforest-alliance.org/articles/empowering-women-is-the-key-to-solving-food-insecurity.

98. Schreinemachers P, et al. Too much to handle? Pesticide dependence of smallholder vegetable farmers in Southeast Asia. Science of The Total Environment. Volumes 593–594, 1 September 2017, Pages 470-477.

99. https://www.latimes.com/opinion/la-xpm-2012-jun-13-la-oe-polakovic-gender-and-the-environment-20120613-story.htmlhttps://.

100. www.theguardian.com/environment/2020/feb/06/eco-gender-gap-why-saving-planet-seen-womens-work

101. https://link.springer.com/article/10.1007/s11199-019-01061-9.

102. Brough A, et al. Is Eco-Friendly Unmanly? The Green-Feminine Stereotype and Its Effect on Sustainable Consumption. Journal of Consumer Research, Volume 43, Issue 4, December 2016, Pages 567–582.

103. https://www.vox.com/2015/5/27/8665401/nuclear-power-gender.

104. https://green.blogs.nytimes.com/2011/10/12/in-nimby-sentiments-a-gender-divide/.

105. Swim J, et al. Gendered discourse about climate change policies. Global Environmental Change. Volume 48, January 2018, Pages 216-225.

106. https://www.newyorker.com/magazine/2021/02/01/the-blackwell-sisters-

References

and-the-harrowing-history-of-modern-medicine.

107. https://www.nytimes.com/2021/01/30/style/mackenzie-scott-prisclila-chan-zuckerberg-melinda-gates-philanthropy.html.

108. https://www.eenews.net/assets/2021/02/04/document_gw_03.pdf.

109. https://www.eenews.net/greenwire/2021/02/04/stories/1063724395?utm_campaign=edition&utm_medium=email&utm_source=eenews%3Agreenwire

110. Ferrell, M., Wang, Z., Anderson, J.T. et al. A terminal metabolite of niacin promotes vascular inflammation and contributes to cardiovascular disease risk. Nat Med 30, 424–434 (2024). https://doi.org/10.1038/s41591-023-02793-8

111. https://www.health.harvard.edu/mind-and-mood/dont-buy-into-brain-health-supplement

Appendix

1. Mehl A, et al. "The effect of trichlorfon and other organiphosphates on prenatal brain development in the guinea pig," Neurochemical Research, 19(5),569-574, 1994.

2. . Lerro CC, Koutros S, Andreotti G, Friesen MC, Alavanja MC, Blair A, et al. Organophosphate insecticide use and cancer incidence among spouses of pesticide applicators in the Agricultural Health Study. Occup Environ Med. (2015) 72:736–44. doi: 10.1136/oemed-2014-102798

3. Davis, J. R., Brownson, R. C., Garcia, R., Bentz, B. J., & Turner, A. 1993. Family pesticide use and childhood brain cancer. Archives of Envi- ronmental Contamination and Toxicology, 24(1), 87-92.

4. Leiss J. K., Savitz D. A. 1995. Home pesticide use and childhood cancer: a case-control study. American Journal of Public Health, 85(2), 249-252

5. Leiss, J.K. and D.A. Savitz. 1995. Home pesticide use and childhood cancer: A case-control study. Amer. J. Publ. Health 85: 249-252. Davis, J.R. et al. 1993. Family pesticide use and childhood brain cancer. Arch. Environ. Contam. T oxicol. 24: 87-92.

6. Davis, J.R. et al. 1993. Family pesticide use and childhood brain cancer. Arch. Environ. Contam. T oxicol. 24: 87-92.

7. Lee GH, Choi KC. Adverse effects of pesticides on the functions of immune system. Comparative Biochemistry and Physiology Part C: Toxicology & Pharmacology Volume 235, September 2020, 108789

8. Lee, M. J. 1977. Inhibition of monocyte esterase activity by organophosphate

insecticides. Blood, 50(5), 947-951.

9. World Resources Institute, Pesticide and the Immune System: The Public Health Risk, 1998.

10. Beaudoin, A.R. and D.L. Fisher. 1981. An in vivo/in vitro evaluation of teratogenic action. T eratol. 23:57-61.

11. Platte Chemical Co. 1995. Dibrom 8 Miscible. Label. www.epa.gov/pesticides.

12. https://www.paneurope.info/old/Archive/About%20pesticides/Banned%20and%20authorised.htm; https://www.miaminewtimes.com/news/florida-department-of-health-incorrectly-says-naled-is-not-banned-in-europe-8766976; https://www.beyondpesticides.org/assets/media/documents/Naled%20ChemWatch%20Factsheet%20Cited.pdf; https://www.latimes.com/nation/la-na-zika-naled-snap-story.html; https://www.latimes.com/nation/la-na-zika-naled-snap-story.html; https://www.miaminewtimes.com/news/pesticide-sprayed-over-wynwood-is-banned-in-europe-may-also-harm-fetuses-8671169; https://www.livescience.com/56039-is-pesticde-naled-used-in-zika-fight-toxic.html

13. . Silver MK, Shao J, Zhu B, Chen M, Xia Y, Kaciroti N, Lozoff B, Meeker JD. Prenatal naled and chlorpyrifos exposure is associated with deficits in infant motor function in a cohort of Chinese infants. Environ Int. 2017 Sep;106:248-256. doi: 10.1016/j.envint.2017.05.015. Epub 2017 Jun 8. PMID: 28602489; PMCID: PMC5533622

14. Berteau, P.E., W.A. Deen, and R.L. Dimmick. 1977. Effect of particle size on the inhalation toxicity of naled aerosols. (Abstract.) Toxicol. Appl. Pharmacol. 41: 183

15. Krzastek, S, et al. Impact of environmental toxin exposure on male fertility potential. Translational Andrology and Urology; Vol 9, No 6 (December 2020): Translational Andrology and Urology

16. Suhartono S, Kartini A, Subagio HW, Budiyono B, Utari A, Suratman S, et al. Pesticide exposure and thyroid function in elementary school children living in an agricultural area, Brebes District, Indonesia. Int J Occup Environ Med. (2018) 9:137–44. doi: 10.15171/ijoem.2018.1207

17. Hertz-Picciotto I, Sass JB, Engel S, Bennett DH, Bradman A, Eskenazi B, Lanphear B, Whyatt R (2018) Organophosphate exposures during pregnancy and child neurodevelopment: Recommendations for essential policy reforms. PLoS Med 15: e1002671 Doi 10.1371/ journal.pmed.1002671

References

18. Gonzalez-Alzaga B, Lacasana M, Aguilar-Garduno C, Rodriguez-Barranco M, Ballester F, Rebagliato M, et al. A systematic review of neurodevelopmental effects of prenatal and postnatal organophosphate pesticide exposure. Toxicol Lett. 2014;230(2):104–21. pmid:24291036; Koureas M, Tsakalof A, Tsatsakis A, Hadjichristodoulou C. Systematic review of biomonitoring studies to determine the association between exposure to organophosphorus and pyrethroid insecticides and human health outcomes. Toxicol Lett. 2012;210(2):155–68. pmid:22020228; Munoz-Quezada MT, Lucero BA, Barr DB, Steenland K, Levy K, Ryan PB, et al. Neurodevelopmental effects in children associated with exposure to organophosphate pesticides: a systematic review. Neurotoxicology. 2013;39:158–68. pmid:24121005; PubMed Central PMCID: PMC3899350; U.S. EPA. EPA Revised Human Health Risk Assessment on Chlorpyrifos. December 2014. Docket ID EPA-HQ-OPP-2008-0850. Available from: http://www.epa.gov/ingredients-used-pesticide-products/revised-human-health-risk-assessment-chlorpyrifos; U.S. EPA. Chlorpyrifos: Revised Human Health Risk Assessment for Registration Review. US Environmental Protection Agency Washington, DC; 2016. Document ID: EPA-HQ-2015-0653-0454. Available from: https://www.regulations.gov/document?D=EPA-HQ-OPP-2015-0653-0454.

19. Liu P, et al. Adverse Associations of both Prenatal and Postnatal Exposure to Organophosphorous Pesticides with Infant Neurodevelopment in an Agricultural Area of Jiangsu Province, China. Environ Health Perspect, doi: 10.1289/EHP196 (2016).

20. Carr R, Alugubelly N and Mohammed A (2018) Possible Mechanisms of Developmental Neurotoxicity of Organophosphate Insecticides Linking Environmental Exposure to Neurodevelopmental Disorders, 10.1016/bs.ant.2018.03.004, (145-188)

21. Ross, S. M., McManus, I. C., Harrison, V., & Mason, O. 2013. Neurobehavioral problems following low-level exposure to organophosphate pesticides: a systematic and meta-analytic review. Critical reviews in toxicology, 43(1), 21-44.

22. Bouchard M, Chevrier J, Harley K, Kogut K, Vedar M, Calderon N, Trujillo C, Johnson C, Bradman A, Barr D, Eskenazi B. Prenatal Exposure to Organophosphate Pesticides and IQ in 7-Year Old Children. Environmental Health Perspectives, 2011; DOI: 10.1289/ehp.1003185

23. Engel S, et al. Prenatal Exposure to Organophosphates, Paraoxonase 1, and Cognitive Development in Childhood. Environmental Health Perspectives, 2011; DOI: 10.1289/ehp.1003183

24. Eskenazi B, Marks AR, Bradman A, Harley K, Barr DB, Johnson C et al.. 2007. Organophosphate pesticide exposure and neurodevelopment in young Mexican- American children.Environ Health Perspect 115:792-798;

doi:10.1289/ehp. 982817520070. Google Scholar

25. Jusko T, van den Dries M, Pronk A, Shaw P, Guxens M, Spaan S, Jaddoe V, Tiemeier H and Longnecker M (2019) Organophosphate Pesticide Metabolite Concentrations in Urine during Pregnancy and Offspring Nonverbal IQ at Age 6 Years, Environmental Health Perspectives, 127:1Jan-2019.

26. Office of Technology Assessment (OTA) of the US Congress, Neurotoxicity: Identifying and Controlling Poisons of the Nervous System.

27. Abreu-Villaca Y, Levin ED. Developmental neurotoxicity of succeeding generations of insecticides. Environ Int. 2017;99:55–77. Epub 2016/12/03. pmid:27908457; PubMed Central PMCID: PMC5285268.

28. Gunier RB, Bradman A, Harley KG, Kogut K, Eskenazi B. Prenatal Residential Proximity to Agricultural Pesticide Use and IQ in 7-Year-Old Children. Environ Health Perspect. 2017;125(5):057002. pmid:28557711.

29. Engel SM, Bradman A, Wolff MS, Rauh VA, Harley KG, Yang JH, et al. Prenatal Organophosphorus Pesticide Exposure and Child Neurodevelopment at 24 Months: An Analysis of Four Birth Cohorts. Environ Health Perspect. 2016;124(6):822–30. pmid:26418669; PubMed Central PMCID: PMC4892910.

30. Sagiv SK, Harris MH, Gunier RB, Kogut KR, Harley KG, Deardorff J, et al. Prenatal Organophosphate Pesticide Exposure and Traits Related to Autism Spectrum Disorders in a Population Living in Proximity to Agriculture. Environ Health Perspect. 2018;126(4):047012. Epub 2018/04/28. pmid:29701446.

31. Gonzalez-Alzaga B, Lacasana M, Aguilar-Garduno C, Rodriguez-Barranco M, Ballester F, Rebagliato M, et al. A systematic review of neurodevelopmental effects of prenatal and postnatal organophosphate pesticide exposure. Toxicol Lett. 2014;230(2):104–21. pmid:24291036.

32. Abreu-Villaca Y, Levin ED. Developmental neurotoxicity of succeeding generations of insecticides. Environ Int. 2017;99:55–77. Epub 2016/12/03. pmid:27908457; PubMed Central PMCID: PMC5285268; Banks CN, Lein PJ. A review of experimental evidence linking neurotoxic organophosphorus compounds and inflammation. Neurotoxicology. 2012;33(3):575–84. pmid:22342984; PubMed Central PMCID: PMC3358519; Bjorling-Poulsen M, Andersen HR, Grandjean P. Potential developmental neurotoxicity of pesticides used in Europe. Environ Health. 2008;7:50. pmid:18945337; PubMed Central PMCID: PMC2577708; Lasram MM, Dhouib IB, Annabi A, El Fazaa S, Gharbi N. A review on the molecular mechanisms involved in insulin resistance induced by organophosphorus pesticides. Toxicology. 2014;322:1–13. pmid:24801903.

References

33. Rauh V. Polluting Developing Brains — EPA Failure on Chlorpyrifos. N Engl J Med 2018; 378:1171-1174. March 29, 2018; Slotkin TA, Seidler FJ. Comparative developmental neurotoxicity of organophosphates in vivo: transcriptional responses of pathways for brain cell development, cell signaling, cytotoxicity and neurotransmitter systems. Brain Res Bull 2007;72:232-274.

34. https://www.nejm.org/doi/full/10.1056/NEJMp1716809

www.ingramcontent.com/pod-product-compliance
Lightning Source LLC
Chambersburg PA
CBHW020624220526
45464CB00001B/10